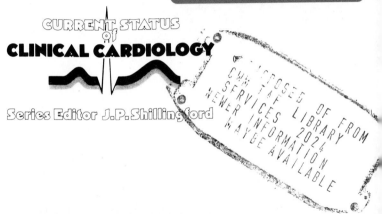

CURRENT STATUS
of
CLINICAL CARDIOLOGY

Series Editor J.P. Shillingford

ISCHAEMIC HEART DISEASE

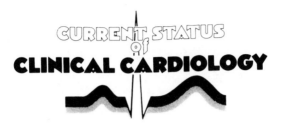

CURRENT STATUS of CLINICAL CARDIOLOGY

Series Editor J.P. Shillingford

ISCHAEMIC HEART DISEASE

Edited by
Kim M. Fox

Consultant Cardiologist
National Heart Hospital
London

 MTP PRESS LIMITED
a member of the KLUWER ACADEMIC PUBLISHERS GROUP
LANCASTER / BOSTON / THE HAGUE / DORDRECHT
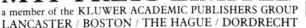

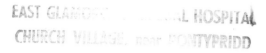
Published in the UK and Europe by
MTP Press Limited
Falcon House
Lancaster, England

British Library Cataloguing in Publication Data
Ischaemic heart disease——(Current
status of clinical cardiology)
1. Coronary heart disease
I. Fox, Kim M.   II. Series
616.1′23   RC685.C6

ISBN 0–85200–871–6
ISBN 0–85200–816–3 Series

Published in the USA by
MTP Press
A division of Kluwer Academic Publishers
101 Philip Drive
Norwell, MA 02061, USA

Library of Congress Cataloging-in-Publication Data
Ischaemic heart disease.

(Current status of clinical cardiology)
Includes bibliographies and index
1. Coronary heart disease. 2. Ischemia. 3. Angina
pectoris. 4 Heart—Infarction. I. Fox, Kim M.
II. Series. [DNLM: 1. Coronary Disease. WG 300 174]
RC685.C61589   1986   616.1′23   86–27593
ISBN 0–85200–871–6

Typeset and printed in Great Britain
by Butler & Tanner Limited,
Frome and London

Contents

Preface

This book attempts to focus on the most important clinical aspects of ischaemic heart disease. Clearly, in no way is it supposed to be a comprehensive review of the subject, but it does attempt to address the most important topics for everyday practising clinicians.

The question of epidemiology is topical both in the lay and medical press and is, therefore, covered in some detail. It is the editor's opinion that proper understanding of the clinical manifestations of the disease and, therefore, subsequent investigation and treatment are based on a detailed understanding of the pathology and pathophysiology, and as a result these subjects have also been covered in detail.

In the last decade there have been considerable advances in our understanding of the mechanisms of angina and also the haemodynamic and metabolic consequences of both angina and myocardial infarction. Again, if appropriate investigations and treatment are to be undertaken, they can only be done with the proper knowledge of the disease being investigated.

Finally, the investigation and management of the various manifestations of ischaemic heart disease have been addressed. In the last ten years there has been an explosion in the drugs available for the treatment of ischaemic heart disease and how they should be used has become much more sophisticated. The place of coronary artery surgery has now been rationalized and angioplasty provides an important adjunct to treatment.

The authors have been asked to give quite extensive references so that if the reader wishes to obtain more detail on any particular aspect, the most important sources should be readily found.

This book is aimed at a wide readership. Anyone involved in the treatment of ischaemic heart disease should, it is hoped, find something of interest or value whether it is in pathophysiology, investigation or treatment of this condition.

Kim Fox
National Heart Hospital
London

Series Editor's Note

The last few decades have seen an explosion in our knowledge of cardiovascular disease as a result of research in many disciplines. The tempo of research is ever increasing, so that it is becoming more and more difficult for one person to encompass the whole spectrum of the advances taking place on many fronts.

Even more difficult is to include the advances as they affect clinical practice in one textbook of cardiovascular disease. Fifty years ago all that was known about cardiology could be included in one textbook of moderate size and at that time there was little research so that a textbook remained up to date for several years. Today all this has changed, and books have to be updated at frequent intervals to keep up with the results of research and changing fashions.

The present series has been designed to cover the field of cardiovascular medicine in a series of, initially, eight volumes which can be updated at regular intervals and at the same time give a sound basis of practice for doctors looking after patients.

The volumes include the following subjects: heart muscle disease; congenital heart disease, invasive and non-invasive diagnosis; ischaemic heart disease; immunology and molecular biology of the heart in health and disease; irregularities of the heart beat; and each is edited by a distinguished British author with an international reputation, together with an international panel of contributors.

The series will be mainly designed for the consultant cardiologist as reference books to assist him in his day-to-day practice and keep him up to date in the various fields of cardiovascular medicine at the same time as being of manageable size.

J.P. Shillingford
British Heart Foundation

Current Status of Clinical Cardiology Series

Drugs in the Management of Heart Disease
Edited by A. Breckenridge

Heart Muscle Disease
Edited by J. F. Goodwin

Congenital Heart Disease
Edited by F. J. Macartney

Invasive and Non-Invasive Diagnosis of Heart Disease
Edited by A. Maseri

Ischaemic Heart Disease
Edited by K. M. Fox

Immunology and Molecular Biology of Cardiovascular Diseases
Edited by C. J. F. Spry

Irregularities of the Heart Beat
Edited by A. J. Camm and D. E. Ward

List of Contributors

M. B. Ablett
Department of Medicine
University of Otago
Dunedin
New Zealand

P. A. Crean
Cardiology Department
National Heart Hospital
Westmoreland Street
London W1M 8BA
UK

H. J. Dargie
Department of Cardiology
Western Infirmary
Glasgow G11 6NT
UK

M. J. Davies
St Georges Hospital Medical
    School
British Heart Foundation
Cardiovascular Pathology Unit
Cranmer Terrace
London SW17 0RE
UK

J. I. E. Hoffman
Department of Pediatrics and
    Physiology
1403 HSE
University of California
San Francisco, CA 94143
USA

C. D. J. Ilsley
Department of Cardiology
Dunedin Hospital
Great King Street
Dunedin
New Zealand

J. I. Mann
Department of Community
    Medicine and General Practice
University of Oxford
Gibson Laboratories Building
Radcliffe Infirmary
Oxford OX2 6HE
UK

M. G. Marmot
Department of Community
    Medicine
University College London
66–72 Gower Street
London WC1E 6EA
UK

P. A. Poole-Wilson
Department of Cardiac Medicine
Cardiothoracic Institute
2 Beaumont Street
London W1N 2DX
UK

A. A. Quyyumi
National Institute of Health
Cardiology Branch, Bethesda
MD 20205 USA

E. Rowland
Department of Cardiac Medicine
Cardiothoracic Institute
Brompton Hospital
Fulham Road
London SW3 6HP
UK

1
Epidemiology of ischaemic heart disease

M. G. MARMOT AND J. I. MANN

Of all the chronic diseases, ischaemic heart disease (IHD) has been the object of the most detailed epidemiological study. We now have much information on possible causes of the disease and, with a reasonable degree of precision, can predict its future occurrence; that is, among an apparently healthy adult population we can distinguish those individuals with a high risk from those with a low risk of subsequently developing IHD. The highest risk group has more than 10 times the risk of the lowest risk group. This epidemiological knowledge has provided the basis for efforts to prevent IHD and to reduce its community burden. This chapter reviews the epidemiology and prevention of IHD, beginning with a consideration of the impact of the disease on the population.

OCCURRENCE OF ISCHAEMIC HEART DISEASE

In most industrialized countries IHD is the commonest cause of death. In England and Wales 30% of all deaths among men and 22% of all deaths among women are the result of IHD[4].

In recent years, in addition to the approximately 156 000 deaths every year in England and Wales there have been, on average, 115 000 hospital discharges with the diagnosis IHD. It should be stressed that in 60% of all fatal myocardial infarctions, death occurs in the first hour after the attack. Most IHD deaths, therefore, occur too rapidly for treatment to influence the prognosis.

International differences

There are marked international differences in the rate of occurrence of IHD. For example, in one study in seven countries[10], among men aged 40–59 years initially free of IHD, the annual incidence rate (occurrence of new cases) varied from 15 per 10000 in Japan to 198 per 10000 in Finland. Mortality statistics show a similar picture. Table 1.1 shows that, even among the industrialized countries, mortality rates vary con-

Table 1.1 Deaths per 100 000 of the population from ischaemic heart disease in people aged 45–49 in 1977

Country	Males	Females
Finland	296	29
Scotland	229	47
Northern Ireland	223	28
United States of America	193	45
Australia	192	41
England and Wales	188	32
New Zealand	175	64
Canada	175	36
Hungary	166	35
Czechoslovakia	157	21
Norway	137	16
Netherlands	135	23
Israel	111	27
Federal Republic of Germany	110	18
Bulgaria	99	21
Italy	97	15
Sweden	94	16
Romania	74	17
France	59	7
Japan	24	6

siderably. Some of the variation between countries is undoubtedly due to differences in diagnostic practice and in coding of death certificates, but numerous studies using comparable methods have confirmed that real differences exist in the frequency of disease. In Europe there is almost a threefold difference between France, Italy and Spain, on the one hand, and such countries as Finland and the United Kingdom on the other.

As shown below, these international comparisons have played an important part in the search for causes. The experience of migrants suggests that the variations between countries are likely to be the result chiefly of environmental or behavioural differences. People who have migrated from a low-risk country (e.g. Japan) to a high-risk country (e.g. United States of America) tend to have rates of IHD approaching that of the host country.

Time trends

In industrialized countries, IHD emerged as the major cause of death in the twentieth century. This resulted both from a decrease in infectious disease mortality and an increase in the age-specific risk of IHD. The same process is now starting in many developing countries.

The heart disease epidemic appears to have reached its peak, and is even declining in some countries. Figure 1.1 shows that since 1968 there has been a substantial decrease in IHD mortality in the United States of America and Finland. By contrast, the rate has remained almost unchanged in England and Wales. This change over a short period of

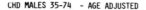

CHD MALES 35-74 - AGE ADJUSTED

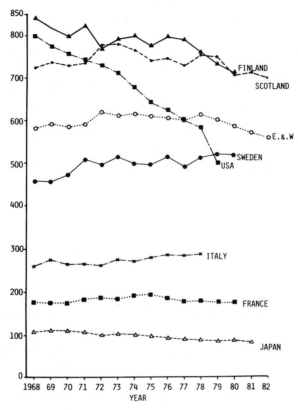

Figure 1.1 Age-adjusted mortality from ischaemic heart disease in men aged 35–74 in England and Wales and other countries. From: Marmot M. G. (1985) Interpretation of trends in coronary heart disease mortality. *Acta Med. Scand.* (Suppl.) **701**, 58–65

time in the United States and Finland and in other countries (Australia and Belgium) encourages us to believe that the disease is preventable, if the causes can be found and modified.

RISK FACTORS

In 1949 Keys[10] suggested that with regard to IHD, 'physico-chemical characteristics of the individual should have predictive value'. It was this idea together with the observation in the early 1950s that IHD showed a strikingly different frequency from country to country that stimulated the search for predictive variables (now referred to rather more loosely as risk factors). The term 'risk factors' has come to include not only physicochemical characteristics of the individual, but also aspects of life style – such as diet, smoking and behaviour pattern. From

3

the very beginning it was believed that the discovery of such predictive variables might point the way to preventive efforts even though identification of such variables does not conclusively establish aetiological relationships.

Increasing age, the masculine gender and a family history of premature IHD are three powerful predictors of IHD but will not be considered here in detail because of their irreversibility. It is of considerable interest that most of the potentially reversible risk factors discussed below are predictive of IHD only in relatively young people (usually under the age of 60 years), suggesting that they relate to speed of development of the disease process. The increased risk in association with a family history of premature IHD is explained at least in part by well established genetically determined conditions (e.g. familial hypercholesterolaemia).

Diet

The evidence provided by epidemiological studies that certain dietary practices may be associated with an increased risk of IHD has been obtained from several different sources:

1. Between-country correlations of IHD rates and food intake;
2. Prospective observation of subjects for whom individual diet histories are available;
3. Associations between diet (and changes in diet) and various measures of lipid metabolism known to be associated with IHD.

Between-country correlations of IHD rates and food intake

Most attempts to study dietary determinants of IHD rates have been based on balance sheets of the Food and Agriculture Organization (or, in the United Kingdom, more reliably on household food surveys), and on national mortality statistics before 1970 during which time IHD was increasing (at least in men) in most affluent societies. Positive associations with saturated fat, sucrose, animal protein and coffee, and negative correlations with flour (and other complex carbohydrates) and vegetables are some of the best described. However, population food consumption data are notoriously unreliable (they are usually derived from local production figures, imports and exports, with no account of quantities not utilized as food), and the accuracy with which mortality is recorded varies from country to country. Consequently, such data do not provide direct evidence concerning aetiology, only clues for further research. Perhaps more interesting are recent studies from the United States of America, the United Kingdom, and Australia, which have examined the downward trend of IHD rates in relation to dietary change. There is certainly some association between the falling IHD rates apparent (particularly in males) in these countries and changes in some nutrients; but in view of the strong correlations (positive and negative) among different dietary constituents it is difficult to be sure which dietary factor is principally involved or indeed whether dietary change is simply occurring in parallel with some other more important environmental factor (e.g. increasing physical activity or a reduction in cigarette smoking).

Actual food consumption by people in 16 defined cohorts (in seven countries) and 10-year incidence rates of IHD deaths form the rather more reliable basis for the correlations tested by Keys and co-workers. A strong positive correlation was noted between mean (for each cohort) saturated fat intake and fatal IHD incidence ($r = 0.84$) (Figure 1.2). A

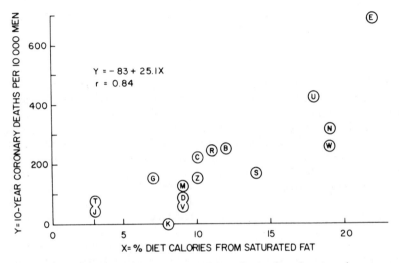

Figure 1.2 Ten-year coronary death rates of the cohorts plotted against the percentage of dietary calories supplied by saturated fatty acids

weaker association was found with dietary sucrose and a later analysis of the data suggested also a positive relationship with intake of polyunsaturated fat. Protein intake appeared to have no effect on IHD incidence and no data were available concerning dietary fibre.

Prospective observation of subjects for whom diet histories are available

In the seven-countries study[10] and several other studies it has not usually been possible to show a relationship between an individual's dietary intake and his subsequent risk of IHD. However, such an association has now been demonstrated in two further studies. In one, male bank staff, bus drivers, and bus conductors in London completed at least one seven-day weighed dietary record, and men with a high intake of dietary fibre from cereals had a lower rate of IHD subsequently than the rest.

A high energy intake (apparently reflecting physical activity) and, to a lesser extent, the presence of a high ratio of polyunsaturated to saturated fatty acids in the diet were also features of men who subsequently remained free of IHD. In another prospective investigation of employees of the Western Electric Company in Chicago[24], the most striking finding was an inverse association between IHD mortality and consumption of polyunsaturated fat. A positive association was also noted between IHD mortality and dietary cholesterol and with the Keys and Hegsted 'scores' (combined measures of the amount of saturated fat, polyunsaturated fat and cholesterol in the diet). No association was found betwen IHD and saturated fat intake considered in isolation. In this study, as in the London study, dietary assessment was carried out very carefully – failure to find similar associations in other prospective studies could be due to insensitivity of their dietary survey techniques.

Diet and lipids

Several measures of lipid metabolism described below have been associated with an increased risk of IHD. Of these, only total cholesterol has been convincingly shown to be associated with diet. For example, in the study of Keys and co-workers, mean concentration of cholesterol in the blood was highly correlated ($r = 0.87$) with percentage of total calories from saturated fat. In the Western Electric Study changes from one year to the next in dietary intake of saturated fatty acids and cholesterol were related to changes in serum cholesterol. In the typical western diet about 40% of energy is provided by fat. A substantial cholesterol reduction is achieved when this is reduced to 30% and the ratio of polyunsaturated to saturated fatty acids increases from 0.2 to 0.8.

The nomadic people of Somalia, Kenya and Tanzania, whose diets consist mainly of meat, milk, and blood have always aroused particular interest since, despite this diet, they have usually maintained low blood cholesterol levels. It has, however, been pointed out recently that their diet is not in fact habitually high in saturated fat but that intake is subject to much irregularity in food supply on a seasonal basis. There are other apparently conflicting results, but Epstein[5] has pointed out that these seemingly inconsistent findings do not exclude type and amount of dietary fat as major determinants of serum cholesterol levels, provided one concedes that these are not the only factors that determine the distribution of serum cholesterol levels within a population. Another factor, which may explain the low cholesterols in East Africa, is the fact that fat content and composition of animals varies widely. In Uganda, wild buffalo meat contains one-tenth as much lipid as beef from British cattle, and only 2% of the British beef fatty acids are polyunsaturated as compared with 30% of the meat fatty acids from woodland buffalo. Man's tissue lipids approximate the pattern of his dietary fat intake, and numerous carefully controlled dietary studies have confirmed the cholesterol-lowering effect of polyunsaturated fatty acids.

In addition to the cholesterol-lowering property of polyunsaturated fatty acids, it is conceivable that the findings from the studies carried out in London and Chicago might be explained by another mechanism: certain long chain essential polyunsaturated fatty acids, such as linoleic acid, are reported to reduce the thrombotic tendency of the blood. A significantly lower proportion of linoleic acid is present in the adipose tissue of healthy Scots compared with similar men in Stockholm[2], where IHD rate is one-third lower than in Scotland. Eskimos who have a high intake of eicosapentaenoic acid have prolonged bleeding times, and laboratory studies suggest that a reduced tendency to platelet aggregation may be explained by the effect of these fatty acids on prostaglandin synthesis.

In summary, epidemiological data do give some credence to the suggestion that diet is related to IHD, possibly via an effect on both atheroma and thrombosis. Certainly IHD seems to occur very infrequently in communities where the 'western diet' is not consumed, although of course features other than diet characterize such communities. IHD is now being diagnosed with increasing frequency among the black people of East and southern Africa amongst whom the disease was previously regarded as exceptionally uncommon, and it is the more affluent sections of the community who are principally involved. Further evidence for an aetiological association between diet and IHD is provided by the single factor intervention studies discussed below.

Abnormalities of lipid metabolism

No other blood constituent varies so much between different people as serum cholesterol. From New Guinea to East Finland, the mean serum cholesterol ranges from 2.6 to 7.02 mmol/l (100–270 mg/100 ml) when estimated by the same method in the same age and sex group. Of the *known* risk factors for IHD, total serum cholesterol appears to be the most important determinant of the geographic distribution of the disease. In the seven-countries study median cholesterol values were highly correlated with IHD death rates ($r = 0.80$), accounting for 64% of the variance in the IHD death rates amongst the cohorts. Amongst individuals within populations the association is equally strong: in over 20 prospective studies in different countries total serum cholesterol has been shown to be related to the rate of development of IHD, the association being dose-related, occurring in both sexes, and being independent of all other measured risk factors. The association in the Framingham study is shown in Figure 1.3[3]. Risk of IHD varies over a fivefold range in relation to serum cholesterol levels found in an average American population. There is no discernible critical value: the risk tends to increase throughout the range. Whilst the absolute risk associated with any given cholesterol value varies in different parts of the world, within almost every population sampled the risk is greater in people with higher than with lower values.

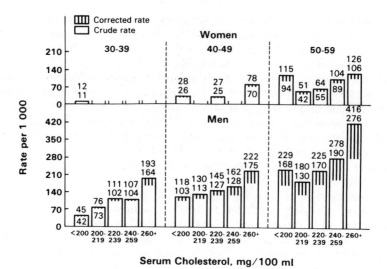

Figure 1.3 Twenty-four-year incidence of myocardial infarction, by serum cholesterol levels in the Framingham study[3]

The association of total cholesterol with IHD mortality and morbidity appears to derive chiefly, if not entirely, from the low density lipoprotein (LDL) fraction with which it is highly correlated. Low levels of total or LDL cholesterol appear to be associated with an increased risk of non-cardiovascular death (chiefly cancer) but studies in two populations – London and Paris – indicate that this inverse association is confined to deaths in the very early years of follow-up. A low cholesterol may be a metabolic consequence of cancer, present but unsuspected at the time of examination.

Increases in total triglycerides and levels of very low density lipoprotein (VLDL) are usually associated in prospective studies with an increased IHD rate. This increased risk is apparent especially when triglyceride levels are higher than 1.7 mmol/l (150 mg/100 ml), but only two studies (both Scandinavian) have suggested that the association is independent of other measures of lipid metabolism.

Table 1.2 Levels of high density lipoprotein (HDL) cholesterol and subsequent incidence of ischaemic heart disease in the Framingham Study

HDL cholesterol level (mg/ml)	IHD incidence	Population at risk	Rate/1000
All levels	79	1025	77.1
<25	3	17	176.5
25–34	17	170	100.0
35–44	35	335	104.5
45–54	15	294	51.0
55–64	8	134	59.7
65–74	1	40	25.0
75+	0	35	—

Recent interest has centred around the possibility that high density lipoprotein (HDL) may be a protective factor. Where HDL has been measured in prospective studies, low levels do seem to be predictive of subsequent IHD (Table 1.2), and in communities where IHD is uncommon HDL levels are high. In people over 50 years of age the predictive value of HDL appears to be stronger than that of LDL. Below the age of 50 it seems that LDL might be the more important predictor.

Other constitutional factors

Blood pressure

Apart from intake of saturated fat and cholesterol levels, blood pressure (both systolic and diastolic) was the only factor measured in the seven-country study[10] which seemed to explain in part geographic variation in IHD[22]; it appeared to be responsible for about 40% of the variance in the 10-year follow-up of IHD mortality. When considering prospective follow-up of a defined cohort, increased blood pressure has been shown consistently to be associated with a subsequent increase in IHD risk (Figure 1.4)[3]. It has usually been assumed that a linear relationship exists

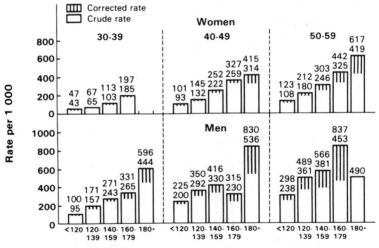

Figure 1.4 Twenty-four-year incidence of coronary heart disease, by systolic blood pressure in the Framingham study[3]

between blood pressure and subsequent IHD risk, implying the most satisfactory outcome for those with lowest levels of blood pressure. Data from the seven-countries study[10], however, suggest that the relationship might not be quite so simple, but there is still no suggestion of a cut-off point by which people might be classified as hypertensive or normotensive. The epidemiological data generally indicate that systolic blood pressure is as good a predictor of subsequent IHD as is the diastolic pressure.

Carbohydrate intolerance

Prospective studies in affluent societies have shown repeatedly that all manifestations of cardiovascular disease occur more frequently in diabetics than in non-diabetics (Figure 1.5). Of particular interest is the fact that diabetic men and women have similar IHD rates, women losing the 'protection' against IHD that is evident in the non-diabetic population. However, observations that diabetics in Africa, East Asia, and Latin America may not experience a similar proneness to atherosclerotic disease raise the question of whether factors other than blood

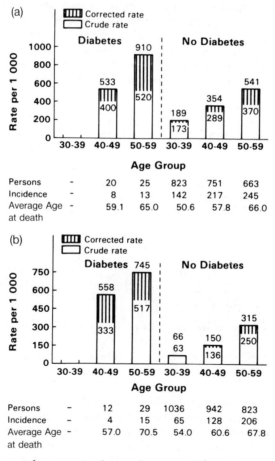

Figure 1.5 Twenty-four-year incidence of coronary heart disease in subjects with diabetes mellitus, aged 30–59 at entry: (a) men, (b) women

glucose levels are important determinants of the increased risk of athero-sclerotic disease in the diabetic. The importance of asymptomatic hyper-glycaemia, based on the study of 15 different populations, has recently been reviewed[25]. There is certainly no clear linear trend between carbo-hydrate intolerance and subsequent development of IHD. There is some evidence of an increased risk in individuals in the top quintiles or deciles of either fasting blood glucose levels or levels one to two hours after a glucose load. It is not conclusively established whether this relationship is an independent one or a consequence of associations between blood glucose and other important risk factors for IHD such as hypertension and hyperlipidaemia which are often associated with carbohydrate intol-erance. If not independent, lowering of blood glucose levels without concomitant change in other factors would be unlikely to lower the risk.

Obesity

Long-term follow-up data of insured individuals published 30 years ago showed that both men and women rated for overweight developed cardiovascular disease more frequently than the non-obese. Data from at least one prospective study have suggested that this observation is valid and independent of other measured factors[21]. However, there is no indication that obesity explains any of the geographic variations in IHD; moreover, other studies have suggested that if obesity is associated with an increased risk of IHD, it is almost certainly due to an association with other factors such as hypertension. Despite this, the clinical sig-nificance of obesity should not be underestimated, since reversal may well improve the risk factors that are causally associated with IHD.

Haemostatic factors

Almost all epidemiological research into the aetiology of IHD has concentrated on factors which are probably associated with athero-genesis and far less on factors which might primarily increase the risk of thrombosis. The Northwick Park Prospective Heart Study included measures of haemostatic function[15]. Compared with survivors, men who died of cardiovascular disease showed, at recruitment, significantly higher plasma levels of Factor VII:$_c$, fibrinogen, and Factor VIII:$_c$. Associations with VIII:$_c$ and fibrinogen were at least as strong as that with cholesterol. Fibrinolytic activity was higher in survivors, but the difference was not statistically significant. There were no differences in platelet count or measures of adhesiveness. The data were also examined for any tendency of the three clotting factors to 'cluster' in individual subjects (clustering being defined as concentrations in the top third of the distribution for at least two of the three factors). Clustering was present in 63% of men who died from cardiovascular disease compared with 23% of survivors. Of 367 men with clustering, 4.6% died of cardiovascular disease as compared with less than 1% without clustering. Although the numbers in the study are rather small, the results are certainly compatible with the idea of 'hypercoagulable state' as a major risk factor for IHD. Recently, data from a prospective study in Sweden have confirmed the importance of fibrinogen as a risk factor[2].

Physical inactivity

In the seven-countries study physical inactivity did not appear to explain the geographic variation in coronary heart disease (CHD)[10]. However, in several prospective studies of defined populations, vigorous exercise at work and in leisure time has been shown to protect against coronary heart disease[17,20]. Perhaps the most publicized study is that of Morris and his colleagues[16] who asked some 18 000 middle-aged British civil servants (on a Monday morning, without notice) to complete a record of how they had spent each five minutes of the previous Friday and Saturday. Men who engaged in vigorous sports, keep fit exercises, and the like had a fatal and non-fatal CHD incidence over the next $8\frac{1}{2}$ years, which was about half that of their colleagues who recorded no vigorous exercise (Figure 1.6). The effect was noted regardless of age and whether

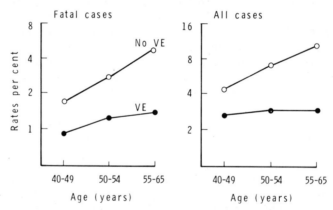

Figure 1.6 Rising incidence of coronary heart disease with age in relation to vigorous exercise

or not other risk factors for CHD were present. Vigorous exercise appeared to reduce the increasing incidence with ageing, so striking in those who did not take vigorous exercise. Vigorous exercise was defined as activity likely to reach peaks of energy expenditure of 31.5 kJ (7.5 kcal) per minute.

To investigate the role of physical activity at work in reducing coronary mortality, some 6000 longshoremen ('dockers') in San Francisco, aged 35–74 years on entry were followed for 22 years or to death or to age 75. Their longshoring experience was compiled in terms of work years according to categories of high, medium and low calorie output. Age-adjusted coronary death rates were 27 per 10 000 work years for the high activity category and 46 and 49 for the medium and low categories respectively. The difference amongst the groups was even more striking with regard to sudden death. Energy expenditure during the type of work defined as 'high output' was in the range of 21.8–31.5 kJ (5.2–7.5 kcal) per minute.

Unfortunately, randomized studies of the effects of vigorous exercise are not feasible, it is difficult to determine whether the observational studies really prove that exercise is beneficial or whether the findings merely reflect a healthier constitution in those who take exercise. There are a substantial number of plausible explanations for a beneficial effect. Physical training is well known to increase the efficiency of cardiac action and to slow the heart. In those who take vigorous exercise a reduced frequency of ectopic beats has been reported. Several other possible 'risk factors' for CHD are favourably influenced by physical activity, including high density lipoproteins, triglycerides, fibrinolytic activity, and obesity. In contemplating possible preventive strategies it should be remembered that epidemiological studies strongly suggest a critical threshold of activity and that near approach to maximal energy output may be more beneficial than overall total output at some lesser intensity of effort.

Smoking

Several longitudinal studies in many countries have shown that people who smoke have a higher incidence of and risk of dying from IHD than non-smokers. Figure 1.7 reproduces data from one such study[23]. It shows there to be a dose–response relationship: the greater the number of cigarettes smoked, the higher the risk.

In countries where other risk factors are lacking and overall level of IHD is low (e.g. in Japan) smoking appears not to be a risk factor for IHD.

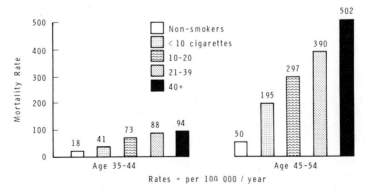

Figure 1.7 Mortality rates from ischaemic heart disease in men by number of cigarettes smoked, in two age groups. (From: Royal College of Physicians and British Cardiac Society (1976) Prevention of coronary heart disease. *J. R. Coll. Physicians* **10**, 1–63, by permission)

It is not clear how smoking harms the cardiovascular system. Smokers have higher levels of carboxyhaemoglobin than non-smokers. Despite earlier speculation, this is not now generally believed to be the mechanism leading to IHD. Cigarette smoke has been shown to cause endothelial damage, and may affect platelet aggregation. These may be mechanisms in the formation of atherosclerosis and thrombosis, and thus lead to clinical disease. The trend towards filter cigarettes in recent years appears to have made little impact on the risk of cardiovascular disease.

The demonstration of an association between smoking and IHD is not in itself proof that smoking is a cause of the disease. It has been argued that smokers may differ from non-smokers in factors apart from smoking which predisposes them to IHD. The judgement that the smoking–heart disease relationship is causal is strengthened by: (a) the consistency of the relationship – it has been demonstrated in many studies in different countries; (b) its strength – a risk approximately threefold greater among heavy smokers than among non-smokers; (c) its independence of other factors – in the presence of high blood pressure and elevated plasma cholesterol there is still a higher risk among smokers than among non-smokers (this is shown for smoking and blood pressure in Figure 1.8); (d) the lower risk of IHD among ex-smokers – the greater

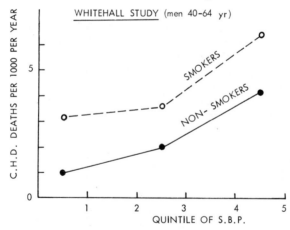

Figure 1.8 Smoking is independent of other risk factors (in this case blood pressure) as a cause of IHD. From: Reid, D. D., Hamilton, P. J. S., McCartney, P., *et al.* (1976) Smoking and other risk factors for coronary heart disease in British civil servants. *Lancet*, **ii**, 979–84 (by permission)

the numbers of years as an ex-smoker, the closer the mortality risk to that of a life-time non-smoker; (e) the time relationship – for example, in England and Wales over the last 20 years, IHD has become more common in working class men than in middle and upper class and at the same time smoking has decreased in middle and upper class men but not in working class men.

Although people who smoke may indeed be different from those who do not, and those who continue to smoke different from those who give up, the balance of evidence indicates that cigarette smoking is an important cause of IHD.

Psychosocial factors[8]

Socioeconomic

In general, IHD is more common in wealthy countries than in poor countries. Paradoxically, in wealthy countries it is the poorer groups who are most at risk. In England and Wales this is a change. In the past, IHD mortality was higher in higher status groups. As shown in Figure 1.9, since the 1950s mortality from IHD in working class men has risen

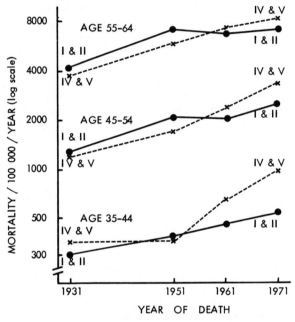

Figure 1.9 Heart disease mortality (ischaemic, degenerative, and hypertensive) in men in England and Wales according to social class. (Registrar-General's classification based on occupation: I-high V-low.) From Marmot, M. G., Adelstein, A. M., Robinson, N. and Rose, G. A., 1978, Changing social class distribution of heart disease. *Br. Med. J.*, ii, 1109–12, by permission

more steeply than in middle and upper class men, overtaking the latter by the 1960s. The reasons for the higher rates in lower income groups and for the change are not completely understood. As indicated above, smoking has become relatively more common in working class men and women – they eat somewhat different diets (but not more fat); they tend to be more overweight; they have higher mean blood pressures; and they report less leisure time physical activity. It is clear that there are other, as yet unidentified, factors which are also involved. It is of interest that more than one report shows a rise in unemployment to be followed by a rise in IHD mortality.

Psychosocial

Many of the great clinicians of history believed that heart disease was related to psychosocial factors. William Harvey ascribed a patient's disease to the fact that he, 'was overcome with anger and indignation which he yet communicated to no one'. John Hunter described his own angina pectoris as brought on by, 'agitation of the mind . . . principally anxiety or anger'. Hunter reportedly died from an attack which was provoked by a particularly irritating hospital board meeting. Osler enquired after the cause of, 'arterial degeneration in the worry and strain of modern life' and described the typical angina patient as the man, 'the indicator of whose engine is at full steam ahead'.

These descriptions accord with much current clinical and lay feeling that an acute coronary event or angina pectoris may be precipitated by psychological factors. The difficulty has been to demonstrate this scientifically. Two main approaches have been taken: (a) to identify potentially stressful situations which may increase the risk of IHD; and (b) to identify a particular 'coronary-prone' behaviour pattern.

Stressful situations

Much interest has centred on the study of stressful life events. Widowers have a higher mortality from IHD in the six months following bereavement than married men of the same age. There is some other evidence that stressful life events may precipitate myocardial infarction, and studies in Sweden, Israel, and Belgium have produced evidence that stress at work may increase the risk of myocardial infarction and angina pectoris. The Israeli study suggested, in addition, that men who received emotional support were less likely to develop angina as the result of their work problems than men without support.

This leads to the hypothesis that the balance between stressful events and the ability to cope with them determines whether a situation increases the risk of disease.

Coronary-prone behaviour patterns

Some of the strongest evidence relating psychosocial characteristics to IHD comes from the studies of 'Type A' or 'coronary-prone' behaviour pattern. The Type A individual is described as aggressive, striving, ambitious, restless, and excessively concerned with time and deadlines. This pattern of behaviour is particularly common where job stress is

16

reported to be high. In longitudinal studies, Type A individuals have greater than twice the risk of developing IHD compared with individuals who do not show this behaviour pattern – Type Bs. This increase in risk is independent of the other coronary risk factors described in earlier sections.

It has been shown by coronary angiography and post-mortem studies that Type As have a greater average degree of atheroma of the coronary arteries than do Type Bs. This suggests the existence of pathological pathways, other than raised lipid levels, which may accelerate athero-sclerosis. The possibility that this behaviour pattern may have adverse effects on the cardiovascular system is strengthened by the finding that Type A individuals react to stressful situations with greater increases in noradrenaline output than do Type Bs.

Much of the work on Type A behaviour has come from the United States of America. Initially, European studies affirmed the importance of Type A behaviour. More recently, doubt has emerged as to whether this can be generalized to different cultures.

In summary, a wide body of research of varying quality has provided evidence that psychosocial characteristics are causally linked to the development of clinical IHD. The exact nature of this link remains to be elucidated, as does a definition of the type of social environmental situation, which may increase the risk of disease. It is not known whether the risk of IHD can be altered by modifying the environment; more evidence is needed on the benefit or otherwise of individual changes in behaviour.

Geographic factors

Climate and season

In England and Wales, the mortality from IHD varies with the season. It is consistently higher in winter months. This winter increase may be related to increased spread of infection and/or an increase in pneumonia leading to a greater risk of death in persons already suffering from IHD. It might also be related to ambient temperature itself. Throughout the year there is an inverse association between temperature and IHD – the lower the temperature, the higher the mortality.

Data from North America show that there is a rise in IHD deaths after heavy snowfalls. The suggestion has been made that the combination of cold and the unaccustomed physical activity entailed in shovelling snow place an acute burden on the heart.

Support for this association with climatic factors comes from a com-parison of IHD mortality rates in different parts of Great Britain[22]. There is a twofold variation in cardiovascular mortality (i.e. IHD, other heart disease and stroke) in Great Britain. The rate is high in Scotland, north-west England, and South Wales, and low in south-east England. The areas with high mortality rates in general have lower average temperatures and more rainy days than the low mortality areas. Although the regional differences in mortality are also negatively correlated with socioeconomic factors and water hardness, there is sufficient variation in all of these factors to disentangle their effects. It has been demonstrated that the negative association between mortality and temperatures is independent of these other factors.

Water hardness

Studies in many countries have shown a negative association between water hardness and IHD mortality. The geographic differences in mortality in Great Britain are highly correlated negatively with water hardness: harder water, lower mortality[22]. The association with water hardness is independent of geographic differences in socioeconomic factors and climate.

It is difficult to determine what substance in hard water may be protective, or in soft water may be harmful; for example, water that is hard tends to have a high content of calcium, of carbonate, of nitrate, and of silica. To date there is no evidence that artificial softening of water increases the mortality from heart disease.

Alcohol

Alcoholics and 'heavy' drinkers of alcohol (variously defined) have an excess mortality from IHD. More recently there have been several reports that non-drinkers have a higher mortality from IHD than people who consume a moderate amount of alcohol (up to three drinks per day). Data from one such study are shown in Figure 1.10[14]. The consistency of

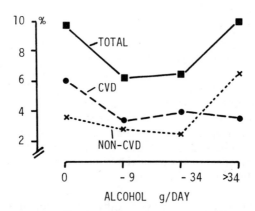

Figure 1.10 Ten-year mortality (age-adjusted percentage) all causes, cardiovascular (CVD), and non-cardiovascular (non-CVD) causes according to daily alcohol consumptions (Whitehall study). From: Marmot, M. G., Rose, G., Shipley, M. J. and Thomas, B. J., 1981, Alcohol and mortality: a U-shaped curve. *Lancet*, **1**, 580–83 (by permission)

this finding in various studies makes it likely that a moderate intake of alcohol is protective against IHD: it is not other characteristics of the non-drinker which put him at higher risk.

An international study comparing IHD mortality rates showed that the apparently protective effect of alcohol was confined to wine. In particular, in the countries of southern Europe, wine consumption is high and IHD mortality low.

Alcohol intake raises the level of plasma HDL cholesterol. This is a possible mechanism by which alcohol exerts its protective effect. It is also possible that a moderate level of alcohol intake is a successful way of dealing with stress and, thereby, lowering risk. It should be remembered, however, that at higher levels, alcohol consumption is associated with a high risk of dying from non-cardiovascular diseases – particularly from cancer.

Possibilities for prevention

Two approaches have been used in studies set up to test the feasibility of preventing premature IHD. The earlier investigations were all aimed at modifying only one factor. These studies, which will be described first, were carried out principally to determine whether the treatment being tested was of benefit in reducing disease frequency. There are several reasons why (with the knowledge of hindsight) these trials could not be expected to produce impressive results. First, the atheromatous process probably starts early in life. Consequently the ideal clinical trial should be started in young people. In fact, very few people under the age of 40 years have been entered into any of the studies and it should not be surprising if such studies fail to demonstrate striking benefit. Secondly, in a disease with multifactorial aetiology it might be expected that modification of only one factor would have little or no effect. Single factor intervention studies can, however, provide useful confirmatory evidence concerning aetiology: modification of a single factor in a randomized study producing reduced frequency of IHD in comparison with the control group is strong evidence that the association between that factor and IHD is causal.

More recently a 'multifactor' approach to prevention has evolved. The approach involves an attempt to modify several risk factors simultaneously, and was initially based on the fact that effects of the factors tend to cumulate. As was shown earlier, a smoker with high blood pressure is at greater risk than a smoker with lower blood pressure. If in addition his plasma cholesterol is high, his risk is increased still further. A pragmatic reason for a multifactor approach in trials of intervention arises from the difficulty in changing one factor at a time. For example, in one study (the United States National Diet Heart Study), 50% of the men who were asked to adhere to a special diet also reduced their cigarette consumption.

Prevention trials may be either primary (carried out in individuals who at the outset have no clinical manifestations of IHD) or secondary (where the subjects already have established disease).

Single factor intervention

Cholesterol reduction by means of diet and drugs

Trials of dietary modification aimed at reduction of cholesterol are not truly single factor trials: changes made in one dietary factor inevitably alter another. A decrease in total fat intake, for instance, will either reduce total energy intake or, if the energy level is maintained, require an increase in carbohydrate or protein. A lowering of the percentage contribution from saturated fatty acids will raise the polyunsaturated to saturated ratio whether or not the intake of polyunsaturated fatty acids is increased. Thus all dietary trials are multifactorial within the diet concept.

There have been three studies of *primary* prevention by dietary means[19]. Usually the main feature of the diet has been an increase in the proportion of fat derived from polyunsaturated sources at the expense of saturated fat in order to achieve a ratio of the former to the latter of 1.5 or 2:1 rather than 0.3:1, which commonly prevails in a typical British or North American diet. Only one (the Los Angeles Veterans Administration Study) has incorporated two essential features of a good clinical trial (random allocation of treatment groups and 'double blind' experimental conditions). This study (with 846 volunteers) showed a significant reduction in atherosclerotic events in the modified diet group compared with the control group and provided evidence that the beneficial effect of the fat-modified diet was via a cholesterol-lowering mechanism (the effect was seen only in those whose cholesterols were high initially and subsequently fell). Deaths from non-atherosclerotic causes occurred more frequently in the experimental group, thus raising the possibility that such a diet may actually be harmful although the difference between groups was not statistically significant (Table 1.3). The fact that the participants in this study were relatively old (average 65 years, range 55–89) and followed for only eight years may explain the failure to reflect in the overall mortality the benefit apparent in atherosclerotic deaths.

The other major primary prevention study was started in 1958 in two Finnish mental hospitals (N and K). During the first six years patients in Hospital K continued their usual diet whereas those in Hospital N were fed on an experimental diet rather similar to that used in Los Angeles. After six years the diets used in the two hospitals were reversed. End-points were assessed by physicians unaware of the dietary allocation, but there are major difficulties in the interpretation of this study. The population was, of course, an unusual one. The patients were not the same throughout the 12 years of the study: some were discharged to other institutions and new admissions were added. How-

Table 1.3 Summary tabulation of deaths and atherosclerotic events in the Los Angeles Veterans Administration Study

Category	Number of cases	
	Control	Experimental
Deaths		
Due to acute atherosclerotic event (sole cause)	60	39
Mixed causes, including acute atherosclerotic event	10	9
Due to atherosclerotic complications without acute event	1	2
Mixed causes, including atherosclerotic complication with acute event	10	7
Other causes	71	85
Uncertain causes	25	32
Total	177	174
Atherosclerotic events (fatal and non-fatal)		
Definite myocardial infarction (ECG)	4	9
Definite overt myocardial infarction	47	33
Sudden death	27	18
Total coronary events	78	60
Definite cerebral infarction	25	13
Ruptured aneurysm	5	2
Amputation	5	7
Miscellaneous	6	3

ever, most of the biases would have tended to have produced a negative rather than a positive result. Consequently the reduction in IHD death rates in the experimental as compared with the control periods together with a reduction in overall mortality (at least in men) is of considerable interest (Table 1.4).

Table 1.4 Age-adjusted death per 1000 person years in the Finnish Mental Hospital Study

	Males		Females	
	Experimental	Control	Experimental	Control
Coronary heart disease	6.6	14.1	5.2	7.9
Cerebrovascular disease	1.7	2.4	2.2	2.0
Other circulatory	3.2	2.5	3.1	2.4
Neoplasms	5.0	4.0	4.1	3.7
Accidents, etc.	2.8	3.5	1.8	1.8
Other causes	15.4	13.0	14.4	11.2
All causes	34.7	39.5	30.8	29.0

There have been six studies of *secondary* prevention by means of dietary modification. These have shown no consistent trends in terms of outcome, but all have been small (100–450 volunteers) and the final results are therefore subject to a considerable margin of error. The data in Figure 1.11, in which confidence limits have been fitted to the results

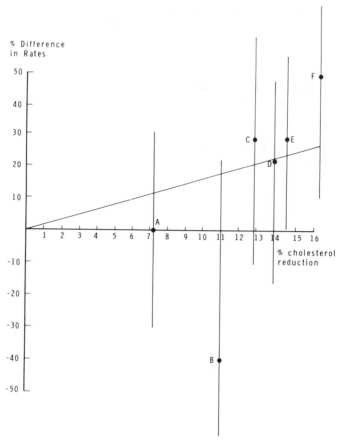

Figure 1.11 The percentages of difference in IHD rates (and confidence limits) between experimental and control groups on the randomized dietary studies of primary and secondary prevention.

A = Research Committee to the Medical Research Council (1965). Low-fat diet in myocardial infarction – a controlled trial. *Lancet, 2,* 500

B = Rose, G., Thompson, W. B. and Williams, R. T. (1965). Corn oil in treatment of IHD. *Br. Med. J.,* 1, 1531

C = Dayton, S., Pearce, M. L., Hashimoto, S., Dixon, W. J. and Tomiyasu, U. (1969). A controlled clinical trial of a diet high in unsaturated fat in preventing complications of atherosclerosis. *Circulation,* 39 and 40 (suppl. II)

D = Research Committee to the Medical Research Council (1968). Controlled trial of soya-bean oil in myocardial infarction. *Lancet, 2,* 693

E = Leren, P. (1970). The Oslo diet-heart study – 11 year report. *Circulation,* 42, 935

F = Turpeinen, O., Karvonen, M. J., Pekkarinen, M., Miettinen, M., Elosuo, R. and Paavilainen, E. (1979). Dietary prevention of coronary heart disease – the Finnish Mental Hospital Study. *Int. J. Epidemiol.,* 8, 99 of all the studies (primary and secondary) which have included a control group, are therefore of particular interest. The best regression line is indicated. It is clear that the confidence limits in each case include this line. The relatively small number of subjects in each study have produced the wide confidence intervals and could explain the apparently conflicting findings. Viewing the data in aggregate, however, it is possible to estimate from the graph that, for example, a 10% reduction in cholesterol confers a $15 \pm 6\%$ reduction in IHD risk ($p < 0.01$). A similar analysis has been carried out for the randomized studies of cholesterol modification by drugs (Figure 1.12). Here a more consistent trend emerges. On the basis of these data a 10% reduction in cholesterol seems to produce a $21 \pm 5\%$ reduction in IHD risk. The consistency between the two data sets is remarkable and provides considerable evidence for the aetiological importance of serum cholesterol in IHD.

Undoubtedly the most impressive of the drug trials is the Lipid Research Clinics Coronary Prevention Trial[11] in which cholestyramine and placebo were compared in 3886 men in whom dietary modification failed to reduce cholesterol below 6.9 mmol/l. The cholestyramine-treated group had a 19% lower rate of fatal and non-fatal IHD. The reduction in IHD incidence was proportional to reduction in total and low density lipoprotein cholesterol. Total mortality was also reduced in the cholestyramine-treated group, although the differences were not quite so striking because of a modest, unexplained, increase in deaths due to accidents in the cholestyramine group. The WHO Clofibrate Study showed a beneficial result in terms of non-fatal and all cardiovascular events (in accordance with the cholesterol-lowering effect) but no reduction in fatal IHD in those taking clofibrate. Indeed, mortality from all causes was significantly higher in the clofibrate than the placebo group; the excess mortality increased progressively over time, leading to the suggestion that clofibrate may have long-term toxic effects.

Blood pressure

Numerous clinical trials have shown a beneficial effect of treating moderate and severe hypertension, but the benefit has invariably been in terms of stroke. However, two recent studies suggest a reduction also in IHD in association with the treatment of hypertension. The Australian National Blood Pressure Study[12] was a controlled trial of antihypertensive drug treatment in men and women aged 30–69 whose diastolic blood pressures were repeatedly 95 mmHg or greater and whose systolic blood pressures were less than 200 mmHg. Eligible subjects were randomized to receive placebo or active treatment – chlorothiazide 500 mg daily initially; methyldopa, propranolol, or pindolol was added if the diuretic alone was inadequate, finally with hydralazine or clonidine if the diastolic blood pressure was still not below 90 mmHg. They were followed for an average of four years; the numbers of trial end-points observed in the various diagnostic categories are given in Table 1.5. By

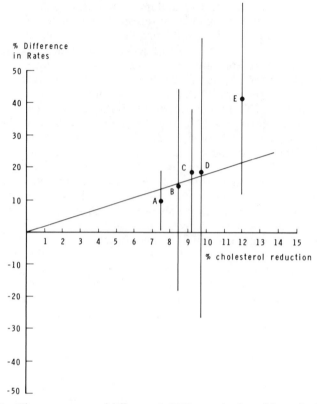

Figure 1.12 The percentages of difference in IHD rates (and confidence limits) between experimental and control groups in the randomized studies of primary and secondary prevention drugs

A = Coronary Drug Project Group (1975). Clofibrate and niacin in coronary heart disease. *J. Am. Med. Assoc.*, **231**, 360

B = Dewar, H. A. and Oliver, M. F. (1971). Secondary prevention trials using clofibrate. A joint commentary on the Newcastle and Scottish trials. *Br. Med J.*, **4**, 784 [Edinburgh sample]

C = Committee of Principal Investigators (1978). A co-operative trial in the prevention of ischaemic heart disease using clofibrate. *Br. Med. J.*, **10**, 1069

D = Dorr, A. E., Gunderson, K., Schneider, J. C., Spencer, T. W. and Martin, W. B. (1978). Colestipol hydrochloride in hypercholesterolaemic patients. Effect on serum cholesterol and mortality. *J. Chron. Dis.*, **31**, 5

E = Dewar, H. A. and Oliver, M. F. (1971). Secondary prevention trials using clofibrate. A joint commentary on the Newcastle and Scottish trials. *Br. Med. J.*, **4**, 784. [Newcastle sample]

Table 1.5   Number of fatal cases in the Australia National Blood Pressure Study

	Intention to treat		On treatment	
	Active	Placebo	Active	Placebo
Ischaemic heart disease	5	11	2	8
Cerebrovascular events	3	6	2	4
Other fatal cases	17	18	5	7

two methods of analysis fewer cases of fatal IHD occurred in the active than in the placebo group. The numbers, however, were small and the difference just short of statistical significance. The study has shown the possible value of treating what would generally be considered quite mild hypertension and also that treating hypertension even in relatively mild degree may produce a reduction of IHD as well as stroke.

The results of the Hypertension Detection and Follow-up Program in the United States were rather similar[7]. Approximately 160 000 people aged 30–69 were screened. Those considered to require treatment for hypertension were randomized to receive either routine ('referred') medical care or treatment in a 'systematic antihypertension treatment program' ('stepped care'). Five-year mortality from all causes was 17% lower for those receiving specialized treatment, which also achieved consistently better blood pressure results. Table 1.6 shows that myo-

Table 1.6   Number of deaths by cause, stepped care (SC) and referred care (RC) in the hypertension detection and follow-up programme

Cause of death (ICDA Codes)	Total		With diastolic blood pressures 90–104 mmHg	
	SC	RC	SC	RC
All cardiovascular diseases	195	240	122	165
Cerebrovascular diseases (430–438)	29	52	17	31
Myocardial infarction (410)	51	69	30	56
Other ischaemic heart disease (411–413)	80	79	56	51
Hypertensive heart disease (402)	5	7	5	5
Other hypertensive disease (400–401, 403–404)	4	7	2	3
Other cardiovascular diseases (390–458 exclusive of above)	26	26	12	19
All non-cardiovascular diseases	154	179	109	126
Total	349	419	231	291

cardial infarction, as well as other cardiovascular conditions, occurred less frequently in this group.

The results of three major multicentre trials were published in 1985: the MRC trial examined the potential benefit of treating mild hypertension and the relative advantages of diuretics and beta blockers. The European Working Party on Hypertension in the Elderly (EWPHE) recruited patients over the age of 60 years with a diastolic blood pressure at entry of 90–119 mmHg. The third study specifically examined the possible beneficial effects of regimens containing a beta blocker. The MRC and EWPHE studies showed similar reductions in the stroke rate (45 and 52%, respectively). When considering only fatal strokes the reduction was not statistically significant. With regard to myocardial infarction the MRC study showed almost identical rates in treatment and placebo groups. In the EWPHE study non-fatal myocardial infarctions were not influenced by treatment but there was a significant reduction in fatal myocardial infarction. This suggests a qualitative difference in the elderly heart as a result of which the combination of myocardial infarction and blood pressure is particularly lethal, although there is no indication from either of these studies that treatment modified the hypertensive patients' predisposition to myocardial infarction. The clinical applications of these trials with regard to when and how to treat hypertension have been extensively reviewed (e.g. Treatment of hypertension: the 1985 results. Leading article, *Lancet*, 1985, **2**, 645–647).

Multiple factor intervention

Because of the substantial number of difficulties associated with single factor intervention studies, more recent interest has focused on the 'multiple factor' approach.

Intervention in subgroups

A multicentre European trial introduced health education into factories randomly selected from pairs, the non-selected member of the pair serving as a control. The health education included advice on diet, the importance of not smoking, of increased physical activity, of weight reduction and information on hypertension. In addition, men with a mean systolic blood pressure above 160 mmHg were started on hypotensive drug therapy. Only small net reductions in risk factors were achieved and the reduction in overall IHD mortality was only 7.4%. However, support that this represented more than a chance improvement came from analysis of the results from individual centres. The United Kingdom had the worst record of risk factor reduction and showed no evidence of a fall in incidence. Belgium and Italy produced the greatest reduction in risk factors with commensurate changes in incidence; for example, in Belgium, there was a highly significant 24% reduction in IHD.

In the Oslo trial[6] men at high risk of CHD (as a result of smoking or having a cholesterol level in the range of 7.5–9.8 mmol/l) were divided into two groups: half received intensive dietary education and advice to stop smoking; the other half served as a control group. An impressive reduction in total coronary events was observed (31 vs 57 per 1000 over a 5-year period) in association with a 13% fall in cholesterol and 65%

reduction in tobacco consumption. There has also been a significant improvement in total mortality. Detailed statistical analysis suggests that approximately 60% of the IHD reduction can be attributed to serum cholesterol change and 25% to smoking reduction.

In the light of these relatively encouraging results the findings of the American Multiple Risk Factor Intervention Trial (MRFIT)[18] were rather disappointing. Men at high risk were chosen on the basis of plasma cholesterol and smoking (similar to Oslo[6]) and also of blood pressure. Intervention against these three risk factors for 6 years in the 'special intervention' group produced a reduction in smoking of 50%, in diastolic blood pressure of 10.5 mmHg, and in serum cholesterol of 5%. However, the control group randomized to 'usual care' also showed changes: reduction of smoking of 29%, in diastolic blood pressure of 7.3 mmHg, and in plasma cholesterol of 3%. Clearly a trial which achieves a reduction in plasma cholesterol in the intervention group only 2% greater than the controls cannot be used to show if a reduction in plasma cholesterol will lead to a reduction in IHD incidence. Furthermore, over the study period IHD mortality in the United States general population declined by 25%. As a result of this and of the risk factor reductions in controls as well as the intervention group, both groups had lower than predicted mortality and there was no significant difference between the groups.

Perhaps the most interesting aspect of the trial is the fact that when considering only hypercholesterolaemic men or men who smoked (i.e. individuals similar to those participating in the Oslo trial) the improvement noted in the special intervention group was comparable with that observed in Oslo[6]. The higher mortality amongst hypertensive men, especially those with ECG abnormalities, has led to the suggestion of adverse effects of the drugs used for treating hypertension. This trial also underlines the near impossibility of achieving an appropriate control group in countries where there is so great an awareness of coronary risk factors and their consequences. It seems most unlikely that further trials will be carried out.

Community approach

A different approach has emphasized intervention to change a whole community. One controlled trial, in North Karelia in eastern Finland, assessed the effect of multiple changes (Table 1.7). As well as health education, there was provision of low fat dairy products and sausages, changed diet in institutions, smoking prohibition in public places and special training of health personnel. These efforts resulted in changes in dietary behaviour and smoking, reduction in blood pressure and a small reduction in plasma cholesterol. There was a reduction in IHD of 18% in North Karelia during the 5 years of study. This seems unimpressive but the duration of the study so far is probably too short to expect much effect on clinical events. Interpretation of the results is made more

Table 1.7 Total mortality and mortality from cardiovascular disease in men and women aged 30–64 in North Karelia and the control area during 1970–1 and 1976–77 showing average annual age-adjusted rate per 1000 people with 95 per cent confidence limits

	Men		Women	
	North Karelia	Control area	North Karelia	Control area
Total mortality				
1970–71	13.8 ± 0.9	13.6 ± 0.7	4.8 ± 0.5	5.0 ± 0.4
1976–77	11.6 ± 0.8	11.4 ± 0.7	3.9 ± 0.5	3.8 ± 0.4
Difference	2.2 ± 1.1	2.2 ± 1.0	0.9 ± 1.3	1.2 ± 0.6
Mortality from cardiovascular disease				
1970–71	7.7 ± 0.6	7.7 ± 0.6	2.5 ± 0.4	2.5 ± 0.3
1976–77	6.3 ± 0.6	5.8 ± 0.5	1.7 ± 0.3	1.6 ± 0.3
Difference	1.4 ± 0.9	1.9 ± 0.7	0.8 ± 0.5	0.9 ± 0.4

difficult by the fact that similar trends were apparent in the control community (and much of the rest of Finland) where, not surprisingly in view of the high IHD mortality rates, the entire population has changed its behaviour. After 10 years, there is a confirmed decline in IHD mortality in many parts of Finland – possibly greater in North Karelia.

A study of similar design in California successfully produced a reduction in smoking, plasma cholesterol and blood pressure in the experimental as compared with the control areas; however, no change in IHD was detected in this small study. Numbers in the trial are currently being expanded in the hope of producing more data with regard to IHD.

The North Karelia project (like the MRFIT trial) confirms the difficulty of any form of controlled study in a population aware of the high risk of IHD and of measures which might reduce the risk. The approach nevertheless remains a promising one for putting prevention into practice.

Intervention for high risk groups or everyone?

There is now reasonable evidence that those at high risk of IHD because of hypercholesterolaemia and smoking will benefit from modification of these risk factors even if the intervention is initiated in middle age. It is not clear whether this applies to those with established clinical IHD nor whether there is an age beyond which a change in life style is no longer of benefit. The trials have not included women, who in general have a lower IHD risk than men. Consensus is gradually emerging concerning the appropriate diet which should be recommended for lowering cholesterol: a reduction in saturated fatty acids, an increase in fibre-rich carbohydrate, and a modest increase in the ratio of polyunsaturated to saturated fatty acids. The MRFIT trial suggests that consideration must be given to the precise hypotensive agent used, but because of the proven benefit in terms of cerebrovascular disease few would dispute the suggestion that those discovered to have moderate or severe hypertension should be treated. Advice to stop smoking, to modify dietary habits, and a consideration of hypotensive drug therapy (if simple life style modifications have failed) are therefore rapidly becoming part of routine clinical practice when individuals are discovered to be smokers or are found to have raised levels of cholesterol or blood pressure. The role of lipid-lowering drugs is less clear but the Lipid Research Clinic's trial[11] of cholestyramine suggests that some individuals with diet-resistant hyperlipidaemia should be considered as candidates for drug therapy.

However, concentration only on high risk individuals has two major disadvantages. First, it entails some form of screening or case finding to detect people at high risk. Secondly, it limits the potential benefit of the intervention to the high risk group. For example, the high risk group might be defined – on the basis of smoking habits, blood pressure, and plasma cholesterol levels – as the top 15% of the distribution of these factors in the population. Of the subsequent IHD events in the total population, one would expect that 30% would occur in this high risk group. If, for example, intervention were successful in achieving a 50% reduction in risk in those who participated, this would lead only to a 15% reduction (50% of the 30% of cases that occur in the high risk group) in the rate of IHD in the whole population. In other words, by concentrating efforts only on the 15% of the population at highest risk, nothing would be done to prevent the 70% of cases that occur in the rest of the population not classified as 'high risk'. Clearly, if it were possible to lower the risk level of the whole population, this could have potentially a much greater impact on the population rate of IHD. Many countries with high IHD rates, including the United Kingdom, now have official recommendations suggesting dietary change for the entire population, a view strongly endorsed by a National Institute of Health Consensus Development Conference in December 1984.

Future research

Further intervention trials are unlikely but perhaps equally helpful epidemiological data will be generated from carefully documented information concerning changing incidence of IHD (in countries where IHD is either increasing or decreasing) in relation to measured changes in environmental factors and to changes in risk factor status. Research is also required concerning simple and acceptable means of modifying risk characteristics. There is as yet not even an established method for persuading people to give up smoking, the advantages of which have been established beyond reasonable doubt.

References

1. Armstrong, B. K., Mann, J. I. and Adelstein, A. M. (1975). Commodity consumption and ischaemic heart disease mortality, with special reference to dietary practices. *J. Chronic Dis.*, **28**, 455–469
2. Carlson, L. A., Bottiger, L. E. and Anfeldt, P. E. (1979). Risk factors for myocardial infarction in the Stockholm Prospective Study. *Acta Med. Scand.*, **206**, 351–360
3. Dawber, T. D. (1980). *The Framingham Study*. Cambridge, Mass.: Harvard University Press
4. Dwyer, J. and Hetzel, B. S. (1980). A comparison of trends of coronary heart disease mortality in Australia, USA and England and Wales with reference to three major risk factors – hypertension, smoking and diet. *Int. J. Epidemiol.* **9**, 65–71
5. Epstein, F. H. (1971). Editorial. *Atherosclerosis*, **14**, 1–2
6. Hjermann, I., Byrne, K. V., Holme, J. *et al.* (1981). Effect of diet and smoking intervention on the incidence of coronary heart disease: report from the Oslo Study Group of randomised trials in healthy men. *Lancet*, **2**, 1303–1309
7. Hypertension Detection and Follow-Up Program Cooperative Group (1979). Five year findings of the hypertension detection and follow-up program. *J. Am. Med. Assoc.*, **242**, 2562–2571
8. Jenkins, C. D. (1976). Recent evidence supporting psychologic and social risk factors for coronary disease (first of two parts). *N. Engl. J. Med.*, **294**, 987–994 and 1033–1038
9. Kannell, W. B. and Castelli, W. P. (1979). Is the serum total cholesterol an anachronism? *Lancet* **2**, 950–951
10. Keys, A. (1980). *Seven Countries*. Cambridge, Mass.: Harvard University Press
11. Lipid Research Clinics Program (1984). The Lipid Research Clinics Coronary Primary Prevention Trial results. I. Reduction in incidence of coronary heart disease. *J. Am. Med. Assoc.*, **251**, 351–364
12. Management Committee (1980). The Australian Therapeutic Trial: mild hypertension. *Lancet*, **1**, 1261–1267
13. Mann, J. I. and Marr, J. W. (1981). Coronary heart disease prevention: trials of diets to control hyperlipidaemia. In N. E. Miller and B. Lewis (eds) *Lipoproteins, Atherosclerosis and Coronary Heart Disease*. Amsterdam: Elsevier/North Holland, Biomedical Press
14. Marmot, M. G. (1984). Alcohol and coronary heart disease. *Int. J. Epidemiol.*, **13**, 160–167
15. Meade, T. W., Chakrabarti, R., Haines, A. P., North, W. R. S. and Stirling, Y. (1980). Haemostatic function and cardiovascular death: early results of a prospective study. *Lancet*, **1**, 1050–1054
16. Morris, J. N., Marr, J. W. and Clayton, D. G. (1977). Diet and heart: a postscript. *Br. Med. J.*, **2**, 1307–1314
17. Morris, J. N., Pollard, R., Everitt, M. G. and Chave, S. P. W. (1980). Vigorous exercise in leisure time: protection against coronary heart disease. *Lancet*, **2**, 1207–1210
18. Multiple Risk Factor Intervention Trial Research Group (1982). Multiple Risk Factor Intervention Trial. Risk factor changes and mortality results. *J. Am. Med. Assoc.*, **248**, 1465–1477
19. Oliver, M. F. (1981). Primary prevention of coronary heart disease: An appraisal of clinical trials of reducing raised plasma cholesterol. In: N. E. Miller and B. Lewis (eds.) *Lipoproteins, Atherosclerosis and Coronary Heart Disease*. (Amsterdam: Elsevier/North Holland, Biomedical Press)
20. Paffenbarger, R. S. and Hale, W. E. (1975). Work activity and coronary heart mortality. *N. Engl. J. Med.*, **292**, 545–550
21. Pelkonen, R., Nikkila, E. A., Koskinen, S., Plenttinen, K. and Sama, S. (1977). Association of serum lipids and obesity with cardiovascular mortality. *Br. Med. J.*, **2**, 1185–1187
22. Pocock, S. J., Shaper, A. G., Cook, D. G., Packham, R. F., Lacey, R. F., Powell, P.

and Russell, P. F. (1980). British Regional Heart Study: geographic variations in cardiovascular mortality, and the role of water quality. *Br. Med. J.*, **280**, 1243

23. Royal College of Physicians of London and British Cardiac Society. (1976). Prevention of coronary heart disease. (Report of a joint working party.) *J. R. Coll. Physicians. Lond.*, **10**, 1–63

24. Shekelle, R. B., Shrycock, A. M., Paul, O., Lepper, M., Stamler, J. *et al.* (1981). Diet, serum cholesterol and death from coronary heart disease: the Western Electric Study. *N. Engl. J. Med.*, **304**, 65–70

25. Stamler, R. and Stamler, J. (1979). Asymptomatic hyperglycaemic and coronary heart disease. *J. Chronic Dis.*, **32**, 683–691

2
Pathology of ischaemic heart disease

M. J. DAVIES

Clinical interest in atheroma, as regards the heart, begins with the asymptomatic patient in whom there is sufficient intimal disease to allow angina, acute infarction or sudden death to occur. The prior detection of such individuals is, however, rarely possible other than they may, but not inevitably, be members of groups identified in epidemiological studies to have certain risk factors[1].

The process of atheroma, which leads to this point, has been progressing slowly over many years since childhood[2,3] but the initiation of symptoms is largely mediated by episodic sudden events – most of which involve thrombosis. This concept that atheroma is a biphasic process is a generalization, which does simplify understanding of the complex morphology of end stage arterial lesions and introduces the possibility that risk factors, or therapeutic interventions, may influence either one or both of these stages.

Atheroma is an intimal disease of arteries in which two components, i.e. connective tissue proliferation and lipid accumulation, are present. Another characteristic is that the process occurs in focal areas of the intima and, with rare exceptions, is not diffuse.

Examination of the intimal surface of an artery, which has been opened longitudinally, shows the smallest atheromatous lesions to be yellow streaks or dots barely raised above the surface. These fatty streaks are focal collections of lipid containing 'foam' cells scattered amid smooth muscle cells within the intima and are regarded as the earliest stage of atheroma. The International Atherosclerosis Project[4] demonstrated that fatty streaks were ubiquitous in all geographic populations, irrespective of whether the clinical manifestations of ischaemic heart disease occurred – thus not all fatty streaks inevitably progress. Study of subjects of different ages from populations with a high incidence of atherosclerotic disease, however, shows that fibromuscular plaques develop at sites where fatty streaks are most common and that the proportional intimal involvement by fatty streaks is higher in such populations. This data suggests there is a precursor–product relation between the fatty streak and raised lesions[5].

In contrast to the fatty streak, the raised fibrous plaque – as seen in a longitudinally opened artery – projects upward from the surface as an oval white hump and is the predominant prevalent lesion in the coronary arteries of populations with a high risk of ischaemic heart disease.

All raised plaques contain varying proportions of lipid, smooth muscle and a connective tissue matrix rich in collagen and glycosoaminoglycans. The proportions of each component vary so widely that plaques are never identical to one another, i.e. there is no 'standard' raised plaque. At one extreme there are lipid rich plaques with a central pool of extracellular cholesterol and its esters; at the other extreme, a plaque may consist almost entirely of collagen with a minimal population of cells containing intracellular lipid.

The developmental relations that exist between the different forms of atheromatous plaque in man have been postulated by comparison of the morphological appearances of lesions of different sizes in an individual at autopsy. The assumption is made that large lesions must develop from smaller lesions, but absolute proof of these transitions is lacking.

The sequence regarded as most credible at the present time (Figure 2.1)

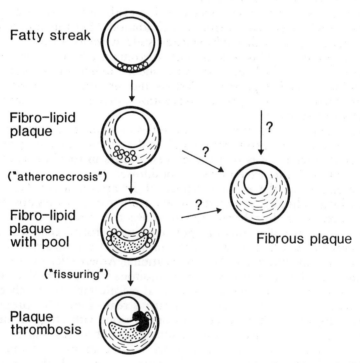

Figure 2.1 Diagrammatic representation of plaque growth seen in cross sections of an artery. Macrophages are shown as open circles, extracellular lipid is stippled, thrombus is black

is that the early fatty streak consists of a focal collection of macrophages containing intracellular lipid immediately beneath the endothelium within the intima. This lesion becomes elevated due to the ingrowth of smooth muscle cells from the media, which then form a layer separating the macrophages from the endothelium. The lesion now enlarges both by proliferation of the connective tissue and by accumulation of more macrophages. In the next stage, there is necrosis of macrophages leading to the formation of a pool of extracellular lipid deep in the intima. The relation of hard fibrous plaques, which consist almost entirely of collagen to this sequence of events is unknown.

Plaques with a pool of extracellular lipid ('atheronecrosis') encapsulated into the basal layer of the intima are very characteristic human lesions but are not a feature of most experimental models of atheroma induced by high lipid diets. The relevance of such animal models must be questioned since the lipid rich plaque is an important substrate for the development of thrombosis and the initiation of symptoms in man.

The morphology of raised atheromatous plaques is seen in a different light in cross sections of arteries distended at physiological pressures during fixation. Lipid rich plaques are seen to contain a crescentic shaped mass of free cholesterol encapsulated within the intima (Figure 2.3). This lipid pool is separated from the arterial lumen by a cap of fibrous tissue which may be quite thin at focal points. The lumen, while often reduced in overall area, remains close to circular in shape since the plaque bulges outward into the media which is thinned. The plaque may involve one quadrant only of the circumference of the artery; the corollary is that the lumen, although it remains approximately circular in shape, is displaced from the centre point of the vessel.

The pathogenesis of the intimal changes that occur in atheroma remain controversial with different views going in and out of fashion. It seems certain that no single mechanism can be responsible for the complexity of the morphological responses in atheroma (Figure 2.2). The focal distribution of the lesions is usually ascribed to localized endothelial injury resulting from haemodynamic forces. The evidence for this view comes from the localization of atheromatous plaques at sites of maximum turbulence and low shear rate[6].

The most essential component of early atheroma is the proliferation of smooth muscle cells, which have migrated into the intima from the media. This proliferation is regarded as a response to intimal injury and current research into the pathogenesis of atheroma concentrates on the nature of this injury[5]. Smooth muscle cells possess specific receptors for a growth factor released from the alpha granules of platelets and a virtually identical factor is released by activated macrophages and damaged endothelial cells.

Smooth muscle cells within the media serve a contractile function responsible for maintaining vascular tone; but following injury to the endothelium smooth muscle cells, they can also migrate into the intima and take on a new 'synthetic' role both proliferating and forming large

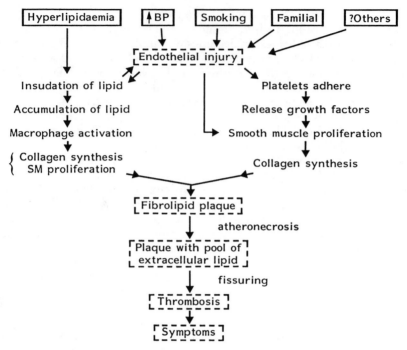

Figure 2.2 Schematic representation of the ways in which risk factors may invoke atheroma and the mechanisms of plaque growth

amounts of connective tissue matrix including basement membrane proteins, elastin, collagen and proteoglycan. The proportion of matrix to cells is so high that it seems unlikely that contraction is an important function and the role of the smooth muscle cell in the intima is more akin to that undertaken by fibroblasts in other tissues. Smooth muscle cells possess receptors for lipoproteins and can take up lipid but the current view is that the majority of foam cells seen within the intima are of macrophage origin[7].

The major lipid present within the intima is cholesterol and its esters believed to have been derived from the plasma lipoproteins but there is a vast literature concerning the equilibrium between low density lipoproteins in the plasma and the normal intima or atheromatous plaque[8]. Macrophages have receptors for both native and modified low density lipoproteins and the formation of foam cells probably represents a normal scavenger function for lipid that has accumulated in the intima. Activation of macrophages could lead to localized tissue damage by the formation of superoxide anions, lysosomal hydrolases and by oxidation products of lipid[9]. Activated macrophages are also known to provide growth factors capable of causing smooth muscle proliferation[5].

Endothelial damage has been linked to underlying smooth muscle proliferation via the production of growth factors, both from endothelial cells and activated platelets[5]. It has been known for a long time that denuding the endothelium in experimental animals exposes the underlying collagen, which in turn causes adherence of platelets and thus the release platelet derived growth factors. Subsequent intimal smooth muscle proliferation is dependent on this growth factor – the release of which can be blocked by antiplatelet drugs[5,10]. It seems unlikely, however, that massive endothelial denudation occurs naturally in man and close attention is now being paid to non-denuding injury of the endothelial cells.

Experimental atheroma induced by high lipid diets leads to changes in the endothelial cells, which result in endothelial retraction allowing platelet adherence as well as increased migration of monocytes into the intima[11]. Damaged endothelial cells may become more permeable allowing greater insudation of lipid, or may themselves release growth factors acting on smooth muscle cells.

The initial growth of atheromatous plaques in man must be a slow progressive proliferation; but there is also a later sudden step-like progression mediated by complications, which include thrombosis[12,13]. This phase of atheroma is not to any appreciable degree simulated in animal models.

CLINICAL EXPRESSIONS OF CORONARY ATHEROMA IN MAN

The clinical expressions of ischaemic heart disease fall into two groups: stable chronic angina and the acute syndromes encompassing unstable angina; acute myocardial infarction and sudden ischaemic death. There is compelling clinical and pathological evidence to believe that the underlying pathology within the arterial wall can similarly be divided into chronic static lesions, or those which are acute and evolving in which thrombosis in some form is present[10].

Stable angina

Pathological studies[14,15] have shown that the great majority of patients with stable angina have one or more segments of coronary artery stenosis greater than 50% by diameter (75% by cross-sectional area) caused by the intimal lesions of atheroma. The relative proportions of single, double and triple vessel disease and the total number of segments involved by high grade lesions varies depending on the source of the patients under study. Any clinical series based on angiography will give more optimistic figures than an autopsy series biased toward end stage disease.

The *morphological appearances* of these areas of high grade stenosis is, at first sight, dauntingly complex; the complexity, however, results from permutations of a small number of variables. The intimal thickening, which comprises the atheromatous plaque, may either be eccentric (i.e. involving one quadrant of the arterial wall only) or concentric

(Figures 2.3, 2.4). In the former, the lumen is displaced from the midline; and in the latter case, the lumen remains more centrally placed. The intimal thickening may either contain large amounts of lipid, both as a free pool of cholesterol and within foam cells (Figures 2.3, 2.6), or virtually no lipid (Figures 2.4, 2.5). In the latter case the intimal thickening is made up of relatively acellular collagen. All these appearances are taken to represent the steady progression of the same processes that lead to the initiation of atheroma.

A proportion of arterial segments with high grade stenosis in patients with stable angina have a different appearance in that the original lumen is obliterated by connective tissue containing several new vascular channels (Figure 2.7). Such morphological appearances are thought to indicate that there has been recanalization of a previous occlusive thrombus.

Post-mortem angiography allows a correlation to be made between the X-ray appearances and the plaque histology. Long diffusely narrowed segments (Figure 2.8) are most consistently associated with concentric intimal fibrosis. Focal areas of high grade stenosis (Figure 2.9) are most consistently related to eccentric intimal thickening, which may or may not contain a free lipid pool. Recanalized segments can be recognized by the multiple channels present within an area of stenosis (Figure 2.10), although the resolution of clinical angiograms may not allow this degree of discrimination.

The widespread publication of histological pictures of cross-sections of arteries that have not been distended during fixation has led to an impression that the lumen, at points of stenosis, may be crescentic, slit like or even star shaped. Examination of arteries, which have been distended at physiological pressures prior to fixation, shows the lumen to be approximately circular in most cases. The intima may be flattened over plaques that only involve one segment of the intima to produce a D shaped lumen; if two such lesions are exactly opposite each other an oval shaped lumen results[16].

Considerable clinical interest has been taken in segments of stenosis that are visible in one plane at angiography but not in another. D or oval shapes of the lumen are one explanation for this phenomenon, but there are other possible explanations. In areas of stenosis in which the lumen is eccentrically placed, the angiogram in one plane shows the lesion to be an indentation in one side of the vessel. A plane at right angles distributes the indentation equally to both sides of the vessel and may be interpreted – within the limitations of the resolution of clinical angiograms – as being less significant. Another explanation suggested by examining artificial stenosis made in glass tubes is that certain planes not exactly at right angles to the *long* axis of the tube are responsible.

Clinical angiograms show that the cross-sectional area of the lumen at points of stenosis due to eccentric plaques can be altered by pharmacological manipulation of vasomotor tone[17]. This variation in lumen size has been linked to the contraction of the medial muscle in the segment

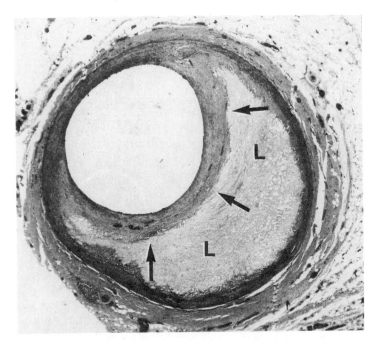

Figure 2.3 Cross section of an artery distended at physiological pressure during fixation. The lumen is circular in shape. There is eccentric thickening of the intima which contains a crescentic pale staining mass of extracellular lipid (L). This lipid is separated from the lumen by a layer of fibrous tissue which forms the cap of the plaque (arrows). *Elastic haematoxylin eosin (EHE) stain*

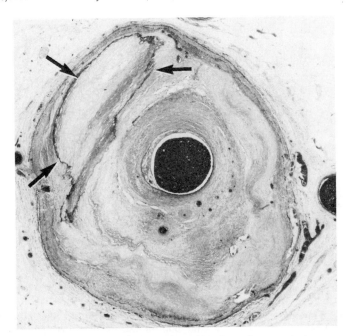

Figure 2.4 Transverse section of an artery with high grade stenosis due to concentric intimal fibrous thickening. The lumen is centrally placed, round, and contains post-mortem angiographic material. Within the intima there is a mass of calcium (arrows). *EHE stain*

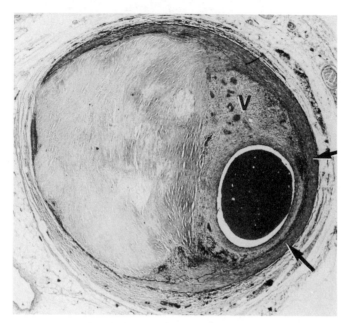

Figure 2.5 Transverse section of high grade stenosis due to eccentric fibrous thickening of the intima. The lumen is displaced from the midline and contains post mortem angiographic media. In relation to the lumen there is an arc of normal vessel wall (arrows). At one point (V) the intima contains a number of new small blood vessels. *EHE stain*

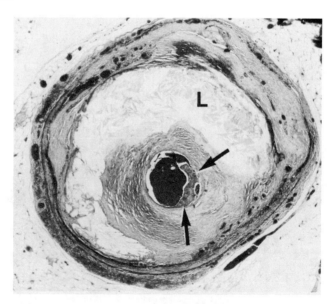

Figure 2.6 Transverse section of an artery with stenosis due to concentric intimal thickening within which there is a large pool of extracellular lipid (L). The lumen contains angiographic media. Attached to the endothelial surface is a small mass of mural thrombus (arrows) but the underlying plaque has an intact cap. *EHE stain*

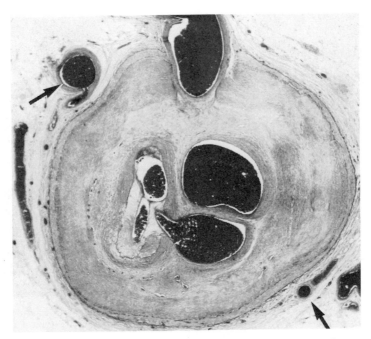

Figure 2.7 Transverse section of a coronary artery in which there are three separate vascular channels containing angiographic media. Adjacent to the artery in the adventitia are well developed collateral vessels also containing angiographic media (arrows). *EHE stain*

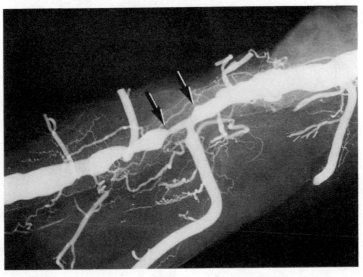

Figure 2.8 Postmortem angiogram in which there is stenosis due to concentric intimal thickening in one segment (arrow). The adjacent arterial segments show eccentric plaques. From a patient with stable angina

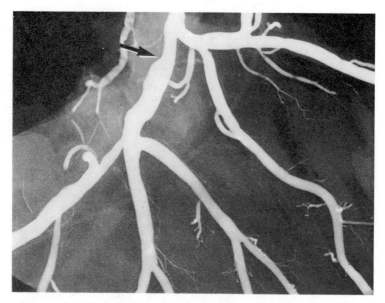

Figure 2.9 Stenosis in the left anterior descending artery due to an eccentric atheromatous plaque (arrows). Smooth edged stenoses of this type are typical of stable angina

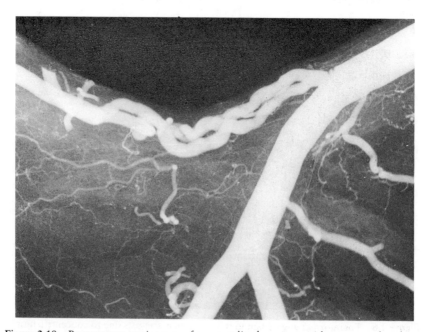

Figure 2.10 Postmortem angiogram of a recanalized segment with two vascular channels within the original arterial lumen

of normal vessel wall opposite the plaque[18–21]. Concentric stenosis does not have the same potential due to the splinting effect of the thickened intima and the loss of medial muscle, which is a constant feature behind plaques (Figure 2.11). It has been calculated that in segments of over 50% stenosis by diameter, if there is an arc of normal media that occupies more than 16% of the perimeter of the residual lumen vaso-constriction then it could reduce flow to a significant degree[19,20]. Segments of stenosis with this vasospastic potential (Figures 2.3, 2.5) have

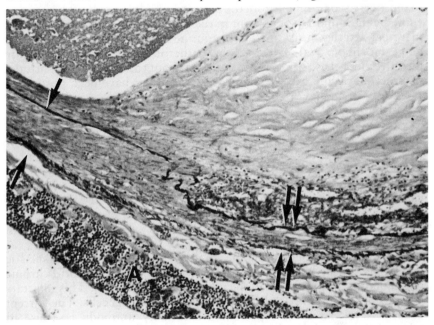

Figure 2.11   The media at the margin of an atheromatous plaque. The media in relation to the normal segment of vessel wall (single arrows) is of normal width. The elastic lamina separating intima from media is intact and straight in distended arteries. Behind the plaque the media (double arrows) is thinned. At the transition between the plaque and normal vessel wall the elastic lamina is broken and coiled. In the adventitia (A) behind the plaque are large numbers of plasma cells. *EHE stain*

been described: at one extreme, to be common making up 70% of all high grade lesions[21,22]; and at the other extreme, being rare in patients with stable angina[23]. The distribution of the types of stenosis in patients with stable angina, however show very wide individual variations. Forty-four per cent of 54 male patients with stable angina (studied personally) were found at autopsy to have no eccentric stenoses with a vasospastic potential; 56% of patients had one or more segments of this type. In three of the 54 patients all their segments of stenosis were of this type, each possessing more than five separate high grade lesions with a vasospastic potential. Any population of patients with stable angina is therefore very heterogeneous with regard to the possession of eccentric stenotic segments; subjects with such segments may be those in whom angina unrelated to exercise occurs[24]. At lesser degrees of stenosis eccentric plaques become much more common – between 30 and 50% diameter stenosis 44% of all lesions are of this type. Many of these lesions will inevitably be in series with adjacent segments of higher grade fixed stenosis.

Myocardial bridging is another postulated cause of labile stenosis[25]. In such arterial segments a band of myocardial muscle passes superficial to the artery separating it from the pericardium. It is a common phenomenon, being found at some point in the left anterior descending and left marginal arteries in up to 50% of routine autopsies in males. There is good morphological evidence that atheromatous plaques are rare directly under these bridges. No absolute proof that intermittent arterial obstruction occurs can be offered, although they have been postulated as a cause of angina or sudden death[25].

Morphological accounts of atheroma give an inordinate importance to *calcification* (Figure 2.4), which is not mirrored by the clinical significance. Calcification develops in the intima close to the media, either as a shell in the connective tissue, or as nodules within the lipid pool of a plaque. There is a tenuous relation between calcification and the degree of stenosis: in older subjects (>65 years of age) the degree of calcification is linked to increasing age and not to the presence of stenosis; while below 65 years of age calcification does correlate to a greater extent with the extent of intimal disease and thus inevitably with the presence of stenosis.

In the adventitia behind plaques that have broken the internal elastic lamina and pushed into the media there often develops a florid chronic inflammatory cell infiltrate in the adventita (Figure 2.11). This infiltrate consists predominantly of B lymphocytes and plasma cells. The current consensus is that these represent a secondary antibody response to released lipoprotein, although the plasma cells have been regarded as indicative of an autoimmune element to the pathogenesis of atheroma itself[6].

ACUTE ISCHAEMIC SYNDROMES IN MAN

In contrast to stable angina in acute infarction, some cases of unstable angina and in sudden ischaemic death there is evidence of an acute evolving arterial lesion. These lesions are plaques, within and on which thrombosis is developing.

Acute myocardial infarction

The pathogenesis of acute myocardial infarction has been in contention for 25 years but data derived from clinical angiography have now largely resolved the matter. Even so, the issues that created the controversy – whether occlusive coronary thrombi were or were not responsible for acute myocardial infarction – are so recent, it is difficult to avoid discussion of the ways in which the pathological world became so divided.

Myocardial infarction is myocardial necrosis consequent upon a reduction or cessation in blood flow and as such, there must be demonstrable necrosis present. Experimental work shows that infarction cannot be recognized by structural changes unless the animal survives a minimum period of 6–8 hours and it is unlikely that the human myocardium differs. Some pathological series made an assumption that sudden ischaemic death in man was due to an early infarct, which would have been recognizable had the patient lived a few more hours. Since only a minority of patients who are resuscitated from sudden death develop acute infarction, this assumption is erroneous[26]. To be valid, any pathological study of the pathogenesis of infarction must therefore be able to positively demonstrate myocardial necrosis. Furthermore, when there is demonstrable infarction there will be very different distributions of the necrosis in relation to the left ventricular anatomy. These different types of infarction have very different pathophysiological causes and must be considered separately.

The pattern of infarction at autopsy can be best recognized by use of the techniques, which demonstrate enzyme loss in tissue slices. When 1 cm thick transverse slices across the ventricles are treated in this way, the outlines of the necrotic muscle can be delineated clearly. Regional infarction (Figures 2.12, 2.13) is confined to the segment of myocardium supplied by one major coronary arterial branch and can be accurately sited by electrocardiography. Regional infarction is further divided into those cases that involve the full thickness of the ventricular wall (transmural) and those which involve the subendocardial layer only (Figures 2.12, 2.13).

Contrasting to regional infarction is necrosis that involves the whole circumference of the left ventricle and is confined to the subendocardial zone (Figure 2.14). The depth to which this necrosis extends through the ventricular wall is variable and in extreme cases its outer border is saw-toothed in outline and approaches the pericardium. In association with diffuse subendocardial necrosis there may be separate foci of necrosis up to 1 cm across scattered throughout the myocardium and also present in the right ventricle. In diffuse circumferential infarction the centre of the papillary muscles are inevitably involved.

The term infarction has also been applied by pathologists to cases where macroscopic abnormality is not present but microscopy reveals multifocal tiny foci of necrosis.

All these patterns must be clearly separated in any valid pathological study of the pathogenesis of infarction and in general have not been.

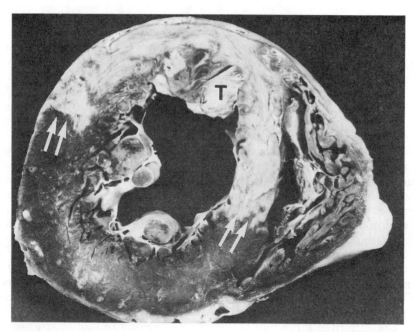

Figure 2.12 Short axis transection of the ventricular myocardium at mid septal level stained to demonstrate normal myocardium by succinic dehydrogenase activity. There is an antero-septal infarct in which the enzyme activity is lost (arrows). Necrosis extends through the full thickness of the ventricular wall. Mural thrombus (T) is present. There was a thrombotic occlusion of the left anterior descending artery

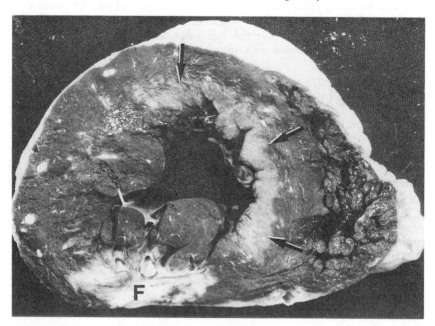

Figure 2.13 Short axis transection of the ventricles stained for succinic dehydrogenase activity. There is a subendocardial regional acute infarct in the antero-septal region (arrows). There is an old full thickness fibrous scar (F) on the posterior wall

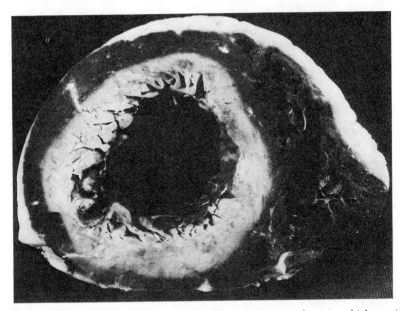

Figure 2.14 Short axis transection of the ventricular myocardium in which succinic dehydrogenase activity is lost throughout the subendocardial zone of the whole circumference of the left ventricle

Regional transmural infarction

The consensus from clinical angiographic studies is that within the first hour the artery subtending a regional infarct is totally occluded but that the vessel re-opens spontaneously over succeeding hours in a proportion of cases[27-29]. By 12 hours, flow has been restored in over 30% of cases and if fibrinolytic therapy is instituted, flow can be restored in the majority of cases. In the reopening phase filling defects in the lumen thought to represent thrombus are often present and a stenotic segment with ragged edges (Type II configuration) is revealed to underly the occlusion[30]. The efficacy of thrombolytic therapy as compared to vasodilator drugs in relieving the occlusion is regarded as confirming the dominant role of thrombosis. For pathologists the message of these clinical studies is that thrombosis is a dynamic process and the findings in a post mortem carried out on a patient who has survived 24 hours or longer from the inception of infarction do not necessarily reflect the earlier state of the artery. Nevertheless, pathological studies which have specifically selected regional full thickness infarcts for study do find that in over 90% of cases the subtending artery is occluded by recent thrombus[31,32] (Figure 2.15). This may indicate that persistent occlusion is associated with larger areas of infarction and death.

Reconstruction of the microanatomy of these occlusive thrombi (Figure 2.16) from serial sections has shown that the majority are associated

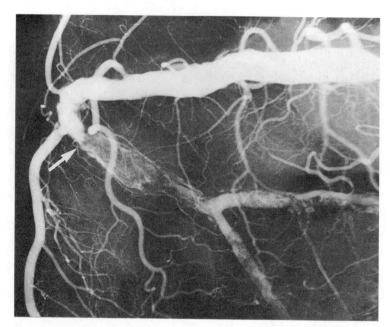

Figure 2.15 Postmortem angiogram of a right coronary artery occluded by recent thrombus (arrow), which has propagated distally. Regional infarction was present

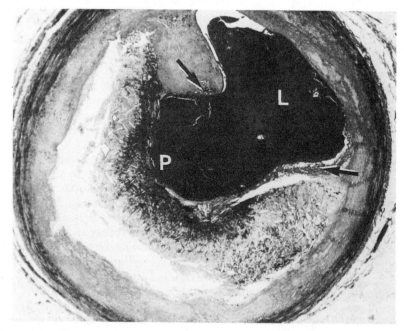

Figure 2.16 Transverse section of an artery occluded by recent thrombosis. The dark staining thrombus is bilobed. One mass occludes the lumen (L). The other lobe lies within a lipid rich plaque (P) and is thus intraintimal. The intraluminal and intraintimal masses of thrombus are contiguous through a large cap or fissure in the cap of the plaque (arrows). *Picro-Mallory trichrome stain*

with plaques which have undergone fissuring[33-38]. The plaques in question are of the lipid rich type in which a fissure or crack develops in the cap. The fissure ranges in size from a few hundred microns across, for which serial histological sections must be used for their demonstration, to loss of the whole cap over a centimetre of vessel. Within the plaque itself there is a mass of thrombus rich in platelets, which is continuous with thrombus within the lumen through the fissure[39]. At the immediate site of fissuring the intraluminal thrombus is rich in platelets and fibrin; but more distally the thrombus predominantly contains fibrin and red cells, suggesting there has been propagation. This tail of thrombus often extends into segments of artery in which atheroma and stenosis are minimal or absent. Clinical work has clearly shown that the intraluminal thrombus does continue to grow after the inception of infarction[40,41] but equally clearly that thrombosis is initiated before infarction occurs[42]. Radiolabelled fibrinogen given to the patient within the first 4 hours of infarction can be found at post mortem in the distal tail of the thrombus but not in its proximal head related to the fissure[42].

While thrombosis related to plaque fissuring is the most important precipitator of transmural infarction, it is not the only cause. In a small proportion of cases, thrombosis develops within areas of high grade stenosis without being triggered by plaque fissuring. Regional infarction mediated by spasm at the site of an eccentric plaque is rare but well documented and infarction due to spasm of normal arteries is also well documented but even rarer[43].

REGIONAL SUBENDOCARDIAL INFARCTION

Although not an uncommon lesion, the pathogenesis of this type of infarction in man is poorly understood and pathological studies are rare. The problem is compounded by growing doubts over the ECG criteria by which the condition is diagnosed in life[44,45]. Traditional electrocardiography regards Q-waves as indicative of full thickness infarction, while subendocardial infarction is associated with ST segment changes without Q-waves. However, recent clinicopathological studies have not born out this simple division[44]. If non Q-wave infarction is compared to Q wave infarction, there are interesting clinical differences[46-48] – the former have a greater development of collateral flow but paradoxically a greater risk of further infarction and sudden death. These facts have led regional subendocardial infarction to be regarded as a halfway house between unstable angina and full thickness regional infarction. Pathological studies do confirm a lower incidence of occlusive thrombi in subendocardial as compared to transmural regional infarction[49]. Two hypotheses are worthy of consideration; the first is that the pathogenesis of subendocardial infarction is identical to transmural infarction but previous collateral development has protected the subpericardial muscle. The second is that the subtending artery was occluded by thrombus, which underwent spontaneous lysis within the

6 hour period it takes for full thickness infarction to develop. This would leave the patient with a potentially unstable plaque at which further events might develop precipitating further infarction.

Diffuse subendocardial necrosis

This form of circumferential infarction commonly occurs in the absence of coronary atheroma, providing proof of its origin in an overall fall in myocardial perfusion due to a number of factors including hypotension, hypoxia, elevated left ventricular end diastolic pressure and increased ventricular wall thickness. Diffuse subendocardial necrosis may be superimposed upon regional infarct in patients with cardiogenic shock. Diffuse subendocardial necrosis may also occur in patients with widespread even stenosis due to atheroma – particularly when small vessels are involved, as in diabetes.

The pathological basis of sudden ischaemic death

Autopsy studies[50-52] have shown a similar distribution and degree of stenosis due to atheroma between stable angina and sudden ischaemic death. However, there have been contradictory results over the presence or absence of coronary thrombi[53,54]. A definition of sudden ischaemic death encompassing cases (1) where death has occurred within 6 hours of the onset of symptoms, (2) where there was demonstrable coronary stenosis of more than 75% by cross-sectional area and (3) where no other cause of death apparent after detailed autopsy, does yield more consistent results. In such patients 95% can be shown, both by post mortem angiography (Figure 2.17) and detailed histological examination (Figure 2.18), to have atheromatous plaques that are undergoing fissuring and that the majority of these have some degree of intraluminal thrombus formation but in only one third of patients is the artery totally occluded[54]. When contrasted to the arterial lesions of acute myocardial infarction, the difference lies in a far lower incidence of total occlusion in sudden ischaemic death. To the clinicians it may seem inconceivable that such simple facts have not been recognized by pathologists for so long. The prime reasons are that angiography is the method most likely to demonstrate the lesions, since it pinpoints exactly what arterial segment should be examined histologically. Without angiography every segment of the whole coronary tree would have to be examined histologically. The majority of cases of sudden death are examined by pathologists, whose main interest lies in the medico-legal field and are not likely to apply either technique. A widely quoted paper[55] is a supreme example of this error, since the techniques used to examine the arteries were never capable of producing data to sustain the conclusion that thrombosis was rare in instantaneous sudden death.

The second cause of confusion lies in the definition of the term ischaemic in relation to sudden death. In up to 10% of sudden natural

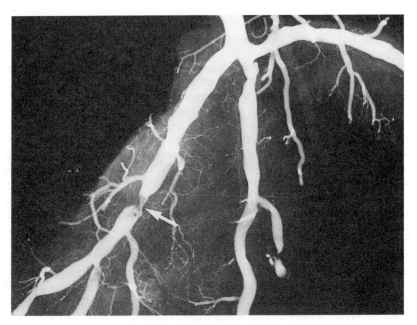

Figure 2.17 Segment of stenosis (arrow) in left anterior descending with ragged edge and an associated intraluminal mass but good filling of the distal vessel. Such stenoses are typical unstable angina and sudden ischaemic death

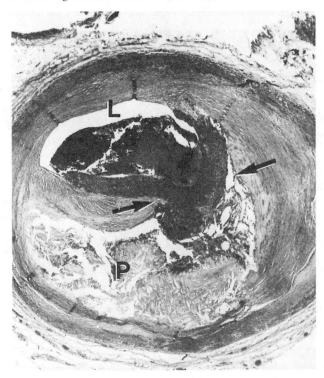

Figure 2.18 Transverse section through a fissured plaque (P) in which thrombus projects into the lumen (L) of the artery but does not occlude. The base of the thrombus is within a fissure (arrows) in the cap of a lipid rich plaque. *EHE stain*

deaths no clear single cause emerges at autopsy – in that even if some coronary atheroma is present, it does not cause significant stenosis. For the pathologist, the least troublesome answer is to include these cases in the ischaemic death group. A proportion of such patients may indeed be ischaemic deaths but must be based on mechanisms such as spasm, which are not capable of morphological confirmation.

If it is accepted that the majority of patients with sudden ischaemic death have an atheromatous plaque undergoing fissuring, what is the mechanism of induction of ventricular fibrillation? All of these plaques have suddenly increased in size due to the formation of a large mass of thrombus within the intima, thus suddenly increasing the degree of obstruction to the lumen. Intimal tearing of this degree, particularly when in association with platelet rich thrombi, may be a cause of local arterial spasm. Many cases have a mass of thrombus within the arterial lumen that acts as a potential source of small platelet emboli into the myocardium. Sudden death would thus be the myocardial analogue of transient cerebral ischaemic attacks, which are firmly established to be due to platelet emboli arising from thrombus on atheromatous plaques in the carotid arteries.

Pathological studies have confirmed that intramyocardial platelet aggregates (Figure 2.19) are present in a significant proportion of patients with sudden ischaemic death[56,57]. These aggregates are almost exclusively

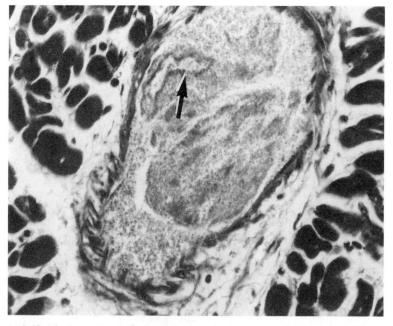

Figure 2.19 An intramyocardial artery whose lumen is completely occluded by a mass of platelets seen as small punctate bodies. A few strands of fibrin are also present (arrow). *Picro-Mallory trichrome stain*

confined to small intramyocardial vessels downstream of a major artery in which there is exposed mural thrombus confirming the embolic nature of the phenomenon. In addition, microscopic foci of myocardial necrosis (Figure 2.20) are associated with these intramyocardial emboli forming a substrate for the onset of ventricular fibrillation and sudden death.

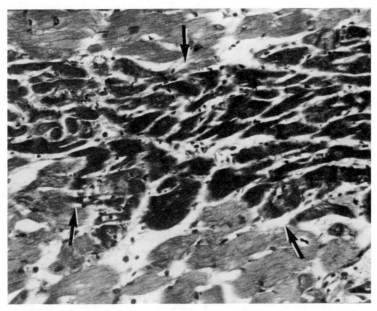

Figure 2.20 Microscopic focus of myocardial necrosis (arrows) in which the muscle cells are deeply eosinophilic and shrunken as compared to adjacent normal viable muscle cells. *Picro-Mallory trichrome stain*

THE PATHOLOGICAL BASIS OF UNSTABLE ANGINA

Clinical angiography rather than autopsy studies has provided most evidence for the basis of unstable angina. The number of vessels in which there is high grade stenosis as well as the degree and distribution of stenosis due to atheroma is not significantly different from patients with stable angina[58]. Review of the clinical angiograms in unstable angina suggests that eccentric areas of stenosis with an irregular outline and intraluminal filling defects (Figure 2.17) suggesting the presence of non-occlusive thrombosis may be found in a high proportion of cases[58,59]. Such angiographic appearances are known from post mortem angiography to indicate fissuring or rupture of atherosclerotic plaques with or without overlying thrombosis[60]. Therefore it seems likely that in unstable angina of crescendo type, the underlying arterial process is not dissimilar from that causing sudden ischaemic death or acute myocardial infarction. The difference lies in the fact that in acute infarction there has been, albeit for a limited period, complete occlusion. In this context, it is relevant that between 5 and 19% of patients with crescendo type of unstable angina will develop acute infarction within 12 weeks and up to 10% will die suddenly. The thrombotic nature of the underlying arterial lesion is also supported by the beneficial effect on prognosis of anti-platelet drugs[61].

An alternative view of unstable angina, well documented in some cases[18], would invoke spasm occurring in relation to plaques in which a normal medial segment has been retained. Such a mechanism may well be responsible for patients who have episodic rest pain, but no overall progression in the severity of symptoms over a period of months or even years.

THE CENTRAL ROLE OF PLAQUE FISSURING IN END STAGE CORONARY ATHEROMA

A firm case can be made for considering that plaque fissuring is the common factor precipitating many of the acute clinical expressions of ischaemic heart disease.

Fissuring occurs in plaques that have a large pool of free lipid within the intima. The fibrous cap separating this pool from the lumen of the artery breaks, fissures or ruptures. The different names reflect that the magnitude of the tear varies from a crack measured in microns to a defect measuring a centimetre or more across. The result is that blood enters the atheromatous plaque leading to the formation of a thrombus formed predominantly of platelets within the intima.

At this stage the plaque may reseal, healing by organization of the thrombus within the fissure track and such a process seems inherently more likely with smaller fissures. Alternatively, thrombosis may develop on the intimal surface over the fissure and begin to project into the arterial lumen waxing and waning in size over hours or days. It is such mural thrombi that can be recognized as filling defects or an irregular outline in association with stenosis in clinical angiograms. The mural thrombus close to the fissure site is rich in platelets but the proportion of fibrin within the thrombus away from this site increases particularly where distal propagation down the vessel has occurred. This propagation of fibrin rich thrombus may reach arterial segments in which atheroma is absent. Once occluded, the artery may reopen by spontaneous lysis and the thrombus steadily diminish in size allowing the plaque to reseal by organization. Alternatively the thrombus may persist, ultimately undergoing some degree of recanalization via the formation of multiple small vascular channels within the original lumen. This form of recanalization occurs particularly with thrombi that have been associated with distal propagation and seem unlikely to restore flow significantly – such segments are seen as chronic total occlusions in clinical angiograms.

Very little is known about the pathogenesis of plaque fissuring other than the fact that a pool of free lipid within the intima is a pre-requisite.

The fibrous cap of such plaques is often thin and mechanical factors including surges in systolic pressure and arterial spasm may be important. Infiltration of the fibrous cap by macrophages leading to weakening of the collagen is also possible. The natural history of a plaque fissure is uncertain but clinical studies of crescendo unstable angina indicates that the majority must reseal without causing occlusion and infarction. Clinical studies of patients with acute infarction who have undergone fibrinolytic therapy show the majority to have residual high grade coronary stenosis[30] illustrating the increase in size of the plaque that has occurred due to incarceration of thrombus within the intima. Thrombolysis may not be effective at reducing this intra-intimal thrombus, which undergoes slow organization by fibrosis. This process may allow some reduction in the degree of obstruction over succeeding weeks, but the undoubted fact is that the formation of intra-intimal thrombosis is a major factor in plaque growth.

Mechanisms of plaque growth

While previous episodes of plaque fissuring and thrombosis may be an important cause of stable angina, it is also considered that an alternative pathway exists of a simple continuation of the first stage of atheroma – i.e. fibro-muscular intimal proliferation. Incorporation of small surface thrombi into the intima within areas of stenosis associated with turbulent flow but not associated with fissuring or breaks in the intima do occur (Figure 2.6) and were championed by Duguid[62] as the prime mechanism of growth of a plaque. It is difficult to assess the relative importance of such slow 'silting up' as compared to the episodic larger thrombi that occur in relation to fissures in the pathogenesis of stable angina. The high proportion of patients with stable angina have recanalized segments of arteries and suggest that the latter process is of major importance. The essence of patients with stable angina is that they have managed to survive several episodes of plaque fissuring and even total coronary occlusion without developing major infarction or dying suddenly.

Plaque haemorrhage

The media of normal coronary arteries is avascular and does not contain vasa vasorum, but behind atheromatous plaques a rich network of small vessels grows into the media from the adjacent adventitia and cross into the intima. A small number of thin walled vessels also enter the intima direct from the lumen of the vessel. This neovascularization of both the intima (Figure 2.5) and media is a consistent feature of intimal thickening, whether diffuse or as focal plaques. The question has been raised as to whether haemorrhage from these thin walled new vessels could lead to significant plaque growth[63]. In the past this process has been confused with the intraplaque thrombosis resulting from breaks in the intimal cap, since a fissure connecting the cavity of the plaque to the lumen goes unrecognized unless the whole lesion is reconstructed. Two facts are certain: first, that many plaques not associated with stenosis or thrombosis contain small numbers of extravasated red cells but not fibrin or platelets; and second, at autopsy plaques that are found to contain large masses of platelets and fibrin when reconstructed from serial sections have a track leading to the lumen. This suggests that plaque haemorrhage when due to bleeding from transmedial vessels is not a major cause of plaque growth or coronary thrombosis.

CORONARY ANGIOPLASTY

The relation between plaque fissuring and coronary thrombosis at first sight suggests that percutaneous coronary angioplasty would be fraught with danger, yet it is successful in many cases. Few studies exist of the pathological effects of angioplasty and the majority are, of necessity, selected to those in which death ensued – a great deal is therefore known[64] about unsuccessful but less about successful angioplasty. The morphology of stenotic areas in particular – whether the lesion is hard and consists entirely of fibrous tissue, or soft and contains a lipid pool – cannot be ascertained in life by current angiographic techniques. Hard and soft lesions may react very differently to dilation and it is possible that the low incidence of thrombosis following angioplasty indicates that many of the lesions undergoing dilatation are predominantly fibrous. Dilation of fibrous strictures may result from actual splitting of the intima (Figure 2.21), extrusion of the whole plaque out into the media or by dilation of the normal quadrant of artery wall remote from the plaque itself. The lipid present in plaques with a pool may be extruded outward through the media or longitudinally redistributed within the intima. Angiography suggests that the intima is torn in a significant number of successful angioplasty procedures and such splits must be thrombogenic by virtue of exposing collagen and/or lipid to platelets. The growth of such thrombi is prevented presumably both by the establishment of high blood flow and by use of anticoagulant cover.

MORPHOLOGICAL CHANGES IN THE MYOCARDIUM IN ISCHAEMIC HEART DISEASE

Complex descriptions of the morphological changes found in acute myocardial infarction exist, which attempt to accurately date the time of onset or link the appearances to specific biochemical and pathogenetic mechanism. In practice, most human infarcts contain areas showing all these morphological appearances.

Timing of the onset of infarction can never be more than a rough approximation since it is clear that, as in the experimental animal, necrosis is not an event killing every myocardial cell at risk at the same

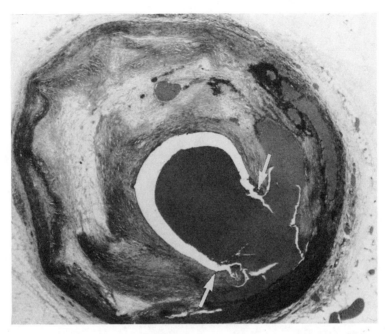

Figure 2.21 Transverse section of right coronary artery after angioplasty, which was successful in relieving stenosis on angiography. Death occurred within a few hours of the procedure. The lumen contains angiographic media, which extends into the intima via a large split (arrows) in the fibrous tissue making up the concentric stenosis. *EHE stain*

moment and the reparative process does not proceed at identical rates throughout the infarcted area.

Coagulation necrosis is the typical appearance found in regional transmural infarction following complete cessation of blood flow to the area. The individual muscle cells become hypereosinophilic but otherwise appear little affected until 24 hours, following which the cross striations vanish and the myofibrils begin to coalesce as granular debris. The earliest recognizable change at 12–24 hours is the accumulation of polymorphs within the interstitial tissue[65].

In contraction band necrosis (Figure 2.22) dense eosinophilic transverse bands are present within the muscle cell. Such cells are often contiguous at the intercalated disc with an apparent normal cell. This form of necrosis is more common in situations where flow is known to have been restored and in man, as in the experimental animal, thought to represent reperfusion[66] of non-viable myocardium.

There is a distinction to be made between areas of necrosis in which the whole tissue is dead, that is including the stroma and vascular component, and where the muscle cells only have died. In the former situation, often known as colliquative necrosis and usually found in the centre of regional transmural infarcts, the reparative process of necessity

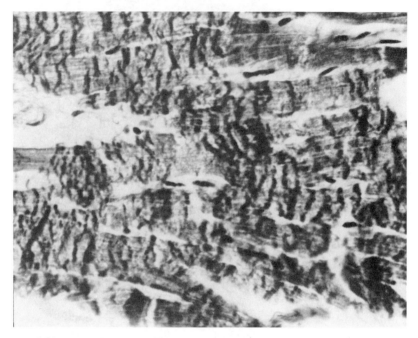

Figure 2.22 Myocardial necrosis in which each muscle cell contains brightly eosinophilic cross bands due to localized hypercontraction of myofibrils. Contraction band necrosis of this type occurs in areas in which ischaemic necrosis has occurred followed by re-establishment of flow within a short period. *Trichrome stain*

only takes place at the margins where the infarct abuts onto tissue with viable stroma and vessels. Amorphous hyaline muscle fibres which have undergone little change other than total loss of the nuclei may persist for many weeks or months incarcerated in the centre of such infarcts. From 3 to 5 days macrophages, fibroblasts and capillaries begin to extend into the infarct from the periphery and although collagen deposition begins by 7–10 days, it may take many weeks to transform the infarct into a fibrous scar. The ingrowth of capillaries into the area of infarction is mediated by release of a myocardial angiogenesis factor closely related in structure to similar factors released by tumour cells.

In areas of infarction where the stroma is not involved, the repair proceeds more rapidly. In part this is due to the foci of necrosis being smaller but also due to the close proximity of viable stromal cells. In such areas, the myofibrillary structure is lost forming hyaline masses within myocardial cells after which macrophages appear to remove the cell debris. The stroma collapses and coalesces followed by proliferation of collagen to leave a small focal scar containing residual lipofuschin derived from the muscle cells. Microscopic focal areas of necrosis in which the stroma has survived (Figure 2.23) are commom in ischaemic heart disease, particularly at the margins of larger areas of necrosis and

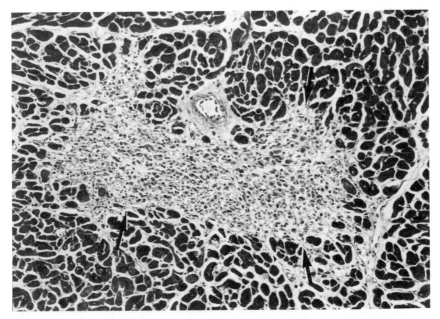

Figure 2.23   A focal area of necrosis (arrows) in which the stroma has survived leaving a lattice of connective tissue in which there are macrophages containing lipofuschin released from dead muscle cells. Such foci ultimately become tiny focal scars. *Trichrome stain*

are also characteristic of those of microembolic origin. Similar foci are found in severe left ventricular hypertrophy, irrespective of the presence of coronary atheroma, and a whole range of other factors – including high catecholamine levels, thyrotoxicosis and potassium deficiency – can lead to identical foci of necrosis.

Myocytolysis is another morphological expression of ischaemic damage to myocardial muscle cells. The cells become large and vacuolated due to the loss of myofibrils but the nuclei persist and mitochondrial enzymes remain. The appearance is often seen immediately beneath the endocardium or around blood vessels within areas which otherwise show conventional coagulative necrosis. The change is thought to indicate muscle cells on the borderline of viability, which have lost the ability to maintain normal ionic gradients with the interstitial fluid and to synthesize intracellular constituents.

Factors influencing infarct size

Thrombotic occlusion of a coronary artery leads to a segment of myocardium 'at risk' of infarction[67]. However, there is evidence that the actual mass of muscle that has undergone infarction by 6–12 hours is significantly less than the mass at original risk. In this context collateral flow is probably the most significant factor. In some instances blood flow is restored in an antegrade manner by spontaneous lysis of the occluding thrombus. This mechanism may be more common than realized in man, particularly in the causation of non-transmural infarction. Collateral flow is also retrograde via anastomotic flow from adjacent coronary arteries. This collateral development varies widely and is probably dependent on a pre-existing pressure gradient between the two arterial beds in question. Collateral development is therefore more likely in patients who have high grade stenosis preceding the episode of thrombosis; and at its extreme, collateral development may completely prevent infarction following an occlusion. Antegrade flow through segments of occluded artery reopened by organization of the thrombus by local collaterals in the adventitia probably develops too slowly to influence infarct size, but may influence the development of post-infarct angina.

Factors influencing prognosis after regional transmural infarction

There is no evidence that arrhythmias are directly linked to the total mass of infarcted muscle but arise in ischaemic but still viable myocardium. By 48 hours, the risk of such arrhythmias is virtually over since the margins of the infarct are defined and ischaemic muscle has either undergone necrosis or recovered. Infarct size, that is the proportion of the left ventricular total muscle that has undergone necrosis, is directly related to the mortality and morbidity of acute infarction from other complications. Cardiogenic shock is a major cause of mortality at the present time and is related to infarcts that involve more than 40% of the total left ventricular muscle mass[68,69]; it is these patients who enter a vicious cycle of hypoperfusion and progressive subendocardial infarction[70]. The remaining causes of mortality and morbidity usually reflect certain specific complications.

PATHOLOGICAL COMPLICATIONS OF ACUTE TRANSMURAL INFARCTION

Infarct expansion

Acute infarcts can undergo stretching and thinning which is associated with a high mortality and may progress to cardiac rupture[71]. Such expansion is a feature of transmural infarcts, which involve more than 10% of the total left ventricular mass. The expansion of the infarct is due to combinations of simple stretching and tearing or sliding of muscle bundles relative to each other. The importance of such expansion is that a permanent globular dilatation of the ventricle results, with detrimental effects, both on left ventricular contraction and mitral valve function.

External cardiac rupture

Pericardial tamponade resulting from external cardiac rupture is responsible for 10–20% of the deaths in acute myocardial infarction and has been estimated to be the most common cause of death after ventricular arrhythmias and cardiogenic shock. Ventricular rupture is a complication of transmural infarction but has no direct relation to infarct size. Cardiac rupture for unknown reasons is relatively more common in older women.

The mechanism of myocardial rupture is not clear, but there are at least two variants[72,73]. In some cases there is a slit-like tear between viable and non-viable muscle in an infarct, which has not undergone expansion; and such rupture can occur within two days of the onset of pain. Other infarcts have undergone expansion and the endocardium is torn with extravasation of blood between the muscle bundles and layers typically leading to rupture at the 5th to 10th day.

Ventricular septal defect

Rupture of a transmural infarction of the interventricular septum leads to a sudden left to right shunt and is a complication of anteroseptal, as well as posteroseptal infarction[74]. In the former case, the arterial occlusion is most often in the left anterior descending coronary artery proximal to the first septal branch in a patient who has not had previous symptoms of angina and in whom collateral flow is minimal. The resulting infarct is large and this fact taken in association with the haemodynamic burden of a shunt ensures a high mortality. The shunt takes place initially through a ragged hole ranging from one to three square centimetres in size. Rare cases who survive, usually those with smaller defects, will develop a smooth edged hole as the infarct heals. In anteroseptal infarction the defect is in the anterior or apical portion of the ventricular septum on the left side and opens either into the right ventricular outflow or to the apex of the right ventricle. In posteroseptal infarction septal defects occur behind the posterior medial papillary muscle on the left side and open posteriorly into the right ventricle close to the septal cusp of the tricuspid valve. Posteroseptal defects are also associated with large infarcts and there is a strong association with aneurysms of the posterior wall of the left ventricle and with right ventricular infarction. External rupture of the same posterior infarct, which induced a shunt a day or two before, is well recognized. Pathological studies of septal defects report approximately equal numbers of anterior and posterior defects, while clinical series stress the preponderance of anterior septal defects. This may reflect selection by the greater ease with which the anterior septal defect can be clinically diagnosed and surgically repaired.

Papillary muscle infarction

Papillary muscle necrosis is common during acute infarction, being present to some degree in from 15 to 30% of anterior and up to 50% of posterior infarcts[75]. The greater frequency of posterior medial papillary muscle infarction reflects the blood supply from the right coronary artery, while the anterolateral group of papillary muscles is predominantly supplied by the left circumflex artery, a rarer site of thrombosis. Papillary muscle infarction complicates both subendocardial and transmural regional infarction and is responsible for transient mitral regurgitation in the acute phase. In a tiny minority, certainly less than 1% of all fatal infarcts, a portion or all of a papillary muscle avulses. In the most severe form, a whole papillary muscle ruptures and the stump attached to the chordae passes in a flail like motion to and fro across the mitral valve orifice leading to torrential mitral regurgitation. Rupture of a subhead, to which one or two chordae only are attached, is less catastrophic and leads to prolapse of a portion of cusp. Partial tears of papillary muscle lead to elongation with a central isthmus of fibrous tissue. Rupture of the posterior papillary muscle is four to seven times more frequent than the anterolateral papillary muscle but in neither case is the infarct usually large or transmural[76,77]. There is also a distinct syndrome of rupture of the anterolateral papillary muscle causing death from rapid onset torrential regurgitation due to a very small localized infarct resulting from thrombosis of the marginal branch of the left circumflex coronary artery.

Ventricular aneurysms

The term aneurysm is used inconsistently in clinical cardiology but a working morphological definition is that of a convex protrusion of the ventricular wall, which comprises collagen throughout its full thickness[78]. Such aneurysms result only from transmural infarction. However, within this definition there is a wide spectrum: from, on one hand, very diffuse bulges with a wide base (Figure 2.24); to, on the other hand, very localized saccular bulges with a narrow neck opening into the ventricular cavity (Figure 2.25). The clinical presentation of these aneurysms is of persistent ventricular arrhythmias, cardiac failure – which may be correctable by resection of the aneurysm sac – and systemic emboli from mural thrombosis within the aneurysm sac. Cardiac rupture occurs but is rare. The presence of mural thrombus is inconstant for unknown reasons – apparently identical aneurysms in different patients may be totally full of thrombus obliterating the sac, contain some mural thrombus, or have no thrombus formation. The wall of these aneurysms is predominantly collagen but calcification may occur particularly where the aneurysm is lined by a thin coat of old thrombus.

The pathogenesis of aneurysm formation has been regarded either as a late expansion of mature collagen, or as collagenous replacement of

62

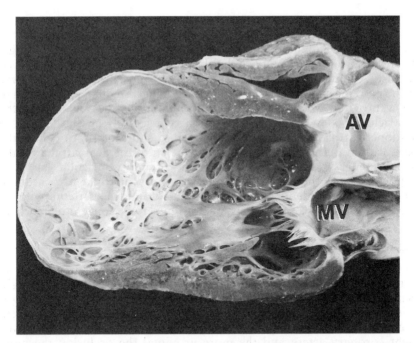

Figure 2.24   Long axis transection of the heart to show an apical diffuse left ventricular aneurysm in which the endocardial surface is white and thickened but no thrombus is present. (AV = aortic valve; MV = mitral valve)

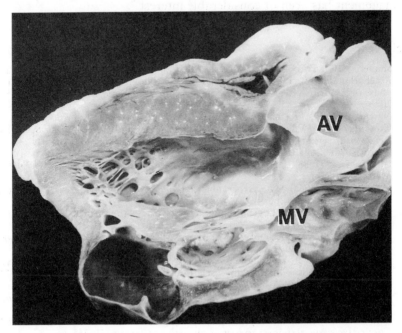

Figure 2.25   Long axis transection of the heart showing a localized aneurysm opening behind the postero-medial papillary muscle by a relatively narrow neck. No thrombus is present

an infarct that had undergone aneurysmal expansion in the acute stage. There is no reason to suppose that both processes do not exist or even coexist. A different pathogenesis has been proposed for the aneurysms at the extreme end of the spectrum, which have a small opening through the ventricular wall leading to a fibrous sac, which is outside the ventricle. The lesion may result from a ventricular tear that has led to a subpericardial haematoma stopping just short of rupture into the pericardium in the acute stage. Organization of the haematoma results in an aneurysm sac to which the name pseudo-ventricular has been applied because the wall did not derive from ventricular myocardium. Aneurysms with identical morphology are found in patients without coronary artery disease and must be presumed to be congenital in origin.

Right ventricular infarction

In isolation right ventricular infarction is very rare but may occur in patients with ischaemic heart disease who have pre-existing severe right ventricular hypertrophy. However, between 20 and 45% of postero-inferior infarcts of the left ventricle have some concomitant right ventricular necrosis. The right ventricular myocardium is supplied by the right coronary artery and the more proximal the occlusion the more likely is infarction to occur in the right ventricle and to spread onto the lateral wall. The effect of right ventricular infarction on clinical management has been of considerable interest[79].

References

1. Shaper, A. G., Pocock, S. J., Walker, M., Phillips, A. N., Whitehead, T. P. and MacFarlane, P. W. (1985). Risk factors for ischemic heart disease: the prospective phase of the British Regional Heart Study. *J. Epidemiol. and Comm. Hlth*, 39, 197–209
2. Newman, W. P., Freeman, D. S., Voors, A. W., Gard, P. D., Sprinivasan, S. R., Cresanta, J. L., Williamson, G. D., Webber, L. S. and Berenson, G. S. (1986). Relation of serum lipoprotein levels and systolic blood pressure to early atherosclerosis: The Bogalusa Heart Study. *N. Engl. J. Med.*, 314, 138–43
3. Glueck, C. J. (1986). Pediatric primary prevention of atherosclerosis. *N. Engl. J. Med.*, 314, 175–6
4. McGill, H. C. (1968). *The Geographic Pathology of Atherosclerosis.* (Baltimore: Williams and Wilkins) pp. 1–193
5. Ross, R. (1986). The pathogenesis of atherosclerosis – An update. *N. Engl. J. Med.*, 314, 488–99
6. Woolf, N. (1982). Endothelial alterations and atherogenesis. In *Pathology of Atherosclerosis.* (London: Butterworth Scientific) pp. 261–78
7. Aqel, N. M., Ball, R. Y., Waldmann, H. and Mitchinson, M. J. (1984). Monocytic origin of foam cells in human atherosclerotic plaques. *Atherosclerosis*, 53, 265–71
8. Mahley, R. W. (1985). Atherogenic lipoproteins and coronary artery disease: concepts derived from recent advances in cellular and molecular biology. *Circulation*, 72, 943–8
9. Baranowski, A., Adams, C. W. M., Bayliss High, O. B. and Bowyer, D. E. (1982). Connective tissue responses to oxysterols. *Atherosclerosis*, 41, 255–66
10. Fuster, V., Steele, P. M. and Chesebro, J. H. (1985). Role of platelets and thrombosis

in coronary atherosclerotic disease and sudden death. *J. Am. Coll. Cardiol.*, 5, 175–84

11. Faggiotto, A., Ross, R. and Harker, L. (1984). Studies of hypercholesterolaemia in the non-human primate. I. Changes that lead to fatty streak formation. *Arteriosclerosis*, 4, 323–40

12. Singh, R. N. (1984). Progression of coronary atherosclerosis. Clues to pathogenesis from serial coronary angiography. *Br. Heart J.*, 52, 451–61

13. Willerson, J. T., Campbell, W. B., Winniford, M. D. *et al.* (1984). Conversion from chronic to acute coronary artery disease: speculation regarding mechanisms. *Am. J. Cardiol.*, 54, 1349–55

14. Roberts, W. C. (1976). The coronary arteries and left ventricle in clinically isolated angina pectoris. *Circulation*, 54, 388–90

15. Roberts, W. C. (1979). The coronary arteries and left ventricle in clinically isolated angina pectoris – a necropsy analysis. *Am. J. Med.*, 67, 792–9

16. Thomas, A. C., Davies, M. J., Dilly, S., Dilly, N. and Franc, F. (1986). Potential errors in the estimation of coronary arterial stenosis from clinical arteriography with reference to the shape of the coronary arterial lumen. *Br. Heart J.*, 55, 129–39

17. Lichtlen, P. R., Rafflenbeul, W. and Freudenberg, H. (1985). Patho-anatomy and function of coronary obstructions leading to unstable angina pectoris – anatomical and angiographic studies. In Hugenholtz, P. G. and Goldman, B. S. (eds.), *Unstable Angina*, (Stuttgart: Schattauer) pp. 81–94

18. Brown, B. G. (1978). Coronary vasospasm. Observations linking the clinical spectrum of ischemic heart disease to the dynamic pathology of coronary atherosclerosis. *Arch. Intern. Med.*, 141, 716–22

19. Brown, B. G., Bolson, E. L. and Dodge, H. T. (1984). Dynamic mechanisms in human coronary stenosis. *Circulation*, 70, 917–22

20. Higgins, D., Santamore, W. P., Walinsky, P. and Nemir, P. (1985). Haemodynamics of human arterial stenosis. *Int. J. Cardiol.*, 8, 177–92

21. Freudenberg, H. and Lichtlen, P. R. (1981). Das nomale Wandsegment bei Koronartstemon, eine post mortale studie. *Z. Kardiol.*, 70, 863–9

22. Saner, H. E., Gobel, F. L., Salomonowitz, E., Erlien, D. A. and Edwards, J. E. (1985). The disease free wall in coronary atherosclerosis: Its relation to degree of obstruction. *J. Am. Coll. Cardiol.*, 6, 1096–99

23. Quyyumi, A. A., Al-Rufaie, H. K., Olsen, E. G. J. and Fox, K. M. (1985). Coronary anatomy in patients with various manifestations of three vessel coronary artery disease. *Br. Heart J.*, 54, 362–6

24. Shea, M. J., Deanfield, J. E., Wilson, R., DeLandsheere, C., Jones, T. and Selwyn, A. P. (1985). Transient ischemia in angina pectoris: frequent silent events with everyday activities. *Am. J. Cardiol.*, 56, 34E–38E

25. Feldman, A. M. and Baughman, K. L. (1986). Myocardial infarction association with a myocardial bridge. *Am. Heart J.*, 111, 784–7

26. Cobb, L. A., Werner, J. A. and Trobaugh, G. B. (1980). Sudden cardiac death. A decade's experience with out of hospital resuscitation. *Mod. Concepts Cardiovasc. Dis.*, 49, 31–6

27. DeWood, M. A., Spores, J. and Notske, R. *et al.* (1980). Prevalence of total coronary occlusion during the early hours of transmural myocardial infarction. *N. Engl. J. Med.*, 303, 897–902

28. Stadius, M. L., Maynard, C. and Fritz, J. K. *et al.* (1985). Coronary anatomy and left ventricular function in the first twelve hours of acute myocardial infarction: the Western Washington randomized intracoronary streptokinase trial. *Circulation*, 72, 292–301

29. Bertrand, M. E., Lefebvre, J. M. and Laisne, C. L. *et al.* (1979). Coronary angiography in acute transmural myocardial infarction. *Am. Heart J.*, 97, 61–69

30. Ambrose, J. A., Winters, S. L. and Arora, R. R. *et al.* (1985). Coronary angiograph morphology in acute myocardial infarction: Link between the pathogenesis of unstable angina and myocardial infarction. *J. Am. Coll. Cardiol.*, 6, 1233–8

31. Chapman, I. (1984). The cause-effect relationship between recent coronary artery occlusion and acute myocardial infarction. *Am. Heart J.*, **87**, 267–71
32. Davies, M. J., Woolf, N. and Robertson, W. B. (1976). Pathology of acute myocardial infarction with particular reference to occlusive coronary thrombi. *Br. Heart J.*, **38**, 659–64
33. Ridolfi, R. L. and Hutchins, G. M. (1977). The relationship between coronary artery lesions and myocardial infarcts: ulceration of atherosclerotic plaques precipitating coronary thrombosis. *Am. Heart J.*, **93**, 468–86
34. Chandler, A. B. (1974). Mechanisms and frequency of thrombosis in the coronary circulation. *Thrombosis Res.*, **4**, 3–23
35. Davies, M. J. and Thomas, A. (1981). The pathological basis and microanatomy of occlusive thrombus formation in human coronary arteries. *Philos. Trans. R. Soc. London (Biological)*, **294**, 225–9
36. Horie, T., Sekiguchi, M. and Hirosawa, K. (1978). Coronary thrombosis in pathogenesis of acute myocardial infarction. Histopathological study of coronary arteries in 108 necropsied cases. *Br. Heart J.*, **40**, 153–161
37. Falk, E. (1983). Plaque rupture with severe pre-existing stenosis precipitating coronary thrombosis. Characteristics of coronary atherosclerotic plaques underlying fatal occlusive thrombi. *Br. Heart J.*, **50**, 127–34
38. Constantinides, P. (1966). Plaque fissures in human coronary thrombosis. *J. Atherosclerosis Res.*, **6**, 1–17
39. Davies, M. J. and Thomas, A. C. (1985). Plaque fissuring – the cause of acute myocardial infarction, sudden ischemic death and crescendo angina. *Br. Heart J.*, **53**, 363–73
40. Erhardt, L. R., Unge, G. and Boman, G. (1976). Formation of coronary arterial thrombi in relation to onset of necrosis in acute myocardial infarction in man. *Am. Heart J.*, **91**, 592–8
41. Henriksson, P., Edhag, O., Jansson, B. et al. (1985). A role for platelets in the process of infarct extension. *N. Engl. J. Med.*, **313**, 1660–1
42. Davies, M. J., Fulton, W. F. M. and Robertson, W. B. (1979). The relation of coronary thrombosis to ischemic myocardial necrosis. *J. Pathol.*, **127**, 99–110
43. Maseri, A., Chierchia, S. and Davies, G. (1986). Pathophysiology of coronary occlusion in acute infarction. *Circulation*, **73**, 233–9
44. Levine, H. D. (1985). Subendocardial infarction in retrospect: pathologic, cardiographic and ancillary features. *Circulation*, **72**, 790–800
45. Spodick, D. H. (1983). Q wave infarction versus ST infarction. Non-specificity of electrocardiographic criteria for differentiating transmural and non-transmural infarction. *Am. J. Cardiol.*, **51**, 913–15
46. Schulza, R. A., Pitt, B. and Griffith, L. S. C. et al. (1978). Coronary arteriography and left ventriculography in survivors of transmural and non-transmural myocardial infarction. *Am. J. Med.*, **64**, 108–13
47. Hutler, A. M., Desanctis, R. W., Flynn, T. and Yeatman, L. A. (1981). Non-transmural myocardial infarction. A comparison of hospital and late clinical course of patients with that of matched patients with transmural anterior and inferior infarction. *Am. J. Cardiol.*, **48**, 591–601
48. Madigan, N. P., Rutherford, B. F. and Frye, R. L. (1976). The clinical course, early prognosis and coronary anatomy of subendocardial infarction. *Am. J. Med.*, **60**, 634–41
49. Erhardt, L. R. (1974). Clinical and pathological observations in different types of acute myocardial infarction. A study of 84 patients deceased after treatment in coronary care unit. *Acta Med. Scand. Suppl.*, **560**, 1078
50. Roberts, W. C. and Jones, A. A. (1979). Quantitation of coronary arterial narrowing at necropsy in sudden coronary death. Analysis of 31 patients and comparison with 25 control subjects. *Am. J. Cardiol.*, **44**, 39–46
51. Warnes, C. and Roberts, W. C. (1984). Comparison at necropsy by age group of amount and distribution of narrowing by atherosclerotic plaque in 2995 five mm

long segments of 240 major coronary arteries in 60 men aged 31–70 years with sudden coronary death. *Am. Heart J.*, **108**, 431–5
52. Davies, M. J. (1981). Pathological view of sudden cardiac death. *Br. Heart J.*, **45**, 88–96
53. Warnes, C. A. and Roberts, W. C. (1981). Sudden coronary death: comparison of patients with to those without coronary thrombus at necropsy. *Am. J. Cardiol.*, **54**, 1206–11
54. Davies, M. J. and Thomas, A. (1981). Thrombosis and acute coronary artery lesions in sudden cardiac ischemic death. *N. Engl. J. Med.*, **310**, 1137–40
55. Spain, D. M. and Bradess, V. A. (1981). Sudden death from coronary heart disease: survival time, frequency of thrombi and cigarette smoking. *Chest*, **58**, 107–10
56. Falk, E. (1985). Unstable angina with fatal outcome: dynamic coronary thrombosis leading to infarction and/or sudden death. *Circulation*, **71**, 699–708
57. Davies, M. J., Thomas, A. C., Knapman, P. A. and Hangartner. (1986). Intramyocardial platelet aggregation in unstable angina and sudden ischemic death. *Circulation*, **73**, 418–27
58. Ambrose, J. A., Winters, S. L., Stern, A. *et al.* (1985). Angiographic morphology and the pathogenesis of unstable angina pectoris. *J. Am. Coll. Cardiol.*, **5**, 609–16
59. Bresnahan, D. R., Davies, J. L., Holmes, D. R. and High, H. C. (1985). Angiographic occurrence and clinical correlates of intraluminal coronary artery thrombus: Role of unstable angina. *J. Am. Coll. Cardiol.*, **6**, 285–9
60. Levin, D. C. and Fallon, J. T. (1986). Significance of the angiographic morphology of localised coronary stenoses. Histopathological correlates. *Circulation*, **66**, 316–20
61. Cairns, J. A. (1985). Aspirin, sulphaphrazone, or both in unstable angine – results of a Canadian multicenter trial. *N. Engl. J. Med.*, **313**, 1369–75
62. Duguid, J. B. (1948). Thrombosis as a factor in the pathogenesis of aortic atherosclerosis. *J. Pathol. Bacteriol.*, **60**, 57–61
63. Barger, A. C., Beeuwkes, R. Lainey, L. L. and Silverman, K. J. (1985). Hypothesis vasa vasorum and neovascularisation of human coronary arteries. A possible role in the pathophysiology of atherosclerosis. *N. Engl. J. Med.*, **310**, 363–73
64. Block, P. C. (1984). Mechanisms of transluminal angioplasty. *Am. J. Cardiol.*, **53**, 69–71
65. Fishbein, M. C., Maclean, D. and Maroko, P. R. (1978). The histopathologic evolution of myocardial infarction. *Chest*, **73**, 843–9
66. Jennings, R. B., Reimer, K. A. (1981). Lethal myocardial ischemic injury. *Am. J. Pathol.*, **102**, 241–55
67. Schuster, E. H. and Bulkley, B. H. (1980). Ischemia at a distance after acute myocardial infarction. A cause of early post-infarction angina. *Circulation*, **62**, 509–15
68. Page, D. L., Caulfield, J. B., Kastor, J. A., DeSanctis, R. W. and Sanders, C. A. (1971). Myocardial changes associated with cardiogenic shock. *N. Engl. J. Med.*, **285**, 133–7
69. Alonzo, D. R., Scheidt, S., Post, M. and K Jillip, T. (1973). Pathophysiology of cardiogenic shock, quantification of myocardial necrosis, clinical pathologic and electrocardiographic correlations. *Circulation*, **48**, 588–96
70. Gutovitz, A. L., Sobel, B. E. and Roberts, R. (1978). Progressive nature of myocardial injury in selected patients with cardiogenic shock. *Am. J. Med.*, **41**, 469
71. Schuster, E. H. and Bulkley, B. H. (1979). Expansion of transmural myocardial infarction: A pathophysiologic factor in cardiac rupture. *Circulation*, **60**, 1532–8
72. Dellborg, M., Held, P., Swedberg, K. and Anders, V. (1985). Rupture of the myocardium – occurrence and risk factor. *Br. Heart J.*, **54**, 11–16
73. Becker, A. E. and Vanmantgem, J. P. (1975). Cardiac tamponade – a study of 50 hearts. *Eur. J. Cardiol.*, **3**, 349–58
74. Vlodaver, Z., Edward, J. E. (1977). Rupture of ventricular septum or papillary muscle complicating myocardial infarction. *Circulation*, **55**, 815–22
75. Sanders, C. A., Armstrong, P. W., Willerson, J. T. and Dinsmore, R. E. (1971).

Aetiology and differential diagnosis of acute mitral regurgitation. *Prog. Cardiovasc. Dis.*, **14**, 129–52
76. Nashimura, R. A., Schaff, H. V., Shub, C., Gersh, B. J., Edwards, W. D. and Takik, A. J. (1983). Papillary muscle rupture complicating acute myocardial infarction – analysis of 17 patients. *Am. J. Cardiology*, **51**, 373–8
77. Wei, J. Y., Hutchins, G. M.. and Bulkley, B. H. (1979). Papillary muscle rupture in fatal acute myocardial infarction: A potentially treatable form of cardiogenic shock. *Ann. Intern. Med.*, **90**, 149–53
78. Tibbutt, D. A. (1984). True left ventricular aneurysm. *Br. Med. J.*, **289**, 450–51
79. Kulbertus, H. E., Rigo, P. and Legrand, V. (1985). Right ventricular infarction: pathophysiology diagnosis, clinical course and treatment. *Mod. Concepts of Cardiovasc. Dis.*, **54**, 1–5

3
Coronary physiology and pathophysiology

J. I. E. HOFFMAN

INTRODUCTION

In order to function as a pump that never stops, the heart uses vast amounts of energy, which it gets by generating large quantities of adenosine triphosphate (ATP) by oxidative metabolism. Testimony to this is the fact that mitochondria, the site of oxidative metabolism, make up 25–40% of the volume of left ventricular myocardial cells – the proportion being higher in species with faster heart rates[103,124]. It is true that ATP can be made anaerobically by glycolysis, but whereas one molecule of glucose produces 36 molecules of ATP by oxidative metabolism it produces only six molecules of ATP by glycolysis. Furthermore, when anaerobiasis is due to ischemia, the end products of glycolysis inhibit key rate-limited enzymes and reduce still more the production of ATP. For these reasons the heart requires a large and continuous supply of oxygen and cannot sustain an oxygen debt for more than a few seconds without becoming severely depressed.

The myocardial demand for oxygen is so great that the heart requires a very high blood supply – the left ventricle uses oxygen and receives blood flow out of all proportion to its mass (Figure 3.1). The left ventricle in an adult human male weighs about 140 g or about 0.2% of body weight, yet at rest it uses about 4–5% of the total body oxygen consumption and receives about 2–3% of the cardiac output. As Figure 3.1 shows, this disparity remains during strenuous exercise. Despite the high blood flow, oxygen extraction from blood passing through the left ventricle is nearly maximal and further extraction soon decreases oxygen tension in capillary blood below acceptable levels. As a result, increased myocardial oxygen consumption has to be met by increases of flow rather than of oxygen extraction.

MYOCARDIAL OXYGEN CONSUMPTION

Accurate measurement of myocardial oxygen consumption can be made only by measuring myocardial blood flow and coronary arterio-venous

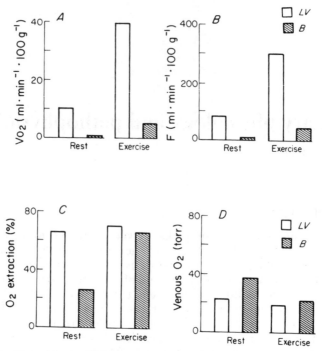

Figure 3.1 Comparison of left ventricular myocardium (open bars) and total body (shaded bars) at rest and during strenuous exercise:
(A) Oxygen consumption per minute per 100 g tissue
(B) Blood flow per minute per 100 g tissue
(C) Oxygen extraction percentage, calculated as 100 times the difference in arterio-venous oxygen content divided by the arterial oxygen content
(D) Venous oxygen tension (mmHg)
Data based on human studies by Ekelund and Holmgren (1967) and Kitamura *et al.* (1972).

oxygen difference. It would nevertheless be useful for many clinical purposes to estimate myocardial oxygen consumption by less invasive methods. Because pressure work and heart rate are major determinants of myocardial oxygen consumption per minute[101], the product of heart rate and systolic blood pressure – the 'double product' – has been used to predict myocardial oxygen demand.

Unfortunately this index is unreliable for measuring changes within or between subjects, unless a very restricted range of changes is induced[55]. This unreliability arises because the double product ignores contractile state, ventricular volume and ventricular mass, all of which are important determinants of myocardial oxygen demand[48,106]. Better predictions can be made by calculating peak systolic wall stress[85,106]. A fairly good estimate of myocardial oxygen demand per minute can be made by multiplying together heart rate, peak wall stress and relative left ventricular mass – echocardiography permits the necessary dimensions to be measured.

Another approach correlates myocardial oxygen consumption with the pressure–volume area of the left ventricle[108,110,111], a relationship that is altered by changes of contractility[109]. This method was found to be better than several other methods for predicting myocardial oxygen consumption within or between dogs[116], but it does not yet incorporate corrections for contractility as other methods may do[97], nor does it allow for ventricular hypertrophy. In general, predictions of myocardial oxygen demand in abnormal states are imperfect[36] and it is important to point out that no predictive formulae have been critically and exhaustively tested in humans[5].

REGULATION OF TOTAL CORONARY BLOOD FLOW

Flow (F) through a vascular bed is a function of the pressure drop $(P_1 - P_2)$ across it and the resistance (R) to flow through it, and the equivalent of Ohm's law for liquids is $F = (P_1 - P_2)/R$. However, in vascular beds R is not constant and will vary with changes in smooth muscle tone, extravascular compression and even the actual transmural pressure. Coronary vascular resistance is minimal when the tone of vascular smooth muscle is abolished and the heart is arrested or in diastole to minimize extravascular forces. The resistance rises when the heart is allowed to beat because extravascular pressures rise in systole; and resistance increases still more when the vascular smooth muscle has tone[67].

Regulation of myocardial blood flow by changes of vascular resistance can be demonstrated in two ways. If cardiac work and oxygen demand are kept constant but coronary perfusion pressure is changed, flow changes transiently but soon returns nearly to its former level. (To do this requires cannulation of the coronary artery so that its pressure can be altered while aortic pressure remains constant.) In other words, vessels dilate when coronary pressure is lowered and constrict when it is raised, so that flow remains relatively constant for a constant myocardial oxygen demand. The maintenance of steady-state flow during pressure changes is termed *autoregulation*, which normally operates over a range of pressures from about 8 to 16 kPa (60 to 120 mmHg) (Figure 3.2a). The second form of flow regulation, termed *metabolic regulation*, is shown by an increase of coronary blood flow while perfusion pressure is constant but myocardial oxygen consumption is increased – the increased oxygen consumption causes vessels to dilate and resistance to decrease. Once a new stable flow level is attained, autoregulation can be demonstrated at this new flow level (Figure 3.2b). Drake-Holland *et al.*[30] have postulated that both types of regulation are mediated by a common mechanism dependent on oxygen supply. Whether this is a direct effect of oxygen or some metabolite that changes when tissue oxygen rises and falls is unknown.

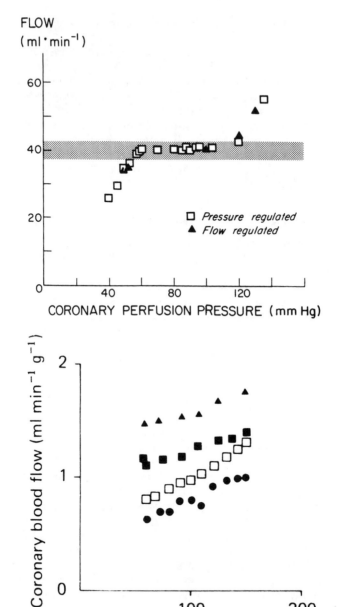

Figure 3.2 Autoregulation.

(a) Autoregulation curve in anaesthetized dog. Flow measured by electromagnetic flowmeter. Reproduced from Rouleau *et al.*, (1978) by permission of the authors and the American Heart Association.

(b) Autoregulation at different levels of metabolic regulation. Reproduced from Drake-Holland *et al.* (1984) with permission of the authors and the Physiological Society.

There are many substances that have been regarded as intermediaries in regulating coronary blood flow, chief among which is adenosine[9,10,93]. The basis of the adenosine hypothesis is that increased cardiac work causes more ATP to breakdown to adenosine monophosphate; this, in turn, is broken down by 5'-nucleotidase to adenosine, which can then dilate blood vessels, increase blood flow and oxygen supply and thus allow more ATP to be produced. Recent studies, however, have cast doubt upon this hypothesis. Infusion of low molecular weight adenosine deaminase has been shown to reduce interstitial adenosine concentrations[53] but does not alter autoregulation[26,53]. Furthermore, DeWitt et al.[24] showed that when increased cardiac work increased coronary flow in the isolated guinea-pig heart – adenosine efflux increased for about two minutes and then returned to normal. They concluded that there was wash-out of adenosine from a pool, after which its steady-state level was unaltered despite the persistent increase in coronary flow. These and many other studies indicate that adenosine can no longer be regarded as the major metabolite responsible for physiological regulation of coronary blood flow, and argue for an alternative or associated metabolite to be considered.

What other agents are involved is unclear. Changes in carbon dioxide tension or the concentrations of hydrogen ions, potassium ions, prostaglandins or vaso-active peptides can all be shown to alter coronary vascular resistance – but only in unphysiological concentrations – or can be shown – by the use of antagonists or inhibitors – to be uninvolved in normal coronary regulation[39,80]. Recently a powerful vasodilator, as yet uncharacterized, has been shown to be released by endothelial cells[44,51], including those of coronary arteries[62,72], but its role in coronary regulation is unknown.

Two other mechanisms for regulation must be considered. Distension of a blood vessel usually causes it to constrict, whereas decreasing pressure in it may make the vessel dilate[31,64]. This effect is termed the Bayliss or myogenic effect and it is independent of nervous or hormonal action. The vascular response may be mediated by changes in calcium flux across the muscle cell membrane. Such a mechanism might explain autoregulation but cannot explain metabolic regulation. Furthermore, Johnson[64] has emphasized that, although a myogenic mechanism may operate in organs with a low metabolic rate, it would be impossible to demonstrate this mechanism in the myocardium with its very high metabolic rate.

The second mechanism to be considered is neural regulation. Coronary vessels contain both adrenergic and cholinergic receptors and have a rich vagal and sympathetic nerve supply. Direct or reflex vagal stimulation dilates coronary vessels, alpha-adrenergic stimulation constricts them and beta-adrenergic stimulation might dilate them[39]. Although these changes may be invoked by drugs or reflexes, there is no evidence that neuro-adrenergic factors play a part in normal coronary regulation. However, they may cause changes in diseased coronary arteries and applying cold to the hands may produce myocardial ischemia in patients with coronary disease[23,89].

CORONARY RESERVE

If an autoregulated pressure–flow line is obtained (as in Figure 3.2), a vasodilator is given to dilate the coronary vessels maximally and then the pressure and flow measurements are repeated – the new pressure–flow line will be higher and steeper (Figure 3.3). The difference between the autoregulated and maximal flows at any pressure is termed the coronary flow reserve. Because the pressure–flow line for maximally dilated vessels is very steep, the coronary flow reserve is very sensitive to the exact pressure at which it is measured. Note that a pressure–flow diagram like that in Figure 3.3 can be obtained only by cannulating the coronary artery so that aortic pressure can be kept constant, while coronary perfusing pressure is changed. It is thus difficult to obtain such a diagram in humans[56] even though flow reserve at specific pressures can be obtained.

Coronary flow reserve will be reduced if the autoregulated flow level increases – as will occur with tachycardia, anaemia, fever, or thyrotoxicosis. Under these circumstances, the pressure–flow line during maximal vasodilatation is not usually altered (but see below). Flow reserve will also be reduced, even at normal autoregulated flows, if the maximal flows achievable at any given pressures are reduced – such reductions occur with marked tachycardia[29,57], greatly increased contractility[83], much increased blood viscosity (as in polycythaemia)[38,112], or small vessel disease[107]. Finally, coronary flow reserve is reduced beyond a coronary stenosis simply because the distal pressure has been lowered (Figure 3.3). Although resting autoregulated flow may be normal beyond a stenosis, the flow is maintained at the expense of vasodilatation and a loss of flow reserve[47,84].

In general, loss of flow reserve implies a limited ability to increase coronary flow when this is needed, as exemplified by the occurrence of angina or ST depression on exercise in patients with coronary artery disease. However, the myocardial ischemia that occurs when flow reserve is exhausted may well affect only a few muscle cells at a time, so that no signs or symptoms of ischemia occur – instead there may be slowly progressive muscle necrosis and fibrosis[59]. Exercise in normal hearts does not cause myocardial ischemia. Although it increases flow it also increases perfusion pressure and so increases the flow reserve, which is not abolished even in severe exercise[6].

CORONARY VASCULAR RESISTANCE

The relationship between coronary pressure and flow has traditionally been assessed by calculating coronary vascular resistance as pressure drop across the vascular bed divided by flow through it. The pressure

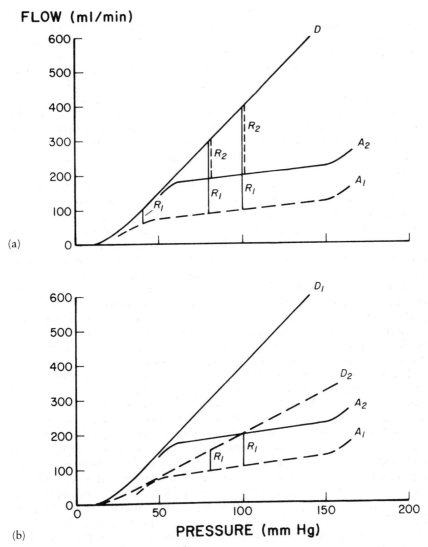

Figure 3.3 Coronary flow reserve diagram.

(a) Two autoregulation curves (A_1, A_2) at two different levels determined by metabolic regulation. Line D is the pressure–flow line after maximal vasodilatation. The vertical lines indicate the coronary flow reserve at a normal perfusing pressure, a lower perfusing pressure, and at a still lower perfusing pressure beyond a coronary stenosis. Note that increasing the myocardial oxygen demand causes flow to rise from A_1 to A_2, thereby decreasing reserve at the two higher perfusing pressures but exhausting it completely beyond the stenosis

(b) The pressure–flow line during maximal vasodilatation (D) has a lower slope, as may occur with a haematocrit of 70%. Even if autoregulated flow is normal (A_1) the coronary flow reserve (R_1) is reduced. Any increase in coronary flow to A_2 may markedly decrease or even abolish reserve at what would seem to be adequate perfusing pressures.

drop is usually taken as the difference between coronary arterial pressure and the right atrial pressure, and flow has traditionally been assessed by calculating coronary vascular resistance as the pressure drop across the vascular bed divided by flow through it. At first mean pressures and flows were used. Then, when in animals phasic coronary flows could be measured by electromagnetic or ultrasonic flowmeters, the concept of measuring late diastolic coronary resistance was introduced[50] in order to eliminate the effects of different degrees and proportions of systolic extravascular compression during the cardiac cycle. In humans, it has recently become possible to measure phasic velocities in the coronary arteries[82,123] but transforming these velocities into flows is not yet possible.

Even with the capability of making phasic flow measurements accurately there are two major problems in assessing late diastolic resistance, or for that matter mean resistance. One is that resistance is not independent of perfusing pressure. In a dilated vascular bed, if the intravascular pressure decreases, then the vessels narrow and their resistance increases[54]. On the other hand, during autoregulation, a fall in pressure causes a fall in resistance. Furthermore, a change in aortic pressure alters myocardial oxygen demand and causes metabolic regulation with consequent change in resistance. Therefore, if an intervention changes perfusing pressure, its effect on resistance is the sum of the changes due to altered passive distension, autoregulation, metabolic regulation and finally the putative vasomotor action of the intervention. It is difficult, if not impossible, to separate these components.

The second problem is that right atrial pressure may not be the correct back pressure to use when calculating the pressure drop across the coronary vascular bed. In 1978, Bellamy[8] published his observations made on conscious dogs chronically instrumented with a flow transducer on the left circumflex coronary artery. During long diastoles there was a gradual decline of coronary artery pressure and flow (Figure 3.4). If flow and pressure were measured every 0.1 second throughout the long diastole, then the resulting pressure–flow points formed a straight line that intersected the pressure axis at 6 to 6.7 kPa (45 to 50 mmHg). This point of intersection represents zero flow and is usually symbolized by P_{zf} or $P_f = 0$. Bellamy also noted that during peak reactive hyperemia the flows were higher at any given pressure and these pressure–flow points formed a higher and steeper line that on extrapolation intersected the pressure axis at about 2.7 kPa (20 mmHg). His tentative explanation was that the intercept at 2.7 kPa (20 mmHg) represented a back pressure to coronary flow, and that the higher intercept observed during autoregulation represented the combination of this back pressure and the effect of vascular tone, the so-called critical closing pressure[16].

These observations are not unique to the heart – they have also, for example, been reported for the femoral vascular bed[34] and the cerebral vascular bed[33]. They have been confirmed many times in the heart, and the only additional finding of more recent studies is that the pressure–

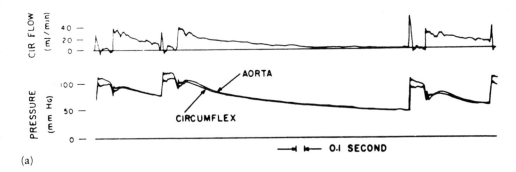

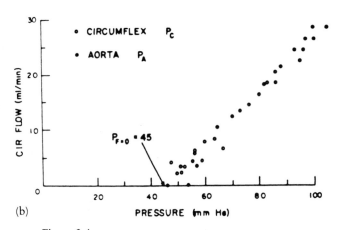

(a)

(b)

Figure 3.4
(a) Measured left circumflex flow (cir. flow) by electromagnetic flowmeter and pressures in aorta and left circumflex coronary artery in a conscious dog with sinus arrhythmia
(b) Pressure–flow relation measured every 0.1 second during several long diastoles. Reproduced from Bellamy (1978) with permission of the author and the American Heart Association.

flow line is usually curved at its lower end[68,86]. This curvature is important because extrapolation from the upper part of the curve usually gives an intercept on the pressure axis that is much higher than the true zero flow pressure[68].

If back pressure really is much higher than right atrial pressure, some important implications follow (Figure 3.5). One is that resistance is constant or relatively constant as perfusion pressure changes, especially if the pressure–flow line is linear. Secondly, resistance is lower if calculated from the difference between coronary arterial and back pressure than between coronary arterial and right atrial pressure. Finally, the concept of a high back pressure implies that the pressure–flow relation can be altered either by altering resistance or by altering back pressure.

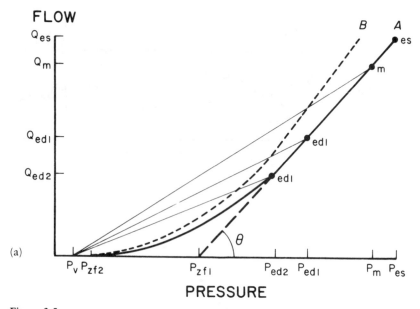

Figure 3.5
(a) Heavy line represents an observed pressure–flow line that curves in its lower portion. Extrapolation from the upper straight portion to the pressure axis (dashed line) produces a pressure intercept (P_{zf1}) that is much higher than the true zero flow pressure (P_{zf2}).

If the pressure–flow line were linear so that the back pressure was indeed P_{zf1}, then the slope of the line would be the vascular conductance (the reciprocal of resistance), and decreasing the perfusing pressure from P_1 to P_2 would not alter the measured conductance, which is the tangent to the angle θ. However, if the back pressure really is venous pressure (P_v), then not only is the conductance of slope $P_1–P_v$ lower than that of slope $P_1 – P_2$, but when pressure falls from P_1 to P_2 the conductance decreases still further. Diagram based on figure by Klocke *et al.* (1985)

For example, if an intervention causes flow to rise at a fixed coronary arterial pressure, then conventionally we would infer that resistance had fallen and that vessels had dilated. However, it is also possible that back pressure was lowered without any change in resistance and this would produce the same findings. Only measuring the pressure–flow line and the P_{zf} would allow separation of these two mechanisms.

What explanation could there be for a back pressure to flow that is much above venous pressure? The most likely mechanism is that there is the equivalent of a waterfall or a Starling resistor in the myocardium. In brief, if there is a collapsible tube within a rigid compartment, then flow through the system depends on the difference between inflow pressure and the pressure around the tube, rather than on the difference between inflow and outflow pressures as long as the outflow pressure is below that around the tube. The subject is reviewed in detail by Permutt and Reilly[95], Conrad[22], Holt[61], Brower and Noordergraff[13], and Fry *et al.*[42].

FLOW

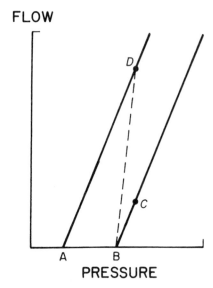

(b)

PRESSURE

Figure 3.5
(b) Two hypothetical straight pressure–flow lines are shown in heavy lines. An increase in flow from C to D could occur either by (i) an increased vascular conductance – dashed line BD is steeper than heavy line BC, or (ii) a shift of P_{zf} from B to A without any change in conductance – heavy lines AD and BC are parallel

In recent years, this approach to thinking about back pressures has undergone some major changes. If decaying pressures and flows are measured, the significant capacitance effects due to compliance of the extramural coronary arteries[18,96] must be considered. Because most studies are done with the flow transducer placed near the origin of the coronary artery, when flow reaches zero at this point it is still continuing downstream because of capacitative discharge of the gradually collapsing coronary arteries. Therefore, at capillary level flow will stop at a lower pressure than that defined by P_{zf} and it will stop at a still lower pressure in the coronary veins[19,104]. Some investigators[37] consider that eliminating the effects of extramural capacitance will abolish virtually all the difference between P_{zf} and right atrial pressure. However, Klocke and his colleagues[68,70], who accept that capacitance does affect the absolute value of P_{zf}, still believe that capacitance free P_{zf} is well above right atrial pressure.

To eliminate capacitance effects we have used steady-state measurements made by (1) constricting the coronary artery to different degrees, (2) waiting for stable pressures and flows to occur at each degree of constriction and (3) then using those values to construct a steady-state pressure–flow curve[115,117]. These still gave high values for P_{zf}. Then more careful studies showed that a major factor responsible for the high P_{zf} was collateral flow from unoccluded arterial branches. The dog has a fairly large collateral coronary flow and this flow enters the artery under study beyond the obstruction. When collateral inflow was prevented, the value of P_{zf} was only slightly above coronary sinus pressure[86]. In support of this hypothesis is the finding that in pigs, which have almost no natural coronary collaterals, P_{zf} is very close to right atrial pressure[94].

Finally, Uhlig et al.[114] were able to demonstrate a waterfall effect – but in the coronary sinus and great cardiac vein, rather than in the myocardium itself. They observed that coronary sinus pressure could be much higher than right atrial pressure and that it tended to rise when left ventricular diastolic pressure rose. Putting all the experimental evidence together, it appears that when allowance has been made for artifacts due to arterial capacitance, collateral flow, and coronary venous waterfalls, there is relatively little difference between P_{zf} and coronary venous pressure. The controversy about high coronary back pressures has recently been reviewed extensively[69,70,104].

TRANSMURAL MYOCARDIAL BLOOD FLOW

Flow across the left ventricular wall is not always homogeneous. For many years it has been known that the subendocardial muscle, particularly of the left ventricle, is vulnerable to ischemic damage[25,59]. This vulnerability could be due either to metabolic differences in different layers so that with equal reductions of flow in all layers the subendocardial muscle will become ischemic first, or to selective subendocardial reductions of flow below the level needed to support tissue viability, or perhaps to both factors together.

There is evidence that subendocardial muscle uses about 20% more oxygen per gram than does more superficial muscle[63,88,120]; this difference may reflect increased local work or metabolic differences. Furthermore, with sudden total cessation of blood flow to the myocardium, lactate is produced most rapidly[32] and necrosis starts first[43,73] in subendocardial muscle – these differences must reflect local differences in metabolism.

Despite these evident differences in metabolism, whenever subendocardial ischemia occurs there is usually a disproportionate reduction in subendocardial blood flow, or else a failure of subendocardial flow to rise as it should to meet an increased myocardial oxygen demand[14]. Normally in animals (for subendocardial flows cannot yet be measured in humans) the innermost quarter or third of the left ventricle has about 30% more flow per gram than does the outermost one-quarter or third in conscious animals and about the same flow in anaesthetized ones. Significant decreases of diastolic aortic pressure or diastolic duration, coronary stenosis, profound anemia or polycythemia, or marked increase of left ventricular diastolic pressure all produce a marked decrease in the subendocardial:subepicardial (also known as the inner: outer, or endo:epi) blood flow ratio, usually associated with signs of subendocardial ischemia[52,59,66,87,112].

The explanation of this disproportionate subendocardial underperfusion is not entirely clear. Early theories that it was related to systolic flow superficial but not deep muscle are disproved by studies that show negligible systolic perfusion of the myocardium of the left ventricle. The 25% of systolic flow, observed in flowmeter tracings from the main left coronary artery, or its major branches, represents mainly or entirely systolic storage of blood in the distensible extramural arteries[18,96]. This finding is compatible with direct observation of blood flow in the superficial myocardial vessels – forward systolic flow is seen in arterioles within the outermost 300 μm but in deeper arterioles flow stops in systole[113].

The possibility that subendocardial ischemia is due to high back pressures in subendocardial muscle is not excluded by the evidence adduced against a high P_{zf} in general. The pressure at which flow stops could well refer to the last layer of muscle to be perfused and does not itself show that in some layers P_{zf} might not be higher. However, investigation of this problem in dogs[40,54] shows similar P_{zf} values in the different layers of the left ventricle and so excludes such differences as a cause of selective subendocardial underperfusion. What is left is some interaction between systole and diastole[58], probably related to the higher tissue pressures generated subendocardially in systole. These systolic pressures have been shown to squeeze blood both anterograde and retrograde during systole[105]. It is likely that because this squeeze is greater in the deeper muscle layers, more blood is moved out of these layers than from more superficial layers in systole. As a result, at the end of systole the deeper vessels are narrower than the more superficial vessels and so offer a greater impediment to reflow of blood in the next diastole.

There are also differences in regional coronary flow reserve[57] in that the reserve is always less in the subendocardial than the subepicardial muscle. A decrease in perfusion pressure while myocardial oxygen consumption remains constant will thus exhaust reserve first in the subendocardial muscle, thereby contributing to the selective subendocardial ischemia. At one time it was thought that before ischemia of a layer occurred its reserve had to be completely exhausted. More recent studies, however, show that even when reduction of perfusion pressure causes marked decreases of subendocardial flow and produces ischemic changes, a vasodilator will cause further vasodilatation – evidently ischaemia is not a maximal vasodilator stimulus[3,17,49].

CORONARY STEAL

This phenomenon is possible only when there is coronary artery stenosis or occlusion that restricts total inflow to a region. With single vessel disease the pressure distal to the obstruction is low and subendocardial flow may be low or else in jeopardy of reduction. As pointed out above, coronary flow reserve is greater in the subepicardium than in the subendocardium, so that a vasodilator may have more effect on subepicardial than subendocardial vessels. If flow through the stenosis or the collaterals cannot increase enough, then the lowered subepicardial resistance may steal blood from the subendocardium[21,45]. In fact, Buffington and Feigl[15] have demonstrated alpha-adrenergic vasoconstriction in subepicardial vessels and concluded that this may protect against the stealing of blood from the subendocardium.

If there is a second distal stenosis on a branch of the artery that already has a proximal stenosis, then the region supplied by that branch may be nearly maximally vasodilated. A vasodilator stimulus will then dilate vessels in all the regions and, because total inflow is restricted by the proximal stenosis, will decrease perfusing pressure and thus divert blood from the region supplied by the distal stenotic branch[7].

RIGHT VENTRICULAR CORONARY BLOOD FLOW

Because the work of the right ventricle is less than that of the left ventricle, right ventricular coronary flow per gram at rest is about 60–70% of that in the left ventricle[1,20,27,76–78]. Oxygen extraction is similar in both ventricles[120,121] or lower in the right ventricle[71] so that right ventricular myocardial oxygen consumption per gram is also about 60–70% or less of that in the left ventricle at rest.

Systolic forces in the right ventricular free wall are lower than those in the left ventricular free wall, so that there is a higher proportion of systolic phasic flow in the right than the left coronary artery. This difference between phasic flows in the two arteries has been noted both in animals[41,74,98] and in humans[82,123].

If right ventricular systolic pressure is raised acutely, the proportion of systolic flow decreases[41], total right ventricular coronary flow rises at first but soon reaches a maximum[2,28,41], and right ventricular failure occurs – as manifested by a raised right atrial pressure, decreased aortic pressure and decreased cardiac output[12,41,46,100,118]. The cause of the failure is right ventricular ischemia[46,118], which can be abolished by raising aortic pressures and thereby increasing right ventricular myocardial flow[12,46,100,118].

VENTRICULAR HYPERTROPHY

Ventricular hypertrophy is a common end result of many forms of heart disease. In the stable phase of hypertrophy, peak wall stress is normal because the increased wall thickness compensates for the increased ventricular pressure or volume[102,106]. For this reason ventricular myocardial blood flow per minute per gram is usually normal[4,106], although total myocardial flow to the ventricle is obviously increased. Because the coronary vascular bed does not enlarge when there is acquired ventricular hypertrophy[79,90,92], the increased total blood flow is achieved by vasodilatation that lowers coronary flow reserve[56,57,60]. As indicated above, the loss of reserve is most marked subendocardially, which may explain why in hypertrophy exercise may cause myocardial damage[122].

In fact, when there is hypertrophy, all other factors that increase coronary flow or decrease maximal flow – such as tachycardia, anemia, or polycythaemia – more readily exhaust coronary flow reserve and produce subendocardial ischemia. Such a loss of reserve has also been observed in left ventricular hypertrophy in humans[81,82,106].

Hypertrophy has similar consequences for the right ventricle, in which it also reduces coronary flow reserve[75,77,82,91]. The one exception to this loss of reserve occurs if the right ventricular hypertrophy begins before or soon after birth, because then the right ventricular coronary vessels grow to keep pace with the hypertrophy of the muscle[1,11,77,119].

Acknowledgement

Supported by US Public Health Service Grant HL-25847.

References

1. Archie, J. P., Fixler, D. E., Ullyot, D. J., Buckberg, G. D. and Hoffman, J. I. E. (1974). Regional myocardial blood flow in lambs with concentric right ventricular hypertrophy. *Circ. Res.*, **34**, 143–54
2. Auckland, K., Kiil, F. and Kjekshus, J. (1967). Relationship between ventricular pressures and right and left myocardial blood flows. *Acta Physiol. Scand.*, **70**, 116–26
3. Aversano, T. and Becker, L. C. (1985). Persistence of coronary vasodilator reserve despite functionally significant flow reduction. *Am. J. Physiol.*, **248**, H403–H411
4. Bache, R. J., Vrobel, T. R., Ring, W. S., Emery, R. W., and Anderson, R. W. (1981). Regional myocardial blood flow during exercise in dogs with chronic left ventricular hypertrophy. *Circ. Res.*, **48**, 76–87
5. Baller, D., Schenk, H., Strauer, B.-E. and Hellige, G. (1980). Comparison of myocardial oxygen consumption indices in man. *Clin. Cardiol.*, **3**, 116–22
6. Barnard, R. J., Duncan, H. W., Livesay, J. J. and Buckberg, G. D. (1977). Coronary vasodilator reserve and flow distribution during near-maximal exercise in dogs. *J. Appl. Physiol.: Respirat. Environ. Exercise Physiol.*, **43**, 988–92
7. Becker, L. C. (1978). Conditions for vasodilator-induced coronary steal in experimental myocardial ischemia. *Circulation*, **57**, 1103–10
8. Bellamy, R. F. (1978). Diastolic coronary pressure–flow relations in the dog. *Circ. Res.*, **43**, 92–101
9. Belloni, R. L. (1979). The local control of coronary blood flow. *Cardiovasc. Res.*, **13**, 63–85
10. Berne, R. M. (1980). The role of adenosine in the regulation of coronary blood flow. *Circ. Res.*, **47**, 807–13
11. Botham, M. J., Lemmer, J. H., Gerren, R. A., Long, R. W., Behrendt, D. M. and Gallagher, K. P. (1984). Coronary vasodilator reserve in young dogs with moderate right ventricular hypertrophy. *Ann. Thoracic Surg.*, **38**, 101–7
12. Brooks, H. L., Kirk, E. S., Vokonas, P. S., Urschel, C. W. and Sonnenblick, E. H. (1971). Performance of the right ventricle under stress; relation to right coronary flow. *J. Clin. Invest.*, **50**, 2176–83
13. Brower, R. W. and Noordergraaf, A. (1973). Pressure–flow characteristics in collapsible tubes: A reconciliation of seemingly contradictory results. *Ann. Biomed. Eng.*, **1**, 333–55
14. Buckberg, G. D., Fixler, D. E., Archie, J. P., and Hoffman, J. I. E. (1972). Experimental subendocardial ischemia in dogs with normal coronary arteries. *Circ. Res.*, **30**, 67–81

15. Buffington, C. W. and Feigl, E. O. (1983). Effect of coronary artery pressure on transmural distribution of adrenergic coronary vasoconstriction in the dog. *Circ. Res.*, 53, 613–21

16. Burton, A. C. (1962). Physical principles of circulatory phenomena: the physical equilibria of the heart and blood vessels. In W. F. Hamilton and P. Dow (eds.) *Handbook of Physiology. Section 2: Circulation.* pp. 85–106. (Bethesda, Maryland: American Physiological Society)

17. Canty, J. M., Jr. and Klocke, F. J. (1985). Reduced regional myocardial perfusion in the presence of pharmacologic vasodilator reserve. *Circulation* 71, 370–7

18. Chilian, W. M. and Marcus, M. L. (1982). Phasic coronary blood flow velocity in intramural and epicardial coronary arteries. *Circ. Res.*, 50, 775–81

19. Chilian, W. M. and Marcus, M. L. (1984). Coronary venous outflow persists after cessation of coronary arterial inflow. *Am. J. Physiol.*, 247, H984–H990

20. Cobb, F. R., Bache, R. J. and Greenfield, J. C., Jr. (1974). Regional myocardial blood flow in awake dogs. *J. Clin. Invest.*, 53, 1618–25

21. Cohen, M. V., Sonnenblick, E. H. and Kirk, E. S. (1976). Coronary steal: Its role in detrimental effect of isoproterenol after acute coronary occlusion in dogs. *Am. J. Cardiol.*, 39, 880–8

22. Conrad, W. A. (1969). Pressure–flow relations in collapsible tubes. *IEEE Trans. Biomed. Eng.*, 16, 284–95

23. Crea, F., Davies, G., Chierchia, S., Romeo, F., Bugiardini, R., Kaski, J. C., Freedman, B. and Maseri, A. (1985). Different susceptibility to myocardial ischemia provoked by hyperventilation and cold pressor test in exertional and variant angina pectoris. *Am. J. Cardiol.*, 56, 18–22

24. DeWitt, D. F., Wangler, R. D., Thompson, C. I. and Sparks, H. V., Jr. (1983). Phasic release of adenosine during steady state metabolic stimulation in the isolated guinea pig heart. *Circ. Res.*, 53, 636–43

25. Dick, M. R., Unverferth, D. V. and Baba, N. (1982). The patterns of myocardial degeneration in nonischemic congestive cardiomyopathy. *Hum. Pathol.*, 13, 740–4

26. Dole, W. P., Yamada, N., Bishop. V. S. and Olsson, R. A. (1985). Role of adenosine in coronary blood flow regulation after reductions in perfusing pressure. *Circ. Res.*, 56, 517–24

27. Domenech, R. J., Hoffman, J. I. E., Noble, M. I. M., Saunders, K. B., Henson, J. R. and Subijanto, S. (1969). Total and regional coronary blood flow measured by radioactive microspheres in conscious and anesthetized dogs. *Circ. Res.*, 25, 581–96

28. Domenech, R. J. and Ayuy, A. H. (1974). Total and regional coronary blood flow during acute right ventricular pressure overload. *Cardiovasc. Res.*, 8, 611–20

29. Domenech, R. J. and Goich, J. (1976). Effect of heart rate on regional coronary blood flow. *Cardiovasc. Res.*, 10, 224–31

30. Drake-Holland, A. J., Laird, J. D., Noble, M. I. M., Spaan, J. A. E. and Vergroesen, I. (1984). Oxygen and coronary vascular resistance during autoregulation and metabolic vasodilatation in the dog. *J. Physiol.*, 348, 285–99

31. Duling, B. R., Gore, R. W., Dacey, R. G., Jr and Damon, D. N. (1981). Methods for isolation, cannulation, and in vitro study of single micro-vessels. *Am. J. Physiol.*, 241, H108–H116

32. Dunn, R. B. and Griggs, D. M., Jr. (1975). Transmural gradients in ventricular tissue metabolites produced by stopping coronary flow in the dog. *Circ. Res.*, 37, 438–45

33. Early, G. B., Dewey, R. C., Pieper, H. W. and Hunt, W. E. (1974). Dynamic pressure–flow relationship of brain blood flow in the monkey. *J. Neurosurg.*, 41, 590–6

34. Ehrlich, W., Baer, R. W., Bellamy, R. F. and Randazzo, R. (1980). Instantaneous femoral artery pressure–flow relations in supine anesthetized dogs and the effect of unilateral elevation of femoral venous pressure. *Circ. Res.*, 47, 88–98

35. Ekelund, L. G. and Holmgren, A. (1967). Central hemodynamics during exercise. *Circ. Res.*, 20, 33–43 (Supplement).

36. Elzinga, G. (1983). Cardiac oxygen consumption and the production of heat and work. In Drake-Holland, A. J. and Noble, M. I. M. (eds.) *Cardiac Metabolism.* pp. 173–94. (Chichester: John Wiley and Sons, Ltd.)

37. Eng, C., Jentzer, J. H. and Kirk, E. S. (1982). The effects of the coronary capacitance on the interpretation of diastolic pressure–flow relationships. *Circ. Res.*, 50, 334–41

38. Fan, F. C., Chen, R. Y. Z., Schuessler, G. B. and Chien, S. (1980). Effects of hematocrit variations on regional hemodynamics and oxygen transport in the dog. *Am. J. Physiol.*, 238, H545–H52

39. Feigl, E. O. (1983). Coronary physiology. *Physiol. Rev.*, 63, 1–205

40. Firmin, R. K., Uhlig, P. N., Baer, R. W., Messina, L. M., Hanley, F. L., Turley, K. and Hoffman, J. I. E. (1982). Transmural pressure–flow (PF) relations in canine left ventricular hypertrophy (LVH). *Circulation*, 66, 44 (Supplement II) (Abstract).

41. Fixler, D. E., Archie, J. P., Jr., Ullyot, D. J. and Hoffman, J. I. E. (1973). Regional coronary flow with increased right ventricular output in anesthetized dogs. *Am. Heart J.*, 86, 788–97

42. Fry, D. L., Thomas, L. J. and Greenfield, J. C., Jr. (1980). Flow in collapsible tubes. In Patel, D. J., Vaishnav, R. M. and Atabek, H. B. (eds.) *Basic Hemodynamics and its Role in Disease Processes.* p. 407–24. (Baltimore: University Park Press)

43. Fugiwara, H., Ashraf, M., Sato, S. and Millard, R. W. (1982). Transmural cellular damage and blood flow distribution in early ischemia in pig hearts. *Circ. Res.*, 51, 683–93

44. Furchgott, R. F. (1983). Role of endothelium in responses of vascular smooth muscle. *Circ. Res.*, 53, 557–73

45. Gallagher, K. P., Folts, F. D., Shebuski, R. J., Rankin, J. H. and Rowe, G. G. (1980). Subepicardial vasodilation reserve in the presence of critical coronary stenosis in dogs. *Am. J. Cardiol.*, 46, 67–73

46. Gold, F. L. and Bache, R. J. (1982). Transmural right ventricular blood flow during acute pulmonary artery hypertension in the awake dog: Evidence for subendocardial ischemia during right ventricular failure despite residual vasodilator reserve. *Circ. Res.*, 51, 196–204

47. Gould, K. L. and Lipscomb, K. (1974). Effects of coronary stenosis on coronary flow reserve and resistance. *Am. J. Cardiol.*, 34, 48–55

48. Graham, T. P., Jr., Covell, J. W., Sonnenblick, E. H., Ross, J., Jr. and Braunwald, E. (1968). Control of myocardial oxygen consumption: relative influence of contractile state and tension development. *J. Clin. Invest.*, 47, 375–85

49. Grattan, M. T., Hanley, F. L., Stevens, M. B. and Hoffman, J. I. E. (1985). Transmural coronary flow reserve patterns in dogs. *Am. J. Physiol.*, 250, H276–H293

50. Gregg, D. E. (1950). *The Coronary Circulation in Health and Disease.* (Philadelphia: Lea and Febiger)

51. Griffith, T. M., Edwards, D. H., Collins, P., Lewis, M. J. and Henderson, A. H. (1985). Endothelium derived relaxant factor. *J. R. Coll. Physicians* 19, 74–9

52. Griggs, D. M. and Nakamura, Y. (1968). Effect of coronary constriction on myocardial distribution of iodoantipyrine-^{131}I. *Am. J. Physiol.*, 215, 1082–8

53. Hanley, F. L., Grattan, M. T., Stevens, M. B. and Hoffman, J. I. E. (1985). Role of adenosine in coronary autoregulation. *Am. J. Physiol.* , 250, H558–H566

54. Hanley, F. L., Messina, L. M., Grattan, M. T. and Hoffman, J. I. E. (1984). The effect of coronary inflow pressure on coronary vascular resistance in the isolated dog heart. *Circ. Res.*, 54, 760–72

55. Hoffman, J. I. E. (1978). Determinants and prediction of transmural myocardial perfusion. *Circulation*, 58, 381–91

56. Hoffman, J. I. E. (1984). Maximal coronary flow and the concept of coronary vascular reserve. *Circulation*, 70, 153–9

57. Hoffman, J. I. E. (1987). A critical view of coronary reserve. *Circulation* . Vol. 75. (Supplement) (In press)

58. Hoffman, J. I. E., Baer, R. W., Hanley, F. L., Messina, L. M. and Grattan, M. T. (1985). Regulation of transmural myocardial blood flow. *J. Biomech. Eng.* 107, 2–9

59. Hoffman, J. I. E. and Buckberg, G. D. (1976). Transmural variations in myocardial perfusion. In Yu, P. and Goodwin, J. F. (eds.) *Progress in Cardiology.* Vol. 5 pp. 37–89. (Philadelphia: Lea and Febiger).

60. Hoffman, J. I. E., Grattan, M. T., Hanley, F. L. and Messina, L. M. (1983). Total and transmural perfusion of the hypertrophied heart. In ter Keurs, H. E. D. J. and Schipperheyn, J. J. (eds.) *Cardiac Left Ventricular Hypertrophy.* pp. 130–51. (The Hague: Martinus Nijhoff).

61. Holt, J. P. (1969). Flow through collapsible tubes and through in situ veins. *IEEE Trans. Biomed. Eng.,* 16, 274–83

62. Holtz, J., Giesler, M. and Bassenge, E. (1983). Two dilatory mechanisms of antianginal drugs on epicardial coronary arteries in vivo: indirect flow-dependent, endothelium mediated dilation and direct smooth muscle relaxation. *Z. Kardiol.,* 72, 98–106 (Supplement)

63. Holtz, J., Grunewald, W. A., Manz, R., von Restorff, W. and Bassenge, E. (1977). Intracapillary hemoglobin oxygen saturation and oxygen consumption in different areas of the left ventricular myocardium. *Pfluegers Arch. Eur. J. Physiol.,* 370, 253–8

64. Johnson, P. C. (1980). The myogenic response. In Bohr, D. F., Somlyo, A. P. and Sparks, H. V., Jr. (eds.) *The Handbook of Physiology, Section 2: The Cardiovascular System.* Vol. 2, pp. 409–42. (Bethesda, Maryland: American Physiological)

65. Kitamura, K., Jorgensen, C. R., Gobel, F. L., Taylor, H. L. and Wang, Y. (1972). Hemodynamic correlates of myocardial oxygen consumption during upright exercise. *J. Appl. Physiol.,* 32, 516–22

66. Kjekshus, J. K. (1973). Mechanism for flow distribution in normal and ischemic myocardium during increased ventricular preload in the dog. *Circ. Res.,* 33, 489–99

67. Klocke, F. J. (1976). Coronary blood flow in man. *Prog. Cardiovasc. Dis.,* 19, 117–66

68. Klocke, J. J., Weinstein, I. R., Klocke, J. F., Ellis, A. K., Kraus, D. R., Mates, R. E., et al. (1981). Zero-flow pressures and pressure–flow relationships during single long diastoles in the canine coronary bed before and during maximal vasodilation. Limited influence of capacitive effects. *J. Clin. Invest.,* 68, 970–80

69. Klocke, F. J., Canty, J. M., Jr. and Mates, R. E. (1984). Evolving concepts of coronary pressure–flow relationships. In Abel, F. L. and Newman, W. H. (eds.) *Functional Aspects of the Normal, Hypertrophied and Failing Heart.* pp. 40–56. (Boston: Martinus Nijhoff Publishing).

70. Klocke, F. J., Mates, R. E, Canty, J. M., Jr. and Ellis, A. K. (1985). Coronary pressure–flow relationships. Controversial issues and probable implications. *Circ. Res.,* 56, 309–23

71. Kusachi, S., Nishiyama, O., Yasuhara, K., Saito, D., Haraoka, S. and Nagashima, H. (1982). Right and left ventricular oxygen metabolism in open chest dogs. *Am. J. Physiol.,* 243, H761–766

72. Lamping, K. G., Marcus, M. L. and Dole, W. P. (1985). Removal of the endothelium potentiates canine large coronary artery constrictor responses to 5-hydroxytryptamine in vivo. *Circ. Res.,* 57, 55–64

73. Lavallee, M. and Vatner, S. F. (1984). Regional myocardial blood flow and necrosis in primates following coronary occlusion. *Am. J. Physiol.,* 246, H635–H639

74. Lowensohn, H. S., Khouri, E. M., Gregg, D. E., Pyle, R. L. and Patterson, R. E. (1976). Phasic right coronary artery blood flow in conscious dogs with normal and elevated right ventricular pressures. *Circ. Res.,* 39, 760–6

75. Manohar, M., Bisgard, G. E., Bullard, V., Will, J. A., Anderson, D. and Rankin, J. H. G. (1978). Myocardial perfusion and function during acute right ventricular systolic hypertension. *Am. J. Physiol.,* 235, H628–H638

76. Manohar, M., Bisgard, G. E., Bullard, V. and Rankin, J. H. G. (1981). Blood flow in the hypertrophied right ventricular myocardium of unanesthetized ponies. *Am. J. Physiol.,* 240, H881–H888

77. Manohar, M., Thurmon, J. C., Tranquilli, W. J., Devous, M. D., Sr., Theodorakis, M. C., Shawley, R. V., Feller, D. L. and Benson, J. G. (1981). Regional myocardial blood flow and coronary vascular reserve in unanesthetized young calves with severe concentric right ventricular hypertrophy. *Circ. Res.*, **48**, 785–96

78. Manohar, M., Parks, C. M., Busch, M. A., Tranquilli, W. J., Bisgard, G. E., McPherron, T. A. and Theodorakis, M. C. (1982). Regional myocardial blood flow and coronary vascular reserve in unanesthetized young calves exposed to a simulated altitude of 3500 m for 8–109 weeks. *Circ. Res.*, **50**, 714–26

79. Marchetti, G. V., Merlo, L., Noseda, V. and Visioli, O. (1973). Myocardial blood flow in experimental cardiac hypertrophy in dogs. *Cardiovasc. Res.*, **7**, 519–27

80. Marcus, M. L. (1983). *The Coronary Circulation in Health and Disease.* pp. 221–241. (New York: McGraw Hill Book Company)

81. Marcus, M. L., Doty, D. B., Hiratzka, L. F., Wright, C. B. and Eastman, C. L. (1982). Decreased coronary reserve. A mechanism for angina pectoris in patients with aortic stenosis and normal coronary arteries. *N. Engl. J. Med.*, **307**, 1362–6

82. Marcus, M., Wright, C., Doty, D., Eastham, C., Laughlin, D., Krumm, P., Fastenow, C. and Brody, M. (1981). Measurement of coronary velocity and reactive hyperemia in the coronary circulation of humans. *Circ. Res.*, **49**, 877–91

83. Marzilli, M., Goldstein, S., Sabbah, H. N., Lee, T. and Stein, P. D. (1979). Modulating effect of regional myocardial performance on local myocardial perfusion in the dog. *Circ. Res.*, **45**, 634–40

84. Mates, R. E., Gupta, R. L., Bell, A. C. and Klocke, F. J. (1978). Fluid dynamics of coronary artery stenosis. *Circ. Res.*, **42**, 152–62

85. McDonald, R. H., Taylor, R. R. and Cingolani, H. E. (1966). Measurement of myocardial developed tension and its relation to oxygen consumption. *Am. J. Physiol.*, **211**, 667–73

86. Messina, L. M., Hanley, F. L., Uhlig, P. N., Baer, R. W., Grattan, M. T. and Hoffman, J. I. E. (1985). Effects of pressure gradients between branches of the left coronary artery on the pressure axis intercept and the shape of steady state circumflex pressure–flow relations in dogs. *Circ. Res.*, **56**, 11–19

87. Moir, T. W. (1972). Brief reviews: Subendocardial distribution of coronary blood flow and the effect of antianginal drugs. *Circ. Res.*, **30**, 621–7

88. Monroe, R. G., Gamble, W. J., LaFarge, C. G., Benoualid, H. and Weisul, J. (1975). Transmural coronary venous O_2 saturations in normal and isolated dog hearts. *Am. J. Physiol.*, **228**, 318–24

89. Mudge, G. H., Jr., Goldberg, S., Gunther, S., Mann, T. and Grossman, W. (1979). Comparison of metabolic and vasoconstrictor stimuli on coronary vascular resistance in man. *Circulation*, **59**, 544–50

90. Mueller, T. M., Marcus, M. L., Kerber, R. E., Young, V. A., Barnes, R. W. and Abboud, F. M. (1978). Effect of renal hypertension and left ventricular hypertrophy on the coronary circulation in dogs. *Circ. Res.*, **42**, 543–9

91. Murray, P. A. and Vatner, S. F. (1981). Reduction of maximal coronary vasodilator capacity in conscious dogs with severe right ventricular hypertrophy. *Circ. Res.*, **48**, 27–33

92. O'Keefe, D. D., Hoffman, J. I. E., Cheitlin, R., O'Neill, M. J., Allard, J. R. and Shapkin, E. (1978). Coronary blood flow in experimental canine left ventricular hypertrophy. *Circ. Res.*, **43**, 43–51

93. Olsson, R. A. and Patterson, R. E. (1976). Adenosine as a physiologic regulator of coronary blood flow. *Prog. Mol. Subcell. Biol.*, **4**, 227–48

94. Pantley, G. A., Ladley, H. D. and Bristow, J. D. (1984). Low zero-flow pressure and minimal capacitance effect on diastolic coronary artery pressure–flow relations during maximum vasodilation in swine. *Circulation*, **70**, 485–94

95. Permutt, S. and Riley, R. L. (1963). Hemodynamics of collapsible vessels with tone: the vascular waterfall. *J. Appl. Physiol.*, **18**, 924–32

96. Reneman, R. S. and Arts, T. (1985). Dynamic capacitance of epicardial coronary arteries in vivo. *J. Biomech. Eng.*, **107**, 29–33

97. Rooke, G. A. and Feigl, E. O. (1982). Work as a correlate of canine left ventricular oxygen consumption, and the problem of catecholamine oxygen wasting. *Circ. Res.*, 50, 273–86
98. Ross, G. (1967). Blood flow in the right coronary artery of the dog. *Cardiovasc. Res.*, 1, 138–44
99. Rouleau, J., Boerboom, L. E., Surjadhana, A. and Hoffman, J. I. E. (1979). The role of autoregulation and tissue diastolic pressures in the transmural distribution of left ventricular blood flow in anesthetized dogs. *Circ. Res.*, 45, 804–15
100. Salisbury, P. F. (1955). Coronary artery pressure and strength of right ventricular contraction. *Circ. Res.*, 3, 633–8
101. Sarnoff, S. J., Braunwald, E., Welch, G. H., Jr., Case, R. B., Stainsby, W. N. and Macruz, R. (1958). Hemodynamic determinants of oxygen consumption of the heart with special reference to the tension time index. *Am. J. Physiol.*, 192, 148–56
102. Sasayama, S., Ross, J., Franklin, D., Bloor, C. M., Bishop, S. and Dilley, R. B. (1976). Adaptations of the left ventricle to chronic pressure overload. *Circ. Res.*, 38, 172–8
103. Sommer, J. R. and Johnson, E. A. (1979). Ultrastructure of cardiac muscle. In Berne, R. M. and Sperelakis, N. (eds.) *Handbook of Physiology Section 2: The Cardiovascular System.* Vol. I, pp. 113–186. (Bethesda, Maryland: American Physiological Society).
104. Spaan, J. A. E. (1985). Coronary diastolic pressure–flow relation and zero flow pressure explained on the basis of intramyocardial compliance. *Circ. Res.*, 56, 293–309
105. Spaan, J. A. E., Bruels, N. P. W. and Laird, J. D. (1981). Diastolic-systolic coronary flow differences are caused by intramyocardial pump action in the anesthetized dog. *Circ. Res.*, 49, 584–93
106. Strauer, B.-E. (1979). Myocardial oxygen consumption in chronic heart disease: role of wall stress, hypertrophy and coronary reserve. *Am. J. Cardiol.*, 44, 730–40
107. Strauer, B.-E., Brune, I., Schenk, H., Knoll, D. and Perings, E. (1976). Lupus cardiomyopathy; cardiac mechanisms, hemodynamics, and coronary blood flow in uncomplicated systemic lupus erythematosus. *Am. Heart J.*, 92, 715–22
108. Suga, H., Hayashi, T., Shirahata, M., Suehiro, S. and Hisano, R. (1981). Regression of cardiac oxygen consumption on ventricular pressure–volume area in dogs. *Am. J. Physiol.*, 240, H320–H325
109. Suga, H., Hisano, R., Goto, Y., Yamada, O. and Igarashi, Y. (1983). Effect of positive inotropic agents on the relation between oxygen consumption and systolic pressure volume area in canine left ventricle. *Circ. Res.*, 53, 306–18
110. Suga, H., Hisano, R., Hirata, S., Hayashi, T. and Ninomiya I. (1982). Mechanism of higher oxygen consumption rate: pressure-loaded vs. volume loaded heart. *Am. J. Phsyiol.*, 242, H942–H948
111. Suga, H., Yamada, P., Goto, Y. and Igarashi, Y. (1984). Oxygen consumption and pressure-volume area of abnormal contractions in canine heart. *Am. J. Physiol.*, 246, H154–160
112. Surjadhana, A., Rouleau, J., Boerboom, L. E. and Hoffman, J. I. E. (1978). Myocardial blood flow and its distribution in anesthetized polycythemic dogs. *Circ. Res.* 43, 619–31
113. Tillmanns, H., Ikeda, S., Hansen, H., Sarma, J. S. M., Fauvel, J.-M. and Bing, R. J. (1974). Microcirculation in the ventricle of the dog and turtle. *Circ. Res.*, 34, 561–9
114. Uhlig, P. N., Baer, J. W., Vlahakes, G. J., Hanley, F. L., Messina, L. M. and Hoffman, J. I. E. (1984). Arterial and venous coronary pressure–flow relations in anesthetized dogs. *Circ. Res.*, 55, 238–48
115. Verrier, E. D., Edelist, G., Consigny, P. M., Robinson, S. and Hoffman, J. I. E. (1980). Greater coronary vascular reserve in dogs anesthetized with halothane. *Anesthesiology* 53, 445–59

116. Vinten-Johansen, J., Duncan, H. W., Finkenberg, J. G., Hume, M. C., Robertson, J. M., Barnard, R. J. and Buckberg, G. D. (1982). Prediction of myocardial O_2 requirements by indirect indices. *Am. J. Physiol.*, **243**, H862–H868
117. Vlahakes, G. J., Baer, R. W., Uhlig, P. N., Verrier, E. D., Bristow, J. D. and Hoffman, J. I. E. (1982). Adrenergic influence in the coronary circulation of conscious dogs during maximal vasodilation with adenosine. *Circ. Res.*, **51**, 371–84
118. Vlahakes, G. J., Turley, K. and Hoffman, J. I. E. (1981). The pathophysiology of failure in acute right ventricular hypertension. Hemodynamic correlations. *Circulation*, **63**, 87–95
119. Vlahakes, G. J., Turley, K., Verrier, E. D. and Hoffman, J. I. E. (1980). Greater maximal coronary flow in conscious lambs with experimental congenital right ventricular hypertrophy. *Circulation*, **62**, 111 (Supplement II)
120. Weiss, H. R., Neubauer, J. A., Lipp, J. A. and Sinha, A. K. (1978). Quantitative determination of regional oxygen consumption in the dog heart. *Circ Res.*, **42**, 394–401
121. Weiss, H. R., Sinha, A. K. (1978). Regional oxygen saturation of small arteries and veins in the canine myocardium. *Circ. Res.*, **42**, 119–26
122. White, F. C., Sanders, M., Peterson, T. and Bloor, C. M. (1979). Ischemic myocardial injury after exercise stress in the pressure overloaded heart. *Am. J. Pathol.*, **97**, 473–88
123. Wilson, R. F., Laughlin, D. E., Ackell, P. H., Chilian, W. M., Holida, M. D., Hartley, C. J., Armstrong, M. L., Marcus, M. L. and White, C. W. (1985). Transluminal, subselective measurement of coronary artery blood flow velocity and vasodilator reserve in man. *Circulation*, **72**, 82–92
124. Wollenberger, A. (1972). Responses of the heart mitochondria to chronic cardiac overload and physical exercise. In Bajusz, E. and Rona, G. (eds.) *Recent Advances in Studies on Cardiac Structure and Metabolism.* Vol. 1, pp. 213–22. (Baltimore: University Park Press)

4
Mechanisms of angina pectoris

A. A. QUYYUMI

The earliest and best description of the syndrome of angina pectoris was by William Heberden in 1772[1]:

'They who are afflicted with it, are seized while they are walking, more especially if it be uphill, and soon after eating with a painful and most disagreeable sensation in the breast, which seems as if it would extinguish life, if it were to increase or to continue; but the moment they stand still, all this uneasiness vanishes.'

The important link between coronary atherosclerosis and angina pectoris was established almost a century later by pathological studies by Herrick and others[2,3]. This led to the theory that angina pectoris was a result of myocardial ischaemia, which was a consequence of myocardial oxygen demand exceeding supply. Strictly speaking, however, the functional and electrocardiographic effects of ischaemia on the myocardium cannot be exactly reproduced by hypoxia alone. It is a combination of deprivation of oxygen, accumulation of ions and metabolites (such as hydrogen, potassium, lactate) and reduction in substrate, which results from inadequate coronary blood flow[4]. The contractile function of the myofibrils is dependent on the availability of adenosine triphosphate (ATP). Adenosine triphosphate production in the mitochondria relies on the availability of oxygen. Thus, myocardial ischaemia can be more accurately defined as a state in which the consumption of ATP exceeds its production resulting in anaerobic cellular metabolism with consequent impairment of myocardial contractile function[5]. This state of affairs is most often produced by the inability of coronary blood flow to deliver oxygen and substrate for the given demand. When this imbalance is transient, ischaemia is limited and is often evident clinically as angina pectoris. If, however, it is prolonged and myocardial neurosis ensues, then the clinical picture is that of myocardial infarction. In this chapter, the mechanisms of transient reversible myocardial ischaemia causing angina pectoris will be reviewed, both from the methodological and clinical view points.

DETERMINANTS OF MYOCARDIAL OXYGEN DEMAND

Essentially, myocardial ischaemia results from an imbalance between myocardial oxygen demand and supply and it is important to delineate the determinants of demand and supply and their interactions in normal and diseased hearts.

Many clinical studies have used the product of heart rate and systolic blood pressure as an index of myocardial oxygen demand, often with sufficient reproducibility for this to be used in assessing the effectiveness of drug therapy (Table 4.1). Sarnoff, Braunwald and co-workers[6,7] have extensively studied the determinants of myocardial oxygen demand in contracting hearts. Apart from heart rate and blood pressure, the development of wall stress in the myocardium was shown to be an essential determinant of myocardial oxygen demand. Wall stress is directly related to the volume and pressure of the left ventricle and is inversely related to wall thickness. Sarnoff defined the tension-time index as the area under the left ventricular pressure curve in systole and demonstrated a close relationship between this and myocardial oxygen consumption[6].

Ventricular dilatation also causes an increase in myocardial oxygen demand[8]. According to the modified Laplace formula, wall stress = (radius × pressure) − twice wall thickness. Thus, for any given pressure and heart rate, a dilated heart will consume more oxygen. Contractility is another very important factor determining myocardial oxygen demand. In an intact heart, sympathetic stimulation not only increases oxygen consumption by increasing contractility; but also reduces the ventricular volume, thereby reducing oxygen demand. It is estimated that these two combined effects increase myocardial oxygen demand by 25% per unit of systolic pressure-time index at maximal sympathetic stimulation[8,9].

Table 4.1 Determinants of myocardial oxygen demand and supply

Myocardial oxygen demand	Myocardial blood flow
Heart rate	Perfusion pressure
Blood pressure	(a) Arterial diastolic blood pressure
	(b) End diastolic left ventricular pressure
Left ventricular volume	(c) Intramyocardial tension
Left ventricular hypertrophy	(d) Diastolic time
Contractility	Coronary resistance
	(a) Blood viscosity
	(b) Size of coronary vasculature (autoregulation)
	(c) Collaterals

DETERMINANTS OF MYOCARDIAL BLOOD FLOW

The basic two determinants of coronary blood flow are the perfusion pressure, which is the driving or inflow pressure for coronary flow and the coronary vascular resistance (Table 4.1). The driving pressure is the difference between the aortic pressure and the intramyocardial pressure, or a difference between inflow and outflow pressures in the coronary circulation[10]. Not only does the aortic pressure vary during systole and diastole; but more importantly, the intramyocardial pressure, which is responsible for compression on intramyocardial collapsible vasculature, also changes during the cardiac cycle. The contraction and relaxation of left ventricular myocardium determines the phasic flow in the left coronary artery. Coronary blood flow is impeded during systole due to both direct contraction of muscle fibres on the intermyocardial vessels and also an indirect compression of the vasculature due to the transmission of the ventricular chamber pressure. The latter effect is considered to be more important[11].

CORONARY VASCULAR RESISTANCE

In normal coronary arteries, according to Poseuille's theorem, coronary vascular resistance is determined by blood viscosity and the diameter and length of the coronary arteries. Thus, the smaller the vessels the greater their contribution to resistance. As viscosity and vessel length do not change normally, the main determinant of vascular resistance is the cross-sectional area of coronary vessels. The coronary arteries are comprised of the large epicardial conductance vessels and smaller, intramyocardial resistance vessels. In normal coronaries, the larger diameter epicardial arteries contribute relatively less to total resistance and the major contributors to coronary vascular resistance are the smaller intramyocardial 'resistance' vessels.

CONTROL OF CORONARY VASCULAR RESISTANCE

The resistance of coronary vessels is autoregulated in the heart[11,12]. As myocardial oxygen demand increases, only a relatively small amount of oxygen can be made available by an increase in oxygen extractions. This is because, even under resting conditions, the heart extracts a relatively high percentage of oxygen and further demand has to be met by means of an increase in delivery and therefore an increase in flow. This results from coronary vasodilation. Indeed, when the myocardium is ischaemic, the coronary vascular resistance is at its minimum in an intrinsic effort to maintain maximal coronary flow, which can increase four- to five-fold. On the other hand, autoregulation also ensures that the changes in perfusion pressures over a substantial physiological range (60 to 110 mmHg) also does not lead to any change in coronary blood flow under circumstances of similar oxygen demand. The control mechanisms for coronary vascular autoregulation have been investigated. It is postulated that a work-dependent release of a metabolite is responsible for changes in vascular resistance. Adenosine, a metabolite of adenosine triphosphate and a power vasodilator, has been hypothesized as being responsible for increasing blood flow during periods of increased myo-cardial work[13]. The importance of neural control on coronary vascu-lature is also debated. Although there is sufficient evidence to suggest the constrictor effect of alpha-adrenoceptor stimulation on the larger epicardial vessels, the role of sympathetic and parasympathetic nerves on the smaller resistance vessels is still uncertain.

Distribution of coronary blood flow in the myocardium

As described above, coronary blood flow distribution is determined by various factors such as the perfusion pressure and the vascular resistance. Although the driving pressure to the coronaries remains constant in the epicardium and endocardium during the cardiac cycle, the opposing 'tissue' pressure varies in these two areas of the myocardium[14]. Thus, during systole, subepicardial flow virtually ceases and this ratio is reversed during diastole under resting conditions. The inner:outer flow ratio does vary between 0.8 and 1.2[8].

Studies in animals using radiolabelled microspheres in myocardium supplied by an artery with high grade stenoses has shown preferential perfusion of the subepicardial tissue[15,16]. As the perfusion pressure to the affected area drops with increasing severity of the stenosis, there are phases within the cardiac cycle when this pressure is exceeded by the opposing 'tissue' or extravascular pressure in the myocardium. In this event, the coronary vessels close. This critical closing pressure is higher for the subendocardium (estimated to be 18 ± 2 mmHg) compared to the subepicardium, where it is estimated to range around 10 ± 2 mmHg[16]. It is therefore logical that in the event of myocardial oxygen demand exceeding supply, the site most likely to become ischaemic first is the subendocardium.

Coronary stenoses and flow

Whatever the cause of luminal narrowing of the major epicardial cor-onary arteries it is the cross-sectional area reduction and the consequent drop in pressure and flow distal to the stenosis that determines the degree of ischaemia that results. When the pressure beyond the stenosis drops below 55 mmHg, subendocardial ischaemia may develop[17]. The more severe the stenotic lesion, the more transmural the ischaemia becomes. McMohen measured the minimum lumen size of coronary lesions in patients with single vessel disease and unstable angina pectoris[18]. Unstable angina was associated with minimum lumen diam-eters averaging 0.88 mm, an area of 0.6 mm^2, representing 72% diameter and 92% area stenosis. Subendocardial myocardial infarction was associated with 78% diameter and 95% area stenosis. They predicted a pressure drop across the stenotic segment of 17 and 50 mmHg respect-ively.

It demonstrates that the relationship between stenosis resistance and the degree of stenosis is non-linear and that the resistance changes rapidly once the stenosis exceeds 50% in internal diameter[19]. Thus, a reduction from 80 to 90% in diameter results in a three fold increase in resistance and a consequent dramatic reduction in blood flow. It is therefore not difficult to visualize that small reductions in the size of already stenosed atherosclerotic segments of coronary arteries whether due to progression of disease, platelet aggregation or increase in tone could result in dramatic reduction in flow distally and precipitation of symptoms[20].

Although the area luminal stenosis of the narrowest point in the coronary artery is the most important determinant of resistance, as recently demonstrated by Sabbah and Stein[21]; the number of obstructions in series and the length of narrowings also contribute to reduction in flow[21]. In an *in vitro* experiment, they demonstrated that the flow reduction across a 6 mm long 50% narrowing of vessel diameter was 8%. However, three 50% diameter narrowings of 2 mm each in series resulted in a flow reduction of 19%. It is presumed that the greater than expected reduction in flow across a series of stenoses is a result of turbulence at each stenotic segment before blood reached the next stenotic segment.

Thus, we have discussed some of the important principles underlying the myocardial oxygen requirements at rest and exercise and those determining the magnitude and distribution of coronary blood flow in normal and stenotic coronary arteries. In the following section we will examine the various mechanisms that have been postulated to account for the clinical manifestations of reversible myocardial ischaemia.

CLINICAL SYNDROMES OF REVERSIBLE MYOCARDIAL ISCHAEMIA

Transient reversible myocardial ischaemia or angina pectoris can present in a number of different clinical settings (Table 4.2). In the most common type, chest pain is precipitated by exertion, emotion or after meals and occurs fairly reproducibly, being exacerbated by cold and relieved by alleviation of the precipitating factors. These symptoms may not only occur on exertion, but in some patients occur also at rest and at night

Table 4.2 Syndromes associated with reversible myocardial ischaemia

With coronary artery disease	With normal coronary arteries
Stable angina on effort	Variant angina
Stable angina on effort and at rest	Syndrome X – reduced vasodilator reserve
Angina with varying threshold	Left ventricular hypertrophy
Variant angina	– aortic stenosis
	– hypertension
Unstable angina	– hypertrophic cardiomyopathy
Painless myocardial ischaemia	Coronary anomalies and arteritis (rare)

causing awakening from sleep. A subgroup of patients with stable angina give a history of variable exercise tolerance. These patients are unable to specify a fixed threshold of exertion, which leads to angina pectoris. It is suggested that the mechanisms for precipitation of myocardial ischaemia in these individuals is multifactorial.

Less commonly, patients may present with an atypical history where typical chest pain suggestive of myocardial ischaemia occurs spontaneously and is not associated with any identifiable precipitating factors. This syndrome is known as variant or Prinzmetal's angina. Patients, some with previous history of stable angina pectoris, may present with a sudden worsening of symptoms. Pain may occur more frequently and readily, with little or no exertion, may last longer and may not be relieved with the usual measures. This syndrome is known as unstable angina pectoris or pre-infarction syndrome. With the advent of newer diagnostic techniques in ischaemic heart diseases, it is being recognized that a number of patients with obstructive coronary artery disease have reversible myocardial ischaemia, which is painfree, and they seldom or never develop angina pectoris. The prevalence of asymptomatic myocardial ischaemia, its haemodynamic accompaniments and its prognostic relevance will be discussed.

INCIDENCE OF VARIOUS ANGINAL SYNDROMES

With recently increasing awareness that angina pectoris may be caused by factors other than simply our increase in myocardial oxygen demand exceeding supply, investigators in the field have tried to subdivide patients into pathophysiological subgroups. Correlation between the history of chest pain and the underlying pathophysiology is, however, fraught with difficulties.

Chest pain typical of angina pectoris can result from unrelated conditions – such as oesophageal spasm[22], mitral valve prolapse, cardiomyopathy etc. In those patients with angina pectoris in whom coronary arteriography was performed it was estimated that up to 75% of Japanese patients had normal coronary arteries, whereas the proportion of these patients was nearer 10% in the United States of America[23]. However, not all these patients had spasm demonstrated. Symptomatic coronary artery spasm with normal coronary arteries is estimated to be very rare. Hempler discovered only 30 (0.1%) cases among 28 000 patients undergoing coronary arteriography[24].

We studied 100 consecutive patients referred to hospital who were undergoing diagnostic coronary arteriography for chest pain[25,26]. A history of typical angina pectoris was given by 91% of these patients and 74 patients had significant coronary artery disease (>70% narrowing). Of the remaining 26 patients with normal coronary arteries, only six had ambulatory ST segment changes and only one of these patients had demonstrable spasm with ergonovine. Thus, of 100 patients studied, 74% had significant coronary artery disease and 4% of those with normal coronary arteries had variant angina. Of the 74 patients with significant coronary artery disease, 11 had nocturnal ischaemia as demonstrated by nocturnal (2400–0600) ST segment changes. Thus 15% of this group of patients had definite evidence of rest/nocturnal ischaemia after 48 hours of monitoring.

Stable exertional angina

This form of angina is by far the most common form of presenting symptom. Typically, patients give a history of precordial discomfort occurring after exertion, emotion, cold or other factors, which are known to increase myocardial oxygen consumption. The symptoms are relieved by removal of the precipitating cause or rest and ischaemia often occurs reproducibly at a specific level of effort.

Pathologically, almost all patients will have atherosclerotic narrowing in one or more of their major epicardial coronary arteries. This stenosis results in a fixed resistance to coronary flow so that an increase in demand results in a decrease in resistance of the smaller distal vasculature, but further increase in flow cannot be achieved because of the fixed obstruction in the epicardial arteries. This results in myocardial ischaemia and chest pain. As discussed earlier, myocardial oxygen demand can be increased by an increase in any of the major determinants of demand – such as heart rate, blood pressure, myocardial tension and contractility.

In the laboratory, myocardial ischaemia can be reproduced in these patients by altering the indices of demand. Thus, by rapid atrial pacing[27,28] heart rate can by increased until ischaemia occurs or by exercise[24,30] which increases the heart rate, blood pressure, contractility and tension developed. Indeed, the development of myocardial ischaemia with exercise in the majority of patients is so reproducible that this test has become a mainstay for the diagnosis and therapeutic assessment of patients with suspected or confirmed coronary artery disease.

Myocardial ischaemia resulting from any cause can be detected by various non-invasive and invasive techniques. Invasive techniques permit earlier recognition of ischaemia than non-invasive tests. Thus, ST segment depression or elevation are widely accepted as reliable indicators of myocardial ischaemia[4]. When myocardial oxygen demand exceeds supply in patients with effort angina, ST segment depression occurs on the electrocardiogram[31]. This is a sign of subendocardial ischaemia. It is only when demand is increased further that ST segment elevation and transmural ischaemia may occur. Rarely, patients with very severe stenosis in the coronary artery may develop ST segment elevation as the first sign of myocardial ischaemia indicating a transmurally ischaemic region. As described earlier, the blood supply to the epicardium is better preserved than the endocardium, as a result of the dynamics of the coronary circulation, and it is not surprising therefore that ischaemia should first develop in the endocardium. Radioisotope markers of myocardial perfusion, such as thallium-201, have been used to demonstrate reproducible areas of decreased uptake in the myocardium in patients with effort angina who had been stressed with exercise or cold to precipitate ischaemia[32]. Regional disturbance of contractile function of the ischaemic myocardium can be detected using radionuclide blood pool scanning[33].

With more invasive means, it can be demonstrated that ischaemia is accompanied almost immediately by a reduction in coronary sinus oxygen saturation[34]. This is followed by a delay in relaxation of the ischaemic myocardium and failure of contractile function. Anaerobic metabolism will become evident as a lactate production occurs instead of lactate extraction. Left ventricular end diastolic pressure rises as a result of reduced compliance of the ischaemic myocardium.

In patients with effort angina, the haemodynamic accompaniments of ischaemia follow an increase in the indices of myocardial oxygen demand. Chest pain is often a late manifestation of myocardial ischaemia, usually following the onset of ST segment change by several minutes[31]. Although it is widely agreed that increases in oxygen demand precede the occurrence of myocardial ischaemia in the majority of patients who complain of stable effort induced angina, there is debate about the pathophysiological basis underlying the development of ischaemia in patients who have effort and nocturnal angina and those who have a variable threshold of exertion before ischaemia occurs. There is increasing evidence that in these subgroups of angina patients, other factors that lead to a primary reduction of myocardial blood flow are responsible for precipitating episodes of ischaemia. The factors proposed include spasm of coronary arteries, platelet aggregation at sites of previous stenoses and reduced vasodilator reserve of distal coronary vasculature.

The role of coronary spasm in stable exertional angina

Two reports in recent years have described a small number of patients with exertional angina who had demonstrable coronary spasm on exertion[35,36]. Two of the four patients described by Yasne[35] had normal coronary arteries and the other two had two or three vessel coronary artery disease. These patients developed ST segment depression and spasm on exercise. Fuller[36] described two patients with ST segment elevation on exercise and spasm in the left anterior descending coronary artery. Both these patients, however, also had rest pain and the occurrence of exercise spasm may have been coincidental. In order to investigate the possibility of spasm during effort angina, Pepine et al. performed a series of studies[37]. After a trial pacing to precipitate ischaemia in 13 patients with varying severity of coronary artery disease and exertional angina, they demonstrated an increase in calibre of eight stenosed segments and 39 normal sections of coronary artery by 7%. They also demonstrated a 21% decrease in coronary diameter during exercise induced angina. Coronary vascular resistance was demonstrated to reduce after stress and exercise induced angina in regions of myocardium supplied by normal and stenosed coronary arteries and small doses of intracoronary (100 μg) nitroglycerin did not relieve the ischaemia. These results confirmed that coronary spasm or sudden reductions in blood flow does not play an important role in patients with stable exertional angina. However, whether such influences are important in patients with a variable history of exertional and rest angina will be considered in later sections.

MECHANISMS UNDERLYING STABLE EFFORT AND NOCTURNAL RESTING ANGINA IN PATIENTS WITH CORONARY ARTERY DISEASE

It is important to recognize two clinically separate types of patients that present with rest and nocturnal angina. One distinct group of patients give a short history of worsening effort angina, which then develops spontaneously at rest lasting for longer duration and worsening in intensity. This group of patients are conventionally labelled as suffering from unstable angina and their pathophysiology will be discussed in detail in later sections. Another group of patients, however, give a longer history of stable effort angina and also chest pain occurring at rest and at night with no recent worsening. These patients are discussed in this section.

There is mounting evidence that primary reduction in myocardial blood flow is an important underlying mechanism for precipitation of ischaemia in not only the unstable angina group, but also the latter group of patients with stable rest angina.

In a recent study by Bertrand[38] where ergonovine provocation tests were performed during coronary arteriography in 1089 consecutive patients, he recorded positive tests in 14% of the patients who had angina at exertion and rest and also in 4% of the patients who complained of angina only on exertion. This contrasts with an 85% positive response in patients with variant angina. They also noted that the test was negative in a large group of patients who had severe obstructive coronary artery disease. De Severi et al[39] reported three patients with effort and rest angina associated with ST segment depression. Coronary spasm could be demonstrated during resting periods of angina but not during exertional episodes suggesting that in some patients two pathogenetic mechanisms may underlie the development of ischaemia. Maseri[40] demonstrated localized coronary artery spasm in 37 patients with a history of rest and exertional angina who developed pain during coronary arteriography. Patients had variable severity of coronary artery disease and this led to a suggestion that rest angina is secondary to localized coronary artery spasm, at least, in a proportion of patients. Thallium-201 scintigrams performed during spontaneous episodes of rest angina demonstrated a primary reduction of coronary sinus oxygen saturation, which was followed by left ventricular functional impairment and development of ST segment elevation, depression or T wave pseudonormalization[34]. In none of the six patients studied was there an increase in any of the determinants of myocardial oxygen demand before the electrocardiographic signs of ischaemia.

There is no doubt from a number of studies[34,40-42], some of which have been described above, that in certain patients with rest and effort angina, factors causing sudden reduction in myocardial oxygen supply are more important than purely an increase in demand. However, in most of these studies, the patients investigated were selected and the selection criteria are uncertain. Furthermore, a number of studies include patients with unstable angina pectoris in whom coronary flow reduction may indeed be an important mechanism. In our study of 100 consecutive patients presenting with chest pain, nocturnal ambulatory ST segment depression or elevation occurred in 12, of whom 11 (15%) had significant coronary artery disease. Furthermore, all these patients had three vessel coronary artery disease or left main stem stenosis and the mean exercise duration during treadmill exercise testing according to the modified Bruce protocol in these patients was 2.2 minutes before ST segment depression occurred[25,26]. It is clear from this that in clinical practice, in patients presenting with chest pain, objective evidence of nocturnal resting ischaemia is often detected in patients with relatively severe forms of coronary artery disease who have extremely limited exercise tolerance. These patients also had frequent and prolonged episodes of daytime, effort related episodes of ST segment change, the majority of which were painfree[43]. Momentary analysis of episodes of ST segment depression during the night in five patients revealed an increase in heart rate before the onset of ST change in nearly all episodes (Figure 4.1)

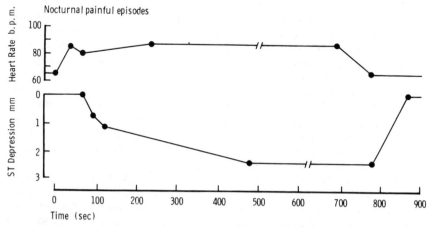

Figure 4.1 Mean changes in heart rate in relation to the development of ST segment depression accompanied by pain during the night. It can be seen that there is an increase in heart rate that precedes the earliest change in ST segment depression. The maximum heart rate occurs shortly before the earliest change in ST segment depression. At the end of the episode, heart rate falls before the ST segment depression resolves. Reproduced with permission from the *Lancet*

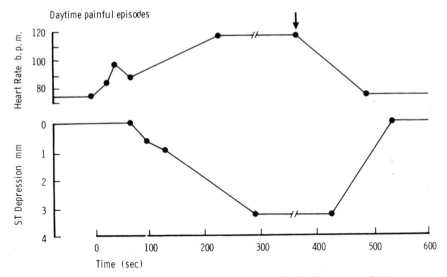

Figure 4.2 Relationship between the heart rate and the development of ST segment depression during the day and accompanied by chest pain. As expected, there is an increase in heart rate that occurs before the earliest change in ST segment depression – resolution of the heart rate to normal precedes the resolution of ST segment changes. Reproduced with permission from the *Lancet*

and was very similar to episodes recorded during the day (Figure 4.2). This highlighted another important problem when one is dealing with angina patients. Many patients develop painfree ischaemia and the absence of pain during similar types of activity at different times of day does not necessarily imply absence of myocardial ischaemia; and detailed objective assessment by such means as ambulatory ST segment monitoring may be warranted to obtain an accurate picture. Indeed, painfree episodes of ST segment depression in angina subjects appears to be very similar to those episodes accompanied by pain (Figures 4.3 and 4.4).

We further investigated ten patients, eight with a positive exercise test and severe coronary artery disease and two with normal coronary arteries and spasm demonstrable at angiography[45]. All patients had multiple episodes of ST segment change during the day and night. Polygraphic sleep studies were performed when continuous recordings of the electrocardiogram, electroencephalogram, electromyogram, electroculogram, chest wall movements, nasal airflow and ear oximeter oxygen saturation were made. Forty-two episodes of transient ST segment depression were recorded in the eight patients with coronary artery disease and 26 episodes of ST segment elevation or depression in the two patients with variant angina. All episodes of ST depression in the former group of patients were preceded by an increase in heart rate (mean 19 ± 12 beats a minute) as a result of (a) arousal and lightening of sleep, (b) bodily movements, (c) REM sleep, and (d) sleep apnoea.

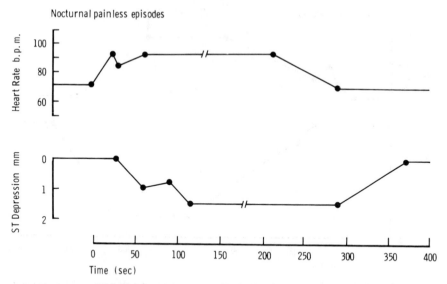

Figure 4.3 Relationship between heart rate and ST segment depression at night but in the absence of chest pain. Heart rate increases before the earliest change in ST segment depression and resolves before the ST segment returns to normal. This pattern is identical with the episodes that occurred at night that were accompanied by chest pain, but tended to be shorter. Reproduced with permission from the *Lancet*

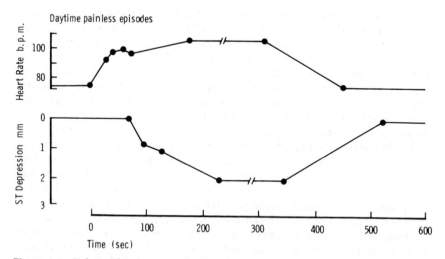

Figure 4.4 Relationship between the heart rate and the development of ST segment depression during the day in the absence of chest pain. The pattern of development is identical with the painful daytime episodes with an increase in heart rate preceding the development of ST segment depression with resolution of the heart rate before the ST segment changes returned to normal. Again these painfree episodes of ST segment depression tended to be shorter than the painful episodes. Reproduced with permission from the *Lancet*

However, in contrast, in patients with variant angina episodes of ST segment change were not preceded by an increase in heart rate, arousal or apnoea in 23 of the 26 episodes. It was therefore evident from this study that increase in myocardial oxygen demand was responsible for precipitating nocturnal resting ischaemia in patients with obstructive coronary artery disease but not in the majority of episodes occurring in patients with variant angina.

Therefore it seems that various studies have shown conflicting results regarding the pathogenesis of myocardial ischaemia occurring at rest and night in patients with obstructive coronary artery disease. It may be possible to reconcile these different view points under one unifying hypothesis that incorporates both explanations – increase in myocardial oxygen demand and reduction in flow due to factors, such as spasm.

Clinical studies in anginal patients have demonstrated a circadian variation in episodes of pain with more frequent attacks in the early morning period and less frequent attacks later in the day. This variation was not only shown in patients with variant angina pectoris[46], but also in two studies in patients with a history of variable anginal threshold and effort and rest angina. Yasue et al.[47] demonstrated that such patients developed a positive exercise test when this was performed in the early morning period (0800) but was negative when performed the same day at 1600. Selwyn et al. have also shown that such patients had more frequent ambulatory ST segment change during the latter part of the night (0400–0600) compared to the daytime period[48]. It has also been demonstrated in patients that coronary arteries were uniformly narrower when arteriography was performed early morning when compared to later on in the day[47].

It has been hypothesized that these findings are a result of intrinsic diurnal variation of coronary artery tone, which may partly be related to the autonomic nervous system activity. It is well known that parasympathetic activity predominates at rest and during the night and acetyl choline is known to cause vasoconstriction of epicardial coronary arteries. Increased parasympathetic activity may be the cause of the diurnal physiological variation in tone of the coronary arteries.

Bearing in mind the effects of physiological increases in tone on already stenosed coronary arteries, it is not difficult to envisage the reasons for variations in threshold to angina that is so often observed in clinical practice. Thus, when coronary tone is low, angina pectoris may occur after moderate exertion from a 60% narrowed lesion in the coronary artery. However, under conditions of increased smooth muscle tone the lesion may well result in 76% area narrowing, which will result in both rest and exertional angina[20]. This theory assumes, however, that medial smooth muscle in the region of intimal atherosclerosis is capable of causing luminal narrowing. This will be possible only if (a) medial smooth muscle is preserved and (b) the intimal lesion is eccentric – that is there is some part of intimal wall, which is not sclerosed or thickened and is capable of constriction[20,49] (Figures 4.5, 4.6).

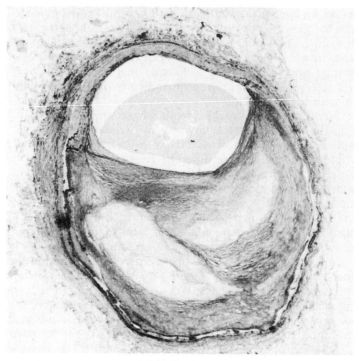

Figure 4.5 Photomicrograph of a section of coronary artery showing eccentric fibro-atheromatous intimal thickening without involvement of the remaining intima and with smooth muscle preservation. Reproduced with permission from the *British Heart Journal*

Increases in coronary vascular tone is just one of the several proposed mechanisms that have been implicated as causes for sudden reductions in coronary blood flow. Evidence in favour of luminal narrowing due to platelet aggregation and small vessel vasocontrictors are considered below.

VARIANT ANGINA PECTORIS

Even in his landmark description of the syndrome of angina pectoris, Heberden[1] described patients whose description of pain differed from that of classical angina of exertion. He stated, 'some have been seized while they are standing still, or sitting, also upon first waking out of sleep ... '. Wilson and Johnston described the occurrence of electrocardiographic changes similar in magnitude and kind to those produced by myocardial infarction and postulated that ischaemia is due to a change in calibre of the coronary arteries rather than to increase in work of the heart alone[50]. However, the full description of the syndrome now known as *variant angina* was reported by Prinzmetal in 1959 when

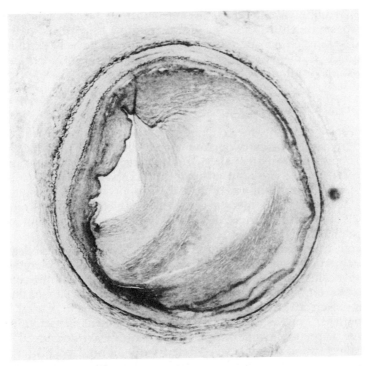

Figure 4.6 Photomicrograph of a section of coronary artery with circumferential fibro-atheromatous intimal thickening where there is no smooth muscle preservation. Reproduced with permission from the *British Heart Journal*

he described a group of 32 patients with angina pectoris, which differed from the conventional angina of exertion[51].

Clinical syndrome

Patients with variant angina typically have chest pain at rest rather than with exertion or emotional disturbance. The episodes of pain recur at roughly the same time each day, often in the early hours of the morning. During chest pain, patients are often found to have ST segment elevation on the electrocardiogram. Sometimes, episodes of pain are accompanied by arrhythmias including atrioventricular block, ventricular extrasystoles, tachycardia or occasionally even ventricular fibrillation. In general, pain responds readily to sublingual nitroglycerin with resolution of electrocardiographic changes. Although the above presentation accounts for many of the patients with classical variant angina, who have subsequently been demonstrated to have complete occlusion of a major epicardial coronary artery during the attack, there are some atypical presentations which have been described in recent years. A small group of patients with normal coronary arteries and history of exertional angina pectoris have been demonstrated to develop coronary artery spasm on effort[46,52,53]. Secondly, a number of patients with documented spasm, either spontaneous or provoked, have been shown to develop ST segment depression or pseudonormalization of T waves during some or all of the episodes of ischaemia[34,39].

Coronary arteriography

Gensini *et al.* were the first to demonstrate angiographically the association of dynamic coronary narrowing and chest pain[54]. During a spontaneous episode of angina, they demonstrated lack of visualization of the greater part of the right coronary artery, which showed complete opacification after sublingual isosorbide dinitrate and resolution of pain. Since then, other investigators[55,56] have clearly demonstrated the presence of epicardial artery occlusion during episodes of pain and ST segment change in these patients.

Several arteriographic features have been described. The degree of atherosclerotic involvement of the coronary arteries that undergo spasm and total occlusion is variable. This ranges from normal calibre coronary lumen to severely stenosed lumen. Also the severity of spasm, its duration and the electrocardiographic changes accompanying it varied in the same patient. Thus with total occlusion, ST segment elevation, peaked T waves or pseudonormalization if inverted T waves occurred[56,57]. At other times, these changes were noted with subtotal occlusion of the lumen by spasm, when the distal vessel could be faintly visualized. Some patients also developed ST segment depression and they were shown to have diffuse but often incomplete spasm of multiple branches with occlusion. Occasionally, patients with diagonal or septal branch spasm have been shown to have ST segment depression in anterior chest leads[58]. Thus, further investigation of patients with a history of variant angina has demonstrated that spasm can occur not only in normal coronary arteries as described by Prinzmetal initially, but also in patients with various degrees of atherosclerotic coronary artery disease.

Haemodynamic studies

Haemodynamic and cardiac metabolic studies in patients with variant angina have demonstrated without doubt that the main underlying cause for ischaemia in these patients is a primary sudden reduction in coronary blood flow to the ischaemic area which coincides with arteriographic occlusion of the epicardial coronary artery.

Maseri *et al.*[56] monitored left and right ventricular pressures in 22 patients with frequent rest angina. They recorded 153 episodes of ST segment elevation, 92 of which were asymptomatic. No consistent increases in heart rate, blood pressure or left ventricular dp/dt were observed before the onset of ST segment change in any patient. The most typical haemodynamic pattern observed was firstly a reduction of relaxation and contraction peak of the left ventricle (dp/dt). This preceded or accompanied the onset of ST segment or T wave change. Left ventricular end diastolic pressure rise followed and some patients had reduction of systolic arterial pressure. Pulmonary artery pressure arose only after ST segment change had occurred. Increase in heart rate and blood pressure was observed some minutes after the onset of ST/T change. The sequence of events was similar in painful and painfree episodes. Several conclusions were reached by the authors: firstly, pain was a late phenomenon during ischaemia and was often absent; secondly, often ST/T wave behaviour was variable in the same patient; and finally, independent of the direction of ST/T wave change, the episodes were never preceded by increases in the indices of myocardial oxygen demand and were consistent with reductions of coronary flow, which caused obvious impairment of left ventricular function.

This group and others have since studied coronary haemodynamics during spontaneous and ergonovine induced episodes of ischaemia in patients with variant angina[59,61]. In these studies, it has been demonstrated that during episodes of ST segment elevation, there was a dramatic decrease in coronary sinus flow[59,60], consistent with an increase in coronary vascular resistance. Lactate extraction in the coronary sinus fell and lactate production was noted[61]. Chierchia et al.[34] demonstrated that the coronary sinus oxygen saturation fell before the onset of electrocardiographic changes and haemodynamic changes of left ventricular impairment in patients with frequent rest angina and ST/T wave changes.

Theoretical mechanisms of spasm in epicardial coronary arteries

Medial smooth muscle can constrict and dilate resulting in luminal change by fixed amounts which are determined by geometric constraints of the artery[49]. The ratio of medial wall thickness to lumen radius is 0.20, which is an average estimate for medium sized arteries. Smooth muscle contraction is accompanied by appropriate thickening of the media. Normal variations in tone of the coronary artery will cause reductions in outer diameter of coronary arteries by 10%, but may reach up to 25% under certain conditions. It is clear from geometrical calculations made by McAlpen and others, that in the absence of medial or intimal thickening, a 25% reduction in outer diameter will reduce the inner diameter of the lumen by 37%[20,49,62]. However, in an artery with intimal thickening, even a smaller increase in tone can result in subtotal or total occlusion of the lumen.

Based on these studies, it has been concluded that in normal sections of coronary artery – that is, where there is no medial hypertrophy or intimal thickening – normal physiological alterations in smooth muscle tone cannot result in total luminal occlusion. For such occlusion to occur, there has to be either medial hypertrophy or intimal thickening. Severe reports have described total occlusion due to spasm, in angiographically normal coronary arteries[54-56]. However, lesions in at least some of these sections of coronary arteries that underwent spasm are rare and often have shown at least partial atherosclerotic involvement. If spasm can result in total occlusion of an entirely normal section of the coronary artery, then one has to postulate the existence of a localized hyper-reactive and hypercontractile segment involving epicardial coronary arteries.

With the evidence currently available to us, we have to consider angiographically demonstrated luminal reduction or obliteration as being a result of two probably separate processes. Firstly, as shown above, it may result from a physiological increase in tone of the medial smooth muscle, which when superimposed on intimal thickening results in severe luminal narrowing. Secondly, there may be pathological increase in tone in a small segment of the epicardial coronary artery, which results in 'spasm' and total occlusion. The first mechanism is a physiological 'variation in tone' and the second a pathological region of spasm.

Triggers causing spasm

No clear trigger factors that precipitate coronary artery spasm have as yet been identified. There may be hypersensitivity to alpha-adrenergic stimulation locally, but studies have not yet demonstrated any increase in receptor density at sites of spasm[20]. There may be local hypersensitivity to and release of vasoconstrictive metabolites, such as thromboxane A_2. Studies in patients with variant angina have demonstrated elevated levels of thromboxane B_2 in coronary venous blood[63]. Other proposed mechanisms are local rise in pH[64], release of histamine[65], calcium activation or platelet aggregation and local release of thromboxane A_2 [63]. The latter mechanism will be discussed in detail in later sections.

Metabolites of arachodonic acid such as prostacyclin and thromboxane are not stored in the body. They are synthesized in various specific sites in response to various stimuli and are readily metabolized. Arachodonic acid is a metabolite of linolic acid, an essentially fatty acid that is available from dietary meat and oils. It is converted to cyclic endopenoxides, that is prostaglandins G_2 (PGG$_2$) and H_2 (PGH$_2$), by the action of the enzyme cycloxygenase. These are then converted to various prostaglandins – including thromboxane A_2, which is synthesized in the platelets and prostacyclin (PGI$_2$), which is formed in the vascular endothelium.

Thromboxane A_2 aggregates platelets and is a powerful endogenous vasoconstrictor[66]. It has a brief half-life of approximately 30 seconds *in vitro* after synthesis and release from aggregating platelets and is degraded to thromboxane B_2 – a stable inert metabolite, which can be quantitated. Prostacyclin on the other hand is a potent inhibitor of platelet aggregation and relaxes vascular smooth muscle and thus has actions diametrically opposite to those of thromboxane A_2[67]. It is synthesized in the endothelial cells and is also extremely unstable with a half-life of two to three minutes *in vivo*. It is degraded to 6-keto-PGF$_1$.

In recent years, many theories have been postulated regarding the role of the thromboxane–prostacyclin balance in the genesis of atherosclerosis. Hypercholesterolaemia has been demonstrated to enhance platelet aggregability and increase thromboxane production, whereas the atherosclerotic arteries have a reduced capacity to produce prostacyclin[68,69]. Recently a family with thromboxane synthetase deficiency has been described, which suggests that genetic control of prostaglandin regulating enzymes may determine the risk of coronary artery disease[70].

THE ROLE OF PLATELETS IN PATHOPHYSIOLOGY OF ISCHAEMIC HEART DISEASE

Experimental evidence

Folts *et al.*, using the dog model, demonstrated cyclic reductions in coronary flow in an artery where a fixed stenosis had been created[71]. These reductions in flow caused ischaemic ST segment changes and premature ventricular extrasystoles and were abolished by pre-treatment with aspirin, a well known platelet inhibitor. Examination of sections of arteries during the low flow periods demonstrated clumps of platelet aggregates, which were present on the narrowed segment of the vessel. The authors concluded that the platelet aggregates had further narrowed the lumen and resulted in ischaemia or the decreased flow was a result of vasospasm and the platelet aggregates were a secondary phenomenon.

In a further series of experiments they demonstrated that the cyclic flow reductions that occurred in coronary arteries that were 60–80% narrowed could be abolished by platelet inhibitors, such as ibuprofen and indomethacin, but not by antifibrin agents, such as heparin[72]. Also, physical interventions – such as pinching of the vessel during low flow periods – resulted in restoration of flow. Vasodilators, such as nitroglycerin and papaverine, did not abolish the cyclic reductions in flow. This suggested a primary role of platelet aggregates in causing sudden reductions in blood flow in an already compromised coronary artery.

Folts *et al.* performed another study in dogs to investigate the role of cigarette smoke on spontaneous reductions of coronary blood flow[73]. Cigarette smoke has been shown to increase platelet aggregation and decrease the production of prostacyclin[73]. In dogs, administration of cigarette smoke resulted in an increased frequency of spontaneous episodes of blood flow reduction, an effect similar to that of intravenous administration of nicotine.

The role of thromboxane–prostacyclin system and platelets in human ischaemic heart disease

There is now plenty of direct and indirect evidence linking the activation of platelets and prostaglandin metabolites to the manifestations of ischaemic heart disease[74].

Stable angina pectoris

Patients with underlying coronary artery disease were demonstrated to have diminished platelet aggregation in coronary venous blood[75]. Endothelial injury to vessels has been shown to result in formation of platelet aggregates and the reduced activity in coronary venous bed is due to entrapment of platelet aggregates in the damaged coronary vasculature, as demonstrated by using indium-111 tagged platelets[76]. Platelet reactivity within the coronary vasculature has been shown to increase after stress, induced either by exercise or rapid atrial pacing[77]. In one study, the level of platelet Factor IV, a platelet specific protein released during platelet activation, was shown to increase in peripheral venous blood in patients with an ischaemic exercise test but not in those with a negative exercise test[78]. These results suggest that activation of platelets and platelet aggregation occurs in patients with obstructive coronary disease and may be related to periods of ischaemia. However, the demonstration of this phenomenon does not imply a causative role of platelets in the precipitation of ischaemia in patients with stable angina pectoris.

Hirsch et al. noted that the ratio of coronary sinus to aorta of thromboxane B_2 was not altered in patients with stable angina either at rest, or after ischaemia was induced by rapid atrial pacing, isometric exercise and cold[79]. Inhibition of platelet aggregability with aspirin does not influence the development of myocardial ischaemia in these patients[80]. Thus, although platelet activation can be demonstrated in patients with exertional angina, neither this, nor the prosta-cyclin/thromboxane system seems to be of pathophysiological import-ance in patients with exertional angina.

Angina at rest and unstable angina

Various studies have shown that metabolites from increased platelet activation are evident in patients with unstable angina pectoris. In separate studies, elevated levels of platelet Factor IV[81,82] and beta-thromboglobulin[81,83] in peripheral venous blood have been detected in patients with unstable angina but not in patients with stable angina pectoris. Sobel et al.[81] demonstrated a close relationship between occur-rence of chest pain and platelet activation products in the venous circulation of patients with unstable angina. Hirsch et al.[79] demonstrated that the transcendial ratio of thromboxane B_2 (coronary sinus/aortic thromboxane B_2) was elevated in patients with unstable angina and not in patients with stable angina pectoris.

Although these studies propose a stronger association between angina occurring at rest, unstable angina and activation of the platelet and prostaglandin metabolic system, the direct causal association between the two is far from proven. Elevated levels of thromboxane B_2 and platelet activation products have been detected in the coronary venous circulation only after episodes of spontaneously occurring myocardial ischaemia and therefore may have been secondary to the ischaemic injury rather than the precipitating cause. In a single sample drawn fortuitously, a minute before ST segment elevation in one patient, the level of thromboxane B_2 was normal. However, the level of thromboxane B_2 remained elevated for 6–10 minutes after ST segment elevation resolved, thus providing presumptive evidence that thromboxane A_2 alone is not sufficient to cause coronary spasm.

Another way to explore whether a casual relationship exists between platelet activation and myocardial ischaemia was to document the effect of anti-platelet agents[84-86]. Use of aspirin alone, or in combination with persantin and sulphinpyrazone, in trials of mortality after myocardial infarction have resulted in conflicting results. In a double-blind study using aspirin and indomethacin in patients with variant angina, the authors failed to show any reduction in attacks of chest pain[87]. However, we know that the effect of aspirin and drugs in its group is dose-dependent. In the conventional doses used in these trials, it not only inhibits thromboxane A_2 production. Thus, the overall effect on the thromboxane A_2 and prostacyclin ratio may remain unaltered, that is the beneficial effects of reducing the vasoconstrictor thromboxane A_2 are offset by a simultaneous reduction of the vasodilator, anti-platelet aggregatory prostacyclin.

A need for more specific anti-platelet agents is clearly justified. Fox et al.[88] used ticlopidine, which does not influence prostacyclin production, but instead acts directly on the platelet membrane to inhibit platelet aggregation. In a double-blind study comparing the effect of ticlopidine with placebo in 10 patients with frequent angina pectoris, they demonstrated a significant reduction in the frequency of chest pain and episodes of ambulatory ST segment change. This effect was more marked in nocturnal episodes and those not preceded by increases in heart rate. This study thus suggested that platelet activation may either play a direct role (by platelet plugging), or indirect role (vasospasm via thromboxane A_2) in the genesis of myocardial ischaemia.

Platelet activation and coronary vasospasm

There is no doubt from the evidence gathered so far that platelet activation and thromboxane A_2 production are temporally related to episodes of ischaemia that occur at rest, in unstable angina and variant angina. Maseri and co-workers and others have also demonstrated that angina at rest is preceded by sudden reductions in coronary blood flow including coronary artery spasm. Could there be a link between vasospasm and platelet activation? If so, which is the precipitating cause? A great deal of experimental evidence links these two mechanisms. Aggregating platelets release thromboxane A_2, a powerful vaso-constrictor that can cause vasospasm. Also, repeated vasoconstriction of coronary arteries can lead to intimal damage. This results in platelet activation, thromboxane A_2 production and further vasospasm. Thus, it has been suggested that thromboxane A_2 may be involved either in triggering off vasospasm or in perpetuating spasm once it has occurred.

UNSTABLE ANGINA PECTORIS

Unstable angina is characterized by an increasing frequency, duration and/or magnitude of pain associated with myocardial ischaemia. Pain may occur with little or no activity, at rest and sometimes at night. The responsiveness of pain to usual anti-anginal medication is often reduced. Several other names have been attributed to this syndrome. These include crescendo angina, preinfarction angina, intermediate coronary syndrome, coronary insufficiency and nocturnal angina.

Pathological features

Patients with unstable angina tend to have severe atheromatous coronary artery disease. In a study of 22 patients who died after coronary bypass surgery was performed for unstable angina, Robert's group examined each 5 mm section of coronary arteries and compared them with con-trols[89]. The found cross sectional narrowing of 76–100% in at least one of the four major coronary arteries in every patient with unstable angina. Over 80% of the arteries examined were narrowed 76–100% in at least one section compared to the control. Thrombus was absent from all arteries. Of the 1049 5 mm sections examined, 41% were 76–100% stenosed (control 1%) and 29% were 51–75% stenosed. The severity and diffuse nature of narrowings observed in patients with unstable angina contrasts with less severe degree of narrowing reported by the same authors when post mortem examination was carried out similarly in patients with sudden coronary death, acute myocardial infarction and old myocardial infarction[90–92].

The presence of severe obstructive coronary artery disease in patients with unstable angina led to the belief that in these patients, pain could occur at rest or during minor activity due to minor increases in the determinant of oxygen demand – such as filling pressure (at night), heart rate and blood pressure (e.g. during REM sleep). However, haemo-dynamic studies that followed in the last 10 years suggested strongly that factors causing decreases in coronary blood flow are probably very important in precipitating ischaemia in unstable angina.

Haemodynamic studies

Early studies using the onset of angina pectoris as an indicator of ischaemia demonstrated that, in some patients, there was an increase in heart rate and blood pressure (determinants of myocardial oxygen demand) before angina whereas in others, there was no such increase[93]; Berndt compared the double and triple products (indices of myocardial oxygen demand) at the onset of spontaneous episodes of angina and at the onset of pacing induced angina. The double product rose by 87% at the onset of pacing angina compared to a 12% increase at the onset of spontaneous angina[94]. It was soon realized that a number of haemodynamic and electrocardiographic changes of ischaemia precede the development of chest pain[95]. Figueras et al.[95] in a study of 23 patients demonstrated a reduction in coronary sinus oxygen as the first change, followed by the onset of left ventricular dysfunction with chest pain following a mean of 8 minutes later. At the onset of electrocardiographic change, the double product had remained unchanged in eight and increased minimally in four patients. These findings were confirmed by Chierchia et al.[34]. These studies strongly suggest that primary reduction of coronary blood flow is the major underlying cause in most patients with unstable angina pectoris.

Angiographic studies

Maseri et al. have demonstrated the occurrence of coronary artery spasm at sites of previous atheromatous narrowing and in normal sections of coronary arteries during both spontaneous and ergonovine induced episodes of ST segment change in patients presenting with unstable angina[55–57]. However, not all patients with rest angina develop discrete spasm with ergonovine[38]. The haemodynamic findings of a primary reduction in coronary flow as a precipitating cause for ischaemia in these patients may be a result of more platelet plugging of already stenosed coronary arteries and activation of local vasoconstrictor metabolites such as thromboxane A_2. The evidence suggesting the role of platelets and prostaglandins and the role of physiologic alterations in coronary tone which may lead to ischaemia have been discussed in the previous section.

SILENT MYOCARDIAL ISCHAEMIA

Historically, patients presenting with reversible myocardial ischaemia have been classified into categories of stable angina, unstable angina, variant angina etc. on the basis of the patient's history of chest pain. With the advent of modern diagnostic techniques, it has come to light that a number of patients – indeed the majority with reversible myocardial ischaemia – have asymptomatic episodes. During exercise testing, up to 40% of patients, who develop a positive test and a perfusion defect on thallium-201 scintigraphy, have no chest pain. Schang and Pepine[96] and Stern and Tzivoni[97] were amongst the first groups to highlight the frequency of painless episodes and ambulatory ST segment change in patients with angina pectoris.

A number of questions regarding the frequency of painless ischaemia, its relationship to underlying coronary artery disease, electro-cardiographic changes and haemodynamic changes have been answered in recent years. We addressed this issue in a recent study of 100 consecutive patients who presented with chest pain of varying severity and frequency and were undergoing diagnostic coronary arteriography[25,26]. All patients had 48 hour ambulatory monitoring performed to detect ST segment changes and kept angina diaries. There was no association between the patients' reported frequency of pain and the frequency of ambulatory ST segment changes recorded[43]. Thus, a history of frequent pain (>1 day) was obtained from 56% of patients with ambulatory ST segment changes and also from 40% of patients with no ambulatory ST changes after 48 hours of monitoring. Almost 90% of patients complaining of nocturnal angina of varying frequency had no nocturnal ST segment changes, whereas 36% of patients with nocturnal ST segment changes during monitoring gave no history of nocturnal pain. This illustrates an import management predicament. Most of our clinical pathophysiological and therapeutic decisions regarding angina are based on the patients' history and the study has highlighted the fact that history is a poor indicator of the frequency and type (rest or exertional) of reversible myocardial ischaemia.

The study also demonstrated a poor relationship between the frequency of pain and the severity of coronary artery disease, but when the frequency of ambulatory ST segment changes was analysed, it was shown that only patients with double or triple vessel disease and those with left main stem stenosis tended to have greater than six episodes of ischaemia per day[26]. Only a mean 30% of all episodes of ST segment change recorded in these patients were accompanied by pain. In patients with coronary artery disease, 27% of patients had painful ST segment changes only, 46% had both painful and painfree episodes and 27% had painfree episodes of ST segment change only during 48 hours of monitoring. Although not statistically significant in this small group of patients, painful episodes tended to be of longer duration and have greater magnitude of ST segment depression compared to painfree episodes[43]. These findings have been supported by other studies[31,98].

That the episodes of painless ST segment change – either elevation, depression or T wave changes recorded during exercise testing, ambulatory monitoring or in the coronary care unit – represent myocardial ischaemia is indisputable[34,41,42,95]. A number of studies have demonstrated that the haemodynamic changes of left ventricular functional impairment that accompany episodes of painless myocardial ischaemia are similar to those that occur during episodes of painful myocardial ischaemia. It has been suggested that the haemodynamic deterioration during pain-free episodes tends to be less in magnitude compared to painful episodes, but there is often wide overlap.

It should therefore be remembered that asymptomatic reversible myocardial ischaemia exists and is common. The perception of pain in the majority of patients may just represent a tip of the iceberg in terms of the frequency of ischaemia suffered by the individuals during normal daily activity. Finally, there is no reason to believe that the prognosis of the patients with asymptomatic ischaemia is any better than those with angina, although no prognostic studies are as yet available to answer this question clearly.

RARE SYNDROMES OF MYOCARDIAL ISCHAEMIA

Reduced vasodilator reserve of small coronary arteries

The coronary vasculature dilates as myocardial work is increased, so that blood flow to the myocardium can be increased. The arterioles account for the main resistive component of the coronary circulation. Under ischaemic conditions, the distal coronary circulation is maximally dilated and it is the failure of maximal dilatation to occur, resulting in myocardial ischaemia, which has been termed 'Reduced vasodilator reserve of small coronary arteries'. In a study of 22 patients with insignificant coronary artery disease and chest pain, Cannon et al. studied the coronary haemodynamics during atrial pacing, cold pressor test and ergonovine provocation[99]. Patients developing chest pain during pacing demonstrated a lesser increase in coronary blood flow and a lesser reduction in coronary resistance than control. After ergonovine and pacing, more patients[12] developed pain and again showed lesser increases in flow, lesser reduction in resistance of coronary arteries and less lactate consumption than control. No epicardial spasm was observed. The authors concluded that these patients with atypical pain and normal coronary arteries have inappropriate coronary arteriolar constriction, which responds inappropriately to atrial pacing. Although feasible in these patients, it is early to extrapolate this hypothesis to patients with angina pectoris and coronary artery disease.

A similar explanation has been put forward to explain the unusual syndrome X. By definition, patients with this syndrome have exertional angina, normal coronary arteries and ST segment depression associated with pain during stress testing. By giving dipyridamole in this group of patients it was demonstrated by Opherx et al. that the maximal coronary blood flow was reduced to 50% of that expected in normal individuals, suggesting a reduction in coronary vasodilator reserve[100]. Ultrastructural examination of myocardial biopsies did not demonstrate physical changes in the intramyocardial 'small' vessels, but degenerative changes were noted in the myocardial cells. During exercise, left ventricular functional impairment was observed using gated blood pool scanning. Lactate production occurred in these patients after stress, indicating development of anaerobic metabolism. Thus, studies suggesting functional disturbance of small, angiographically invisible coronary arteries, which may be the cause of ischaemia in certain patients with angina have been described and the picture will no doubt clarify in the next few years.

Non-atheromatous pathology of coronary arteries

Although by far the most important cause of angina pectoris is coronary atherosclerosis, it is not the only pathological process involving the coronary vasculature that can cause angina pectoris. Coronary dissection, vasculitis[27-29], and congenital abnormalities (such as fistulae and aneurysms[76-79]) have all been described and may cause reduction in coronary blood flow and precipitate angina. Acquired diseases – such as syphilis, which causes ostial stenosis – are now a rare cause of angina pectoris.

Abnormal increase in myocardial oxygen demand

Any condition leading to myocardial hypertrophy may cause ischaemia, as oxygen consumption of the hypertrophied myocardium is higher at the same workload compared to a non-hypertrophied myocardium. Thus, it is not unusual to have patients with hypertrophic cardiomyopathy, aortic stenosis and rarely severe hypertension to present with angina pectoris, even though the coronary arteries are normal in calibre.

References

1. Heberden, W. (1772). Some account of a disorder of the breast. *Med. Trans. Coll. Physicians (London)* **2**, 59
2. Herrick, J. B. and Nuzum, F. R. (1918). Angina Pectoris: Clinical experience with 200 cases. *J. Am. Med. Assoc.*, **70**, 67
3. Zoll, P. M., Wessler, S. and Blumgart, H. L. (1951). Angina Pectoris: Clinical and pathological correlation. *Am. J. Med.*, **11**, 331
4. Holland, R. P. and Brooks, H. (1977). TQ-ST segment mapping: critical review and analysis of current concepts. *Am. J. Cardiol.*, **40**, 110–29
5. Poole-Wilson, P. A. (1983). Angina: pathological mechanisms, clinical expression and treatment. *Postgrad. Med. J.*, **59**, 11
6. Sarnoff, S. J., Braunwald, E. and Welch, G. H. *et al.* (1958). Haemodynamic determinants of oxygen consumption of the heart with special reference to the tension time index. *Am. J. Physiol.*, **192**, 148
7. Braunwald, E, Sarnoff, S. J., Case R. B. *et al.* (1958). Hemodynamic determinants of coronary flow. Effect of changes in aortic pressure and cardiac output on the relationship between oxygen consumption and coronary flow. *Am. J. Physiol.*, **192**, 157
8. Hoffman, J. E., Buckberg, G. D. (1978). The mycardial supply: demand ratio – a critical review. *Am J. Cardiol.*, **41**, 327
9. Krasnow, N., Rolett, E. L., Yurchak, P. *et al.* (1964). Isoproterenol and cardiovascular performance. *Am. J. Med.*, **37**, 514–25

10. Downey, J. M. and Kirk, E. S. (1975). Inhibition of coronary blood flow by a vascular waterfall mechanism. *Circ. Res.*, **36**, 753
11. Downey, J. M., Downey, H. F. and Kirk E. S. (1974). Effects of myocardial strains on coronary blood flow. *Circ. Res.*, **34**, 286
12. Weber, K. T. and Janicki, J. S. (1979). The metabolic demand and oxygen supply of the heart. Physiologic and clinical considerations. *Am. J. Cardiol.*, **44**, 722
13. Rubio, R. and Berne, R. M. (1975). Regulation of coronary blood flow. *Prog. Cardiovasc. Dis.*, **18**, 105
14. Downey, J. M. (1900). The extravascular coronary resistance. In Kalsner, S. (ed.). *The Coronary Artery.* pp 268–91. (London and Canberra: Croom Helm)
15. Bache, R. J. and Schwartz, J. S. (1982). Effect of perfusion pressure distal to a coronary stenosis on transmural myocardial blood flow. *Circulation*, **65**, 928
16. Sabbah, H. N. and Stein, P. D. (1982). Effect of acute regional ischaemia air pressure in the subepicardium and subendocardium. *Am. J. Physiol.*, **242**, H240
17. Wyatt, H. L., Forrester, J. S., Tyber J. V. *et al.* (1975). Effect of graded reductions in regional coronary perfusion on regional and total cardiac function. *Am. J. Cardiol.*, **36**, 185
18. McMohan, H. H., Brown, B. G., Cukingnan, R. *et al.* (1979). Quantitative coronary arteriography: Measurement of the 'critical' stenosis in patients with unstable angina and single vessel disease without collaterals. *Circulation*, **60**, 106–113
19. Klocke, F. J. (1983). Measurement of coronary blood flow and degree of stenosis: current clinical implications and continuing uncertainties. *J. Am. Coll. Cardiol.*, **1**, 31
20. Brown, B. G. (1981). Coronary vasospasm: Observations linking the clinical spectrum of ischemic heart disease to the dynamic pathology of coronary atherosclerosis. *Arch. Intern. Med.*, **141**, 716
21. Sabbah, H. N. and Stein, P. D. (1982). Hemodynamics of multiple versus single 50% coronary arterial stenoses. *Am. J. Cardiol.*, **50**, 278
22. Tibbling, L. and Wranne, B. (1976). Oesophageal dysfunction in male patients with angina like pain. *Acta Med. Scand.*, **200**, 391
23. Maseri, A., L'Abbate, A. and Chierchia, S., *et al.* (1979). Significance of spasm in the pathogenesis of ischaemic heart disease. *Am. J. Cardiol.*, **44**, 788
24. Heuplar, F. A. (1980). Syndrome of symptomatic coronary arterial spasm with nearly normal coronary arteriograms. *Am. J. Cardiol.*, **45**, 873
25. Quyyumi, A. A., Wright, C., Mockus, L. and Fox, K. M. (1985). The role of ambulatory ST segment monitoring in clinical practice. *Br. Heart. J.*, **53**, 96
26. Quyymi, A. A., Mockus, L. J., Wright, C. M. and Fox, K. M. (1985). The morphology of ambulatory ST segment changes in patients with varying severity of coronary artery disease. Investigation of the frequency of nocturnal ischaemia and coronary spasm. *Br. Heart. J.*, **53**, 186
27. Helfant, R. H., Forrester, J. S., Hampton, J. R. *et al.* (1970). Coronary heart disease: Differential hemodynamic, metabolic and electrocardiographic effects in subjects with and without angina pectoris during atrial pacing. *Circulation*, **42**, 601
28. Parker, J. O., Chiang, M. A., West, R. O. *et al.* (1969). Sequential alterations in myocardial lactate metabolism, ST segments and left ventricular function during angina induced by atrial pacing. *Circulation*, **40**, 113
29. Faris, J. V., McHenry, P. L. and Morris, S. N. (1978). Concepts and application of treadmill exercise testing and the exercise electrocardiogram. *Am. Heart. J.*, **95**, 102
30. Goldschlager, N., Selzer, A. and Cohn, K. (1976). Treadmill tests as indicators of presence and severity of coronary artery disease. *Ann. Intern. Med.*, **85**, 277
31. Davies, A. B., Balla Subramanian, V., Cashman, P. M. M. and Raftery, E. B. (1983). Simultaneous recording of continuous arterial pressure, heart rate and ST segment in ambulent patients with stable angina pectoris. *Br. Heart J.*, **50**, 85
32. Pitt, B. and Strauss, H. W. (1976). Myocardial imaging in the non-invasive evaluation of patients with suspected ischaemic heart disease. *Am. J. Cardiol.*, **37**, 797

33. Borer, J. S., Bacharach, S. L., Green, M. V. *et al.* (1977). Real time radionuclide cineangiography in the non-invasive evaluation of global and regional left ventricular function at rest and during exercise in patients with coronary artery disease. *N. Engl. J. Med.*, **296**, 839

34. Chierchia, S., Brunelli, C., Simonetti, I., Lazzari, M. and Maseri, A. (1980). Sequence of events in angina at rest: primary reduction in coronary flow. *Circulation*, **61**, 759

35. Yasue, H., Omote, S., Takizawa, A. *et al.* (1979). Exertional angina pectoris caused by coronary arterial spasm: Effects of various drugs. *Am. J. Cardiol.*, **43**, 647

36. Fuller, G. M., Raizner, A. E., Chahine, R. A. *et al.* (1980). Exercise induced coronary arterial spasm: Angiographic demonstration, documentation of ischaemia by myocardial scintigraphy and results of pharmacologic intervention. *Am. J. Cardiol.*, **46**, 500

37. Pepine, C. J., Feldman, R. L. and Conti, C. R. (1980). Observations on the role of coronary artery spasm in stress induced angina. *Circulation*, **62**, 99

38. Bertrand, M. E., LaBlanche, J. M., Tilmant, P. Y. *et al.* (1982). Frequency of provoked coronary arterial spasm in 1089 patients undergoing coronary arteriography. *Circulation*, **65**, 1299

39. deServi, S., Specchia, G., Ardissino, D. *et al.* (1980). Angiographic demonstration of different pathogenetic mechanisms in patients with spontaneous and exertional angina associated with ST segment depression. *Am. J. Cardiol.*, **45**, 1285

40. Maseri, A., Severi, S., De Nes, M. *et al.* (1978). 'Variant' angina: one aspect of a continuous spectrum of vasospastic myocardial ischaemia. Pathogenetic mechanisms, estimated incidence and clinical and coronary arteriographic findings in 138 patients. *Am. J. Cardiol.*, **42**, 1019

41. Parodi, O. (1977). Angina pectoris at rest: regional myocardial oxygen perfusion during ST segment elevation or depression. *Circulation*, **56**, 229

42. Guazzi, M., Polese, A., Fiorentini, C., Magrini, I., Olivari, M. T., Bartorelli, C. (1975). Left and right heart haemodynamics during spontaneous angina pectoris. *Br. Heart J.*, **37**, 401

43. Quyyumi, A. A., Wright, C., Mockus, L. and Fox, K. M. (1985). How important is the history of pain in determining the degree of ischaemia in patients with angina pectoris? *Br. Heart J.*, **54**, 22

44. Quyyumi, A. A., Wright, C. A., Mockus, L. J. and Fox, K. M. (1984). Mechanisms of nocturnal angina pectoris: importance of increased myocardial oxygen demand in patients with severe coronary artery disease. *Lancet*, **1**, 1207

45. Quyyumi, A. A., Efthimiou, J., Anees *et al.* (1984). Mechanisms of rest angina evaluated during sleep. *Br. Heart J.*, **57**, 693

46. Yasue, H., Omote, S., Takizawa, A. and Tanaka, S. (1979). Circadian variation of exercise capacity in patients with Prinzmetal's variant angina: role of exercise induced coronary arterial spasm. *Circulation*, **59**, 938

47. Yasue, H., Omote, S. Takizawa, A. and Nagao, M. Circadian variation in angina pectoris. In: Julian, D. G., Lie, K. I. and Wilhelmson, L. *What is Angina?* pp. 102–110

48. Selwyn, A. P., Fox, K., Eves, M., Oakley, D., Dargie, H. and Shillingford, J. (1978). Myocardial ischaemia in patients with frequent angina pectoris. *Br. Med. J.*, **2**, 1594

49. Freedman, M. B., Richmond, D. R. and Kelly, D. T. (1982). Pathophysiology of coronary artery spasm. *Circulation*, **66**, 705

50. Wilson, F. and Johnston, F. (1941). The occurrence in angina pectoris of electrocardiographic changes similar in magnitude and in kind to those produced by myocardial infarction. *Am. Heart J.*, **22**, 64

51. Prinzmetal, M., Kemnamer, R., Merliss, R. *et al.* (1959). The variant form of angina pectoris. *Am. J. Med.*, **27**, 375

52. Specchia, G., De Servi S., Falcone, C. *et al.* (1979). Coronary arterial spasm as a cause of exercise induced ST segment elevation in patients with variant angina. *Circulation*, **59**, 948

53. Freedman, B., Dunn, R. F., Richmond, D. et al. (1981). Coronary artery spasm during exercise treatment with verapamil. *Circulation*, **64**, 68
54. Gensini, G. C., Di Giorgi, S., Murad-Netto, D. et al. (1963). The coronary circulation: An experimental and clinical study. In: *Memorias del IV Congres. Mondial de Cardiologie IA Mexico*, 325
55. Oliva, R. B., Potts, D. E. and Pluss, R. G. (1973). Coronary arterial spasm in Prinzmetal angina: documentation by coronary arteriography. *N. Engl. J. Med.*, **788**, 745
56. Maseri, A., Severi, S., Denes, M. et al. (1978). 'Variant Angina': One aspect of a continuous spectrum of vasospastic myocardial ischaemia. *Am. J. Cardiol.*, **42**, 1019
57. Maseri, A., Pesola, A. and Marzilli, M. et al. (1977). Coronary vasospasm in angina pectoris. *Lancet*, **1**, 713
58. Weiner, L. (1976). Spectrum of coronary arterial spasm: clinical angiographic and myocardial metabolic experience in 29 cases. *Am. J. Cardiol.*, **38**, 945
59. Goldberg, S., Lam, W. and Mudge, G. (1979). Coronary hemodynamic and metabolic alterations accompanying coronary spasm. *Am. J. Cardiol.*, **43**, 481
60. Ricci, D. R., Orlick, A. E., Cipriano, P. et al. (1979). Altered adrenergic activity in coronary artery spasm. Insight into mechanism based on study of coronary hemodynamics and the electrocardiogram. *Am. J. Cardiol.*, **43**, 1073
61. Curry, R. C., Pepine, C. J., Sabour, M. B. et al. (1978). Hemodynamic and myocardial metabolic effects of ergonovine in patients with chest pain. *Circulation*, **58**, 648
62. Macalpin, R. N. (1980). Relation of coronary arterial spasm to sites of organic stenosis. *Am. J. Cardiol.*, **46**, 143
63. Levy, R. I., Smith, J. B., Silver, M. J. et al. (1979). Detection of thromboxane B2 in the peripheral blood of patients with Prinzmetal's angina. *Prostaglandins Med.*, **2**, 243
64. Weber, S., Pasquier, G., Guiomard, A. et al. (1981). Clinical applications of alkalosis stress testing for coronary artery spasm. *Arch. Mal. Coeur*, **74**, 1389
65. Ginsburg, R., Bristow, M. R., Kantrowitz, N. et al. (1981). Histamine provocation of clinical coronary artery spasm: implications concerning pathogenesis of variant angina pectoris. *Am. Heart J.*, **102**, 809
66. Gorman, R. R. (1980). Biochemical and pharmocological evaluation of thromboxane synthetase inhibitors. *Adv. Prostagl. Thromb. Res.*, **6**, 417
67. Moncada, S., Gryglewski, R., Bunting, S. et al. (1976). An enzyme isolated from arteries transforms prostaglandin endoperoxides to an unstable substance that inhibits platelet aggregation. *Nature*, **263**, 663
68. Shattil, S. J., Anaya-Galindo, R., Bennett, J. et al. (1975). Platelet hypersensitivity induced by cholesterol incorporation. *J. Clin. Invest.*, **55**, 636
69. Stuart, M. J., Gerrard, J. M. and White, J. G. (1980). Effect of cholesterol on production of thromboxane B2 by platelets in vitro. *N. Engl. J. Med.*, **302**, 6
70. Machin, S. J., Carreras, L. O., Chamone, D. A. F. et al. (1980). Familial deficiency of thromboxane synthetase. *Acta Therapeutica*, **6**, 34
71. Folts, J. D., Crowell, E. B. Jr and Rowe, G. G. (1976). Platelet aggregation in partially obstructed vessels and its elimination with aspirin. *Circulation*, **54**, 365
72. Folts, J. D., Gallagher, K. and Rowe, G. G. (1982). Blood flow reductions in stenosed canine coronary arteries: vasospasm or platelet aggregation? *Circulation*, **65**, 245
73. Folts, J. D. and Bonebrake, B. S. (1982). The effects of cigarette smoke and nicotine on thrombus formation in stenosed dog coronary arteries: inhibition with phentamine. *Circulation*, **65**, 465
74. Mehta, P., Mehta, J., Pepine, C. J. et al. (1979). Platelet aggregation across the myocardial vascular bed in man. Normal versus diseased coronary arteries. *Thromb. Res.*, **14**, 423
75. Moschos, C. B., Lahiri, K., Manskopf, G. et al. (1973). Effect of experimental coronary thrombosis upon platelet kinetics. *Thromb. Diath. Haem.*, **30**, 339

76. Davis, H. H., Siegel, B. A., Joist, J. H. *et al.* (1978). Scintigraphic detection of atherosclerotic lesions and venous thrombi in man by indium-111 labelled autologous platelets. *Lancet*, **1**, 1185
77. Mehta, J., Mehta, P., Pepine, C. J. *et al.* (1980). Platelet function studies in coronary artery disease. VII Effect of aspirin and tachycardia stress on aortic and coronary venous blood. *Am. J. Cardiol.*, **45**, 945
78. Green, L. H., Seroppian, E. and Handin, R. I. (1981). Platelet activation during exercise induced myocardial ischaemia. *N. Engl. J. Med.*, **302**, 193
79. Hirsh, P. D., Hillis, L. D., Campbell, W. B. *et al.* (1981). Release of prostaglandins and thromboxane into the coronary circulation in patients with ischemic heart disease. *N. Engl. J. Med.*, **304**, 685
80. Frishman, W. H., Christodoulou, J., Weksler, B. *et al.* (1976). Aspirin therapy in angina pectoris. Effects on platelet aggregation, exercise tolerance, and electrocardiographic manifestations of ischaemia. *Am. Heart. J.*, **92**, 3
81. Sobel, M., Salzman, E. W., Davies, G. C. *et al.* (1981). Circulating platelet products in unstable angina pectoris. *Circulation*, **63**, 300
82. Ellis, J. B., Krentz, L. S. and Levine, S. P. (1978). Increased plasma platelet factor 4(PF4) in patients with coronary artery disease. *Circulation*, **58**, 116
83. Smitherman, T. C., Milam, M, Wood, J. *et al.* (1981). Elevated beta-thromboglobulin in peripheral venous blood of patients with acute myocardial ischaemia: Direct evidence for enhanced platelet reactivity *in vivo*. *Am. J. Cardiol.*, **48**, 395
84. Stratton, J. R., Malpass, T. W., Ritchie, J. L. *et al.* (1982). Studies of platelet factor 4 and beta thromboglobulin release during exercise: lack of relationship to myocardial ischaemia. *Circulation*, **66**, 33
85. Elwood, P. C. and Sweetman, P. M. (1979). Aspirin and secondary mortality after myocardial infarction. *Lancet*, **2**, 1313
86. The Anturan Reinfarction Study Research Group (1978). Sulphinpyrazone in the prevention of cardiac death after myocardial infarction. *N. Engl. J. Med.*, **298**, 289
87. Robertson, R. M., Robertson, D., Roberts, L. C. *et al.* (1981). Thromboxane A$_2$ in vasotonic angina pectoris. *N. Engl. J. Med.*, **304**, 998
88. Fox, K. M., Jonathan, A. and Selwyn, A. P. (1982). Effects of platelet inhibition on myocardial ischaemia. *Lancet*, **2**, 722
89. Roberts, W. C. and Virmani, R. (1979). Quantification of coronary arterial narrowing in clinically isolated unstable angina pectoris. An analysis of 22 necropsy patients. *Am. J. Med.*, **67**, 792
90. Roberts, W. C. and Jones, A. A. (1980). Quantification of coronary arterial narrowing at necropsy in sudden coronary death. Analysis of 31 patients and comparison with 25 control subjects. *Am. J. Cardiol.*, **44**, 39
91. Roberts, W. C. and Jones, A. A. (1980). Quantification of coronary arterial narrowing at necropsy in acute transmural myocardial infarction. Analysis and comparison of findings in 27 patients and 22 controls. *Circulation*, **61**, 786
92. Virmani, R. and Roberts, W. C. (1980). Quantification of coronary arterial narrowing and in left ventricular myocardial scarring in myocardial infarction with chronic, eventually fatal, congestive cardiac failure. *Am. J. Med.*, **68**, 831
93. Canndom, D. S., Harrison, D. C. and Schroeder, J. S. (1974). Hemodynamic observations in patients with unstable angina pectoris. *Am. J. Cardiol.*, **33**, 17
94. Berndt, T. B., Fitzgerald, J., Harrison, D. C. *et al.* (1977). Hemodynamic changes at the onset of spontaneous versus pacing-induced angina. *Am. J. Cardiol*, **39**, 784
95. Figueras, J., Singh, B. N., Ganz, W. *et al.* (1979). Mechanism of rest and nocturnal angina: Observations during continuous hemodynamic and electrocardiographic monitoring. *Circulation*, **59**, 995
96. Schang, S. J. and Pepine, C. J. (1977). Transient asymptomatic ST segment depression during daily activity. *Am. J. Cardiol*, **39**, 396
97. Stern, S., Tzivoni, D. and Stern, Z. (1975). Diagnostic accuracy of ambulatory ECG monitoring in ischemic heart disease. *Circulation*, **52**, 1045
98. Cecchi, A. C., Dovellini, E. V., Marchi, F., Pucci, P., Santoro, G. M. and Fazzini,

F. (1983). Silent myocardial ischaemia during ambulatory electrocardiographic monitoring in patients with effort angina. *J. Am. Coll. Cardiol.*, **1**, 934

99. Cannon, R. D., Watson, R. M., Rosing, D. R. and Epstein, S. E. (1983). Angina caused by reduced vasodilator reserve of the small coronary arteries. *J. Am. Coll. Cardiol.*, **1**, 1359

100. Opherx, D., Zebe, H., Weihe, E. *et al.* (1981). Reduced coronary dilatory capacity and ultra-structural changes of the myocardium in patients with angina pectoris but normal coronary arteriograms. *Circulation*, **63**, 817

5
Haemodynamic and metabolic consequences of angina and myocardial infarction

P. A. POOLE-WILSON

INTRODUCTION

The biochemistry and physiology of the normal and diseased heart have been extensively studied in the last 20 years. Early work was founded on the belief that an understanding of the underlying biochemistry of ischaemic heart muscle would show the way to the development of new therapies for coronary artery disease. The use of cardioplegic solutions during cardiac surgery emerged from this work. So did the calcium antagonists. But perhaps the greatest advance has not been in the dramatic resolution of medical problems but in improved understanding of how the heart is impaired in ischaemia and more appropriate use of already available drugs and interventions.

The concepts of 'limitation of infarct size' and 'prevention' or 'early intervention' in myocardial infarction have been of less obvious benefit. Whilst clinical trials have shown that some interventions, notably the administration of beta-blockers[1] or thrombolytic agents[2-4], can reduce mortality after myocardial infarction and prevent the recurrence of a heart attack, the concept of altering 'infarct size' by preservation of the 'border-zone' has been shown to be illfounded[5-7].

The advent of angioplasty and thrombolytic therapy has renewed interest in the causation of myocardial infarction and the early metabolic events following the onset of myocardial infarction. These techniques, early resuscitation of patients, the availability of coronary ambulances and the partial success of coronary care units indicate that acute interventions can reduce mortality from coronary artery disease. The understanding of metabolic changes early in ischaemia may be particularly relevant to the genesis of arrhythmias at that time and the clinical problem of sudden death, which accounts for a high proportion of those dying of coronary artery disease.

THE NORMAL HEART

The average human heart weights $300\,g$ and coronary flow at rest is $0.8\,ml\,min^{-1}g^{-1}$. The arterial blood content of oxygen is $188\,ml\,l^{-1}$ $(PO_2 = 100\,mmHg$, 98% saturated). The oxygen content of coronary sinus blood is substantially lower than that of mixed venous blood being $68\,ml\,l^{-1}$ $(PO_2 = 25\,mmHg$, 30% saturated). Thus, the oxygen consumption of the heart is $27\,ml\,min^{-1}$ or $0.09\,ml\,min^{-1}g^{-1}$. The normal cardiac output of the heart is approximately $5\,l\,min^{-1}$ and can increase on exercise to $25\,l\,min^{-1}$. The increase in cardiac output is achieved by more than a three fold increase in heart rate and a smaller increase in stroke volume. The heart is critically dependent on the supply of oxygen and substrate. Unlike other tissues, the availability of oxygen cannot be greatly increased by a widening of the arterio-venous difference. When heart rate increases there is a transient fall in the oxygen content in the coronary sinus, but this returns to normal within approximately 15 seconds in the absence of coronary artery disease. This is the time taken for the coronary resistance to be reduced. Increased availability of oxygen to the heart is provided primarily by an increased coronary blood flow. Coronary blood flow can increase by as much as four fold. With increasing heart rate, the proportion of time that the heart is in systole increases and blood flow to the left ventricle of the heart only occurs during diastole. Thus, the true resistance to blood flow must be reduced proportionally more than the overall increase of blood flow.

The major and overriding determinant of coronary blood flow is the myocardial oxygen consumption (*metabolic regulation*) (Figure 5.1). Over a wide range of diastolic blood pressure coronary flow increases only slightly with blood pressure (*autoregulation*). Neural and hormonal mechanisms appear to be secondary control mechanisms of coronary blood flow to the heart[8,9].

DEFINITION OF ISCHAEMIA

Myocardial ischaemia has traditionally been defined as the state of the heart when there exists an imbalance between oxygen supply and demand. Such a definition has great conceptual appeal to the clinician but little if any practical value, since it is difficult to measure both these entities. Metabolic poisoning, where there is an obvious imbalance between so-called supply and demand, would be regarded as ischaemia. Furthermore, the heart never demanded oxygen nor is the sole function of the coronary circulation to provide oxygen. The removal of metabolites, particularly heat and carbon dioxide, is as an important function of myocardial blood flow as the supply of substrate and oxygen.

A more precise definition of ischaemia would be that it is characterized by an imbalance of ATP (adenosine triphosphate) consumption and blood flow (Figure 5.2). Ischaemia occurs either when ATP consumption

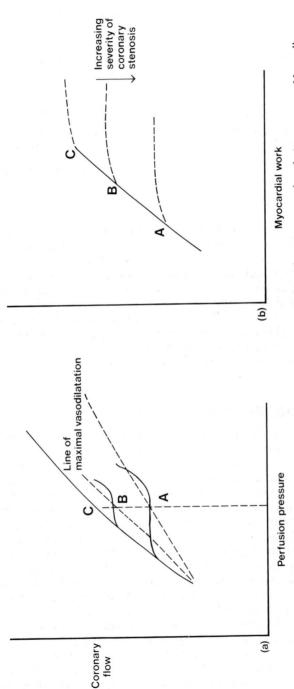

Figure 5.1 (a) At maximal vasodilatation coronary flow increases progressively with an increase of perfusion pressure. Normally over a range of perfusion pressures, flow changes little with pressure (autoregulation). At a given perfusion pressure, flow can increase as a result of metabolic vasodilatation (line ABC).

(b) Metabolic vasodilatation occurs with increasing myocardial work at constant perfusion pressure and when vasodilatation is maximal, flow cannot be increased further and angina results.

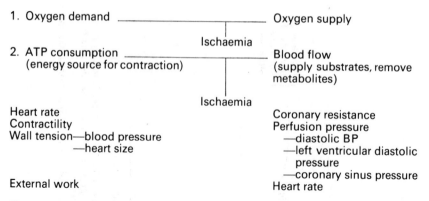

1. Oxygen demand ———————————— Oxygen supply

Ischaemia

2. ATP consumption ————————————— Blood flow
   (energy source for contraction)   (supply substrates, remove
                                                  metabolites)

Ischaemia

Heart rate   Coronary resistance
Contractility   Perfusion pressure
Wall tension—blood pressure   —diastolic BP
              —heart size   —left ventricular diastolic
                                                      pressure
                                                     —coronary sinus pressure
External work   Heart rate

Figure 5.2 Two concepts of myocardial ischaemia

increases above the rate of ATP production that can be sustained by a given blood flow, or when blood flow is reduced so that the existing rate of ATP consumption cannot be maintained. In the first minute of ischaemia, flux through the glycolytic pathway is stimulated but is subsequently inhibited by the development of an acidosis and the accumulation of citrate, NADH (reduced nicotinamide-adenine dinucleotide) and lactate[10–12] (Figure 5.3). Inadequate oxygen is available to permit oxidative phosphorylation and pyruvate (the end-product of the glycolytic chain) instead of passing into the Krebs cycle is converted to lactate. Ischaemia may be simply defined as a state characterized by the flow related accumulation of lactic acid.

EARLY CONSEQUENCES OF ISCHAEMIA

Following the total occlusion of a coronary artery, sufficient oxygen is available in the tissue to supply energy for 2–3 heart bearts[13]. High energy phosphates (ATP and CP, creatine phosphate) within the myocardium can provide energy for a further 6–10 beats. The total tissue content of ATP within the tissue does not fall for several minutes, whereas the tissue content of creatine phosphate falls rapidly so that at the end of 2–3 minutes it is reduced by almost 80%[14–16]. Creatine phosphate is believed in part to be a back-up system within the heart providing immediate energy for contraction by donation of its high energy phosphate group to ADP to produce ATP and creatine.

Contraction declines rapidly and developed tension ceases within approximately 90 seconds[17,18]. In patients the surface electrocardiagram is altered after approximately 30 seconds and pain is experienced at about one minute. More recent studies have shown that the monophasic action potential is altered after approximately 16 beats of the heart[19] and at the same time both contraction and relaxation of heart muscle are altered[20]. The function of the whole heart is difficult to evaluate because that is determined by the sum of regional abnormalities of

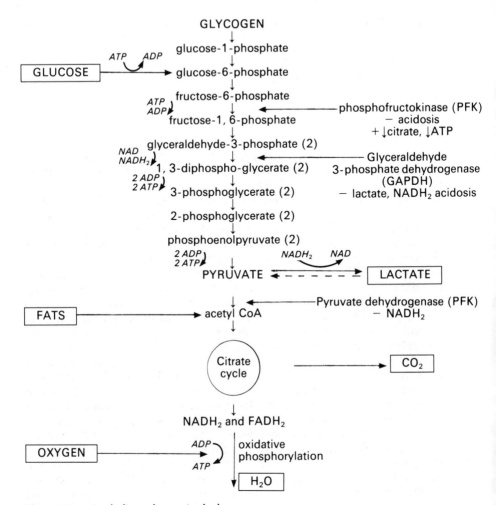

Figure 5.3 Metabolic pathways in the heart

contraction. During systole the ischaemic muscle may develop reduced tension but is stretched by the interventricular pressure generated by normal myocardial tissue. Furthermore, contraction of ischaemic muscle may be more prolonged than the contraction of normal muscle.

The mechanisms of many of these events has now been established, though controversies still exist[21]. Several causes have been put forward for the early failure of myocardial contraction (Table 5.1). An immediate consequence of the occlusion of a coronary artery is that the pressure within the distal part of the artery is no longer present to splint and distend the myocardial tissue. This leads to a reduction in sarcomere length of the muscle and a fall in contraction. The effect is known as the *erectile effect* or *garden hose* effect[22,23]. This phenomenon is

Table 5.1 Causes of early contractile failure in ischaemia

Acidosis

Reduced sensitivity of contractile proteins to calcium

Intracellular accumulation of phosphate

Intracellular accumulation of lipid

Loss of erectile effect of coronary arteries

Reduced free energy for contraction

---

accentuated in isolated muscle preparations perfused at high flow with physiological fluids. It appears to be a less important mechanism in man. The consequences of this phenomenon are evident within 2–3 heart beats. The decline in the development of systolic tension beginning at about the 16th beat has been ascribed to intracellular acidosis, an accumulation of phosphate and a lack of energy for contraction[21].

For any explanation to be tenable it is necessary to show that the change of the putative factor occurs sufficiently early and is of sufficient magnitude. Although under some experimental conditions the contractile tension can be shown to fall in the absence of an acidosis during ischaemia[24], the fall of developed tension is usually accompanied by a fall of pH[25]. In intact dogs, the acidosis is evident within less than 20 seconds[26] and recent observations (Crake and Poole-Wilson, 1986, unpublished) show this to be true in man. Several hypotheses have been put forward to account for the acidosis. Early during ischaemia the oxygen in the tissue is converted to carbon dioxide. The glycolytic pathway is stimulated and lactate is generated from the small amount of glucose within the tissue and from tissue stores of glycogen. Because of lack of oxygen, oxidative phosphorylation cannot proceed and citrate increases in the tissue. The increase of citrate and fall of ATP stimulate the enzyme phosphofructokinase in the glycolytic pathway to increase the glycolytic flux (the Pasteur effect, see Figure 5.3). After approximately 30 seconds of ischaemia glycolysis is reduced because acidosis inhibits the activity of phosphofructokinase and because acidosis, lactate and the accumulation of NADH inhibit the activity of glyceraldehyde-3-phosphate dehydrogenase, a later enzyme in the pathway. The generation of lactic acid and conversion of oxygen to carbon dioxide are probably the major causes for the early development of acidosis, although hydrogen ions are also generated by the breakdown of ATP. Early in ischaemia the tissue content of ATP does not fall[14,15]. The conversion of creatine phosphate to creatine absorbs a proton and under some circumstances a transient alkalosis has been reported. This does not appear to occur during ischaemia in the intact animal[26] or man (unpublished observations). Thus acidosis occurs sufficiently early to explain some of the early fall of developed tension. The mechanism by which acidosis reduces contraction is less certain. Acidosis is known to effect the transport of calcium across the sarcolemma, to alter the slow calcium current, to effect the uptake of calcium by the sarcoplasmic reticulum and to alter the interaction of calcium with the contractile proteins. Recent work has shown that during an imposed acidosis the cytosolic calcium increases[27]. This suggests that the major reason for the negative inotropic effect of an acidosis in the heart is a direct effect on the contractile proteins.

Another cause of early contractile failure is the accumulation of tissue phosphate. The breakdown of creatine phosphate early in ischaemia will lead to the accumulation of phosphate within the tissue[28]. Experiments on isolated muscle show that a raised cytosolic phosphate will reduce the development of tension by isolated myocardial fibres[29].

The molecule directly providing energy for contraction of the myocardium is ATP. The tissue content of ATP does not fall early during ischaemia[14,15]. Nevertheless, since creatine phosphate does fall it has been argued that ATP in the tissue is compartmentalized and that the ATP in the compartment providing energy for contraction is diminished[15]. This hypothesis remains contentious and unproven[30,31]. The energy for contraction does not depend solely upon the amount of ATP in the tissue but also on the concentrations of the end products of the reaction. It is the free energy of the reaction that is critical to the muscle. The increase in phosphate and ADP in the ischaemic tissue will reduce the free energy available for contraction. The free energy falls early in ischaemia at the same time as the fall in contraction and the two have been related although the causal link is disputed.

The second major consequence of acute myocardial ischaemia is an alteration in the configuration of the action potential and the subsequent development of arrhythmias. Changes in the conduction velocity, rate of depolarization, resting membrane potential and duration of the action potential can be accounted for by the known changes of pH and extracellular potassium[32]. Using potassium sensitive electrodes several groups[33-37] have shown in the last few years that early following the onset of ischaemia there is accumulation of potassium in the extracellular space. The loss of potassium is rapid, occurring almost instantaneously in isolated tissues. In man, potassium loss is evident after about the 16th heart beat[38]. The extracellular potassium reaches a concentration of approximately $10 \, \text{mmol} \, l^{-1}$ after three minutes and after 15 minutes reaches a concentration of $15 \, \text{mmol} \, l^{-1}$. It remains at this concentration for up to 25 minutes. Subsequently there is a further rise in the extracellular potassium concentration which can reach $40 \, \text{mmol} \, l^{-1}$ (Figure 5.4). The secondary rise is thought to be due to destruction of myocardial cells and the outward movement of intracellular potassium, which is at a high concentration. The early rise of potassium must have a different explanation, since if the tissue is reperfused the function of the tissue returns to normal and the myocardium takes up potassium, so restoring the loss during the period of ischaemia. The timing and magnitude of the change in extracellular potassium is sufficient to account for alterations in the configuration of the action potential and other electrophysiological effects, particularly if the change

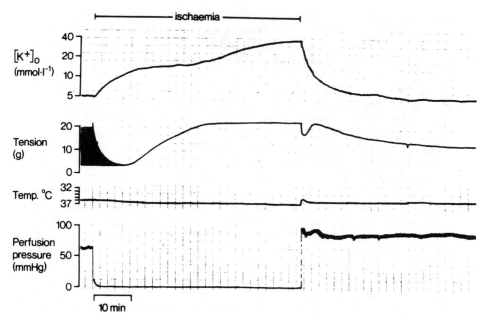

Figure 5.4 Changes in the extracellular concentration of potassium in the total and globally ischaemic myocardium of the rabbit. Note that the increase occurs in two phases. The early rise is due to reversible mechanisms and the later rise is associated with cell disruption

in pH is also taken into account[32]. Several mechanisms have been put forward to account for the early loss of potassium (Table 5.2). The loss is not due to a reduced influx of potassium but to an increased efflux[39,40]. The sodium potassium pump has been shown to be functional even if

Table 5.2 Mechanism for the early loss of potassium from the ischaemic myocardium

Increased K^+ conductance (?due to low ATP)

Intracellular accumulation of permeant anions

Acidosis

Reduced activity of sodium pump ($Na^+–K^+–ATPase$)

Intracellular hyperosmolarity

inhibited[39,41]. The intracellular sodium activity of the myocardium is not changed at least for the initial 15 minutes of ischaemia[42]. The loss of potassium may be partly accounted for by the outward movement of permeant anions, such as lactate and phosphate[40], which accumulate rapidly in the ischaemic myocardium and partly due to alterations in membrane permeability to potassium, particularly during the action potential.

LATE BIOCHEMICAL CONSEQUENCES OF ISCHAEMIA

During prolonged ischaemia many biochemical changes occur in the myocardial cell. In myocardium of dog subjected to total ischaemia little recovery of function will occur if the tissue is reperfused after 40 minutes[43]. The state of the ischaemic myocardium has been described as 'irreversibly' damaged[44]. The use of this phrase can be most misleading. In general it is not possible to test whether damage is irreversible except by reperfusing the myocardium. Many events occur at the time of reperfusion (see below) and it could be and is probable[45–47] that the degree of recovery might be altered by manipulation of conditions at the time of reperfusion. That is 'irreversible' damage can only be demonstrated by study of the myocardium after reperfusion. There is currently no method of determining with certainty whether muscle is irreversibly damaged during a period of ischaemia. There is one clear exception to this argument and that is when gross disruption of the cell membrane is present. Then and only then undoubtedly the cell will eventually necrose. The use of the phrase 'irreversible' damage during ischaemia should be limited to those situations where gross disruption of the cell membrane is present.

Study of cell function during ischaemia has shown that by approximately 30 minutes of total global ischaemia ATP in the cell has fallen substantially[43]. Abnormalities can be demonstrated in the function of sarcoplasmic reticulum, the mitochondria and the cell membrane. Lipids accumulate within the myocardial cell. Abnormalities are evident under the electron miroscope. Mitochondrial swelling and aggregation of nuclear chromatin are early changes. At about 30 minutes the myofibrils shorten ('contracture' or 'rigor') probably due to a low ATP rather than an increased cytosolic calcium concentration. This shortening of the myofibrils is a feature of total global myocardial ischaemia. In regional low flow myocardial ischaemia the myofibrils tend to be pulled apart by the contraction of the adjacent normal muscle. Eventually, blebs form in the cell membrane, discontinuities develop and gross disruption follows.

Changes in ion concentrations within the myocardial cell during prolonged ischaemia are not well described. There is an early loss of potassium which increases later when cells break down (see above and Figure 5.4). Intracellular sodium does not accumulate for at least 15 minutes[42] and although the sodium pump may be inhibited it has been demonstrated to be functional[39,41,42]. Cytosolic calcium concentration appears not to rise early in hypoxia but may increase later as contracture develops[48].

Phospholipases are activated in the cell membrane but gross changes in the lipids of the cell membrane appear to be a feature of late ischaemia[49].

During total and global ischaemia it is self evident that there can be no change in the total tissue content of ions or of any other non metabolizable substance. Such a situation rarely exists in man and is rare in dogs. Collateral flow allows a small residual flow even at the centre of the infarcted muscle[50,51]. In the presence of a continuing low flow ion exchange can occur and there is a loss of enzymes. These enzymes are used as a marker of myocardial infarction by the clinician (see below).

REPERFUSION OF ISCHAEMIC MYOCARDIUM

Reperfusion is accompanied by a variety of well characterized phenomena[52–54]. If reperfusion occurs early during ischaemia full recovery results. After about 30 minutes of total global ischaemia complete functional recovery of the muscle does not occur. Often in isolated tissues there may be an increase in the resting tension and this may be linked to the inward movement of large quantities of calcium[56,57]. Enzymes are released from the myocardium. A very similar phenomenon occurs on reoxygenation of the myocardium after a period of hypoxia[58]. This has been called the 'oxygen paradox' and the phenomenon 'reoxygenation damage'. After a period of ischaemia the phrase 'reperfusion damage' has been used.

Reperfusion of the myocardium is not always possible. After a short period of ischaemia reperfusion is associated with an increase of blood flow, the phenomenon being referred to as the hyperaemic response. However, after a period of approximately 15 minutes, the blood flow on reperfusion is less than the blood flow expected in the maximally vasodilated normal myocardium. That is, tissue changes have occurred, which result in an increase in resistance. The mechanisms include oedema of the endothelial cells, contraction of the smooth muscle in the arterioles by an altered ionic environment and by other factors, and increased pressure of the capillaries by contracture of the adjacent myocardium[22,59]. After a prolonged period of ischaemia, reperfusion is not possible and this is called the 'no reflow' phenomenon[60–62]. Reperfusion may also be associated with haemorrhage into the myocardium. Sudden reperfusion rather than slow reperfusion results in greater long-term damage to the myocardium[63].

There is a dispute as to whether so-called 'reperfusion damage' is: (a) the result of events occurring during the period of ischaemia, but which are only manifest at the time of reperfusion; or (b) whether they are events associated with reperfusion with the reintroduction of oxygen and the removal of metabolites; or (c) whether the reperfusion damage is an immediate manifestation of changes, which would inevitably occur after prolonged reperfusion[7]. Many interventions, which are known to reduce the effects of ischaemia – such as hyperthermia, cardioplegia or the calcium antagonists – are in general only effective if applied to the myocardium prior to the period of ischaemia[57]. They have no benefit if they are applied at the time of reperfusion. Recently some interventions, particularly a lowering of the extracellular calcium concentration[47] or the introduction of oxygen scavengers[46], have led to an improved recovery of the myocardium. These experiments do seem to suggest that some of the events occurring at the moment of reperfusion are damaging to the myocardium and alteration of these events can lead to greater recovery of the muscle. A major problem is whether this increased recovery of the muscle is merely a hastening of recovery, which would have occurred if the muscle had been reperfused for a prolonged period of time. At present that depressing proposition seems unlikely to be correct.

CAUSE OF CELL DEATH

It is a truism, which needs emphasizing, that the myocardium will inevitably necrose if blood flow is not restored. The phrase 'reperfusion damage' is therefore rather misleading, in that without reperfusion cell necrosis becomes inevitable. Reperfusion is always beneficial in terms of potential recovery of heart muscle. The causes of cell death in myocardium that is reperfused are a matter of considerable controversy[45,53,55]. Table 5.3 summarizes some of the present hypotheses.

Table 5.3 Mechanisms of cell death in reperfused myocardium

Loss of ionic homeostosis (calcium overload)

Disruption of cells by increased intracellular osmolality

Disruption of cells by contracture forces

Damage by oxygen radicals

Activation of proteases

Lack of energy

Although an appealing hypothesis, it is difficult to link cell necrosis with a lack of energy in the form of high energy phosphates (CP and ATP)[64]. Many experiments have shown that the degree of necrosis does correlate with the fall of high energy phosphates. Such a correlation would inevitably be found between any variable that declined or increased during ischaemia because recovery is linked closely to the duration of ischaemia. In order to demonstrate a causal relationship a mechanism must be identified and that mechanism must be shown to be the critical event. The recovery of the ischaemic myocardium can be improved without alteration of high energy phosphates. In many tissues high energy phosphates can reach very low levels but the tissue recovers. Although ATP consumption is undoubtedly a necessary requirement for recovery it does not seem to be a key requirement.

Some authors have argued that at the time of reperfusion there is an increase of contracture of the myocardial cells and that this force pulls apart adjacent cells disrupting the cell membrane at the intercalated disc where one cell is joined to its neighbours[65]. The disruption of the cell membrane is said to cause the inward movement of calcium and destruction of the ionic gradients, which are essential to the cell's survival. However, there are experimental conditions in which the rise in resting tension is either absent or very small and yet recovery does not occur[66]. Although this mechanism may be a factor in cell necrosis it does not appear to account for all the known findings.

A further hypothesis is that late in ischaemia there is a fall in intracellular pH and a rise in cytosolic calcium. These changes activate phospholipases in the cell membrane, which break down the lipids to form lysophosphoglycerides and other lipid moieties, which alter the function of the cell membrane. Recent measurements in the heart indicate that such changes occur very late in ischaemia, long after the time at which reperfusion leads to no recovery whatsoever[49].

Ischaemia is known to give rise to a variety of metabolic events, which lead to an increased concentration of small ions (such as lactate) within the myocardial cell. The accumulation of these substances leads to an increase in osmotic pressure. Some authors suggest that this increase in osmotic pressure in association with a weakness or abnormality of the cell membrane occurring during ischaemia results in rapid cell swelling on reperfusion and rupture of the cell membrane[61].

A popular hypothesis in the last few years has been called the 'calcium hypothesis'. For many years it has been known that at the moment of reperfusion there is a rapid uptake of calcium into the heart and that this is due to an increased influx[56,57,68,69]. The calcium crosses the cell membrane from the extracellular space and is taken up in the mitochondria where it can be seen as small dark opacities under the electron microscope. In the heart the cytosolic calcium is carefully controlled and calcium is a key ion for normal contracture, many enzyme reactions[70], the stability of the cell membrane and the generation of ATP by the mitochondria[71]. When mitochondria become overloaded with calcium they are no longer able to generate ATP in the normal manner[71,72]. If this hypothesis is correct, then it is important to understand the mechanism by which the increased calcium influx occurs. The calcium influx appears not to be through the slow calcium channel, is not always associated with disruption of the cell membrane and may or may not be linked to sodium efflux[66]. The calcium influx has been supposed to be the result of an increased permeability of the cell membrane, so that calcium passes down the concentration gradient from the extracellular fluid to the intracellular fluid. Alternatively it may result from sodium–calcium exchange or more complex ionic exchange mechanisms[73]. Certainly the degree of calcium overload can be related to the functional recovery of the myocardium[57] and alteration of the calcium concentration in the extracellular fluid at the time of reperfusion has been shown to lead under some circumstances to an increased recovery of function[47].

The final current hypothesis for damage to the myocardium on the reperfusion is that it is due to the increased generation of oxygen radicals[44,74,75]. This hypothesis is attractive because it would account for the similarity between the events occurring on reoxygenation of the myocardium with those observed on reperfusion. Radicals may be formed by the infiltration of white cells into the ischaemic myocardium or may be formed in the endothelial cell by the action of xanthine dehydrogenases, which are often called 'oxidases', during the period of ischaemia[75]. Radicals may also be formed in the mitochondria of the heart. Mechanisms that normally exist in the heart to limit the formation of oxygen radicals are reduced during ischaemia[76] and oxygen radicals have been shown to be generated during ischaemia and particularly at the time of reperfusion. The source of the radicals may vary with time after reperfusion and between different experimental models. This hypothesis has led to some important observations – such as treatment with allopurinol can reduce infarct size in some animal species[77] (allopurinol inhibits xanthine dehydrogenases); and that the use of radical scavengers, such as superoxide dismutase and catalase, can limit the damage occurring at the moment of reperfusion[46].

LONG TERM EFFECTS OF ISCHAEMIA

Although after short periods of ischaemia the partial recovery of the function of the heart is rapid, careful measurements have shown that further recovery occurs over days and even weeks[78]. Despite restoration of flow and the absence of ischaemia, the consequences of ischaemia to the myocardium can last for several weeks. Cardiac function remains depressed after periods of up to four weeks. The mechanism is by no means certain. One proposal is that during ischaemia high energy phosphates are broken down to xanthine and hyperxanthine and that these moieties are lost from the myocardium. The normal energy of the state of the myocardium is not restored until these high energy phosphates have been resynthesized. The process may take up to a week[79,80]. There is evidence both for and against this hypothesis[79,80]. The loss of potassium, which is known to occur during short periods of ischaemia, is not restored for up to 30 minutes so that repeated episodes of ischaemia may well lead to an accumulative loss of ions from the heart. These observations have led to the concept of the 'stunned myocardia'[81]. This phrase has rather similar connotations to 'chronic ischaemia'. The term chronic ischaemia was used to imply that the myocyte could exist in a state in which the metabolic derangements observed during ischaemia could persist over a long period of time or perhaps indefinitely. There are biochemical reasons for supposing that that is unlikely and the cell either recovers or dies. Nevertheless, the consequences of ischaemia do persist for up to several weeks. These effects include abnormal ionic homeostatis, coronary flow and myocardial contractile function.

MECHANISM OF MYOCARDIAL INFARCTION

Although the symptoms and clinical picture of myocardial infarction had been described earlier, it was only in 1912 that the entity was clearly described by Herrick[82]. The cause of myocardial infarction has long been debated. The debate centred on the issue of whether thrombosis in a coronary artery occurred prior to the infarction and was the cause of that infarction or occurred subsequent to the infarction and was therefore a consequence. Recent evidence and popular opinion strongly favours the view that thrombosis occurs prior to infarction and is a causal mechanism but this view may be overstated[83,84].

Myocardial infarction has no single cause and a list of mechanisms is shown in Table 5.4. If causes, such as emboli, are put aside the central

Table 5.4 Nature of 'dynamic stenosis'

Physiological vasoconstriction

Pathological vasoconstriction
  (a) localizing factor
  (b) trigger factor

Passive changes
Intravascular plugging
Compression by extramuscle forces

issue is the origin of the myocardial infarction in the presence of coronary artery disease. According to one scheme there is rupture and/or haemorrhage into an atheromatous plaque. Collagen in the wall of the artery is brought into contact with the blood stream. Platelets adhere to the collagen and a thrombus is formed. The thrombus finally occludes the coronary artery and infarction ensues. Vasoconstriction of the coronary artery may occur, if it is anatomically possible as a result of the release of vasoconstricting substances by the platelets in the developing thrombus. There are other causes of a variable obstruction in a coronary artery (Table 5.4). The key evidence in favour of this hypothesis is that unstable atheromatous plaques are commonly found in patients dying with coronary artery disease[85] and that total occlusion of coronary arteries has been demonstrated in more than 70% of patients between one and four hours after the onset of chest pain[86]. Subsequently, the prevalence of coronary occlusion declines, presumably due to the spontaneous dissolution of the thrombus by natural thrombolytic mechanisms.

This is not the only possible mechanism and some alternatives are shown in Tables 5.5 and 5.6 and in Figure 5.5. As indicated above, after one hour of total coronary occlusion an infarct will be established and very little of the myocardium would recover were reperfusion established. The observation that there is a high proportion of thrombotic occlusions of coronary arteries between one and four hours after the onset of chest pain, in no way resolves the problem of whether thrombosis occurs prior to or after the development of myocardial infarction. This evidence merely moves the time window of interest to the first hour. It is possible and even probable that unstable plaques are

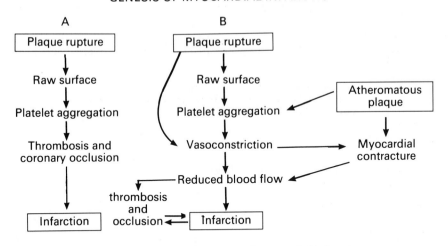

Figure 5.5 Hypotheses concerning the origins of myocardial infarction

a rare event in individual patients with coronary artery disease, but since many persons have coronary artery disease they occur quite frequently. Not all unstable plaques will lead to myocardial infarction. Indeed it is possible that myocardial infarction causes splinting and changes in the coronary artery, which contribute to the development of so called plaque rupture. Evidence on the incidence of thrombosis from the studies on patients with sudden death is conflicting[85,87] and does not contribute greatly to the debates, since the causes of sudden death may differ substantially from the causes of acute myocardial infarction. Several alternative hypotheses exist for the origin of myocardial infarction. These include platelet emboli, vasoconstriction and compression of the myocardial capillaries by contracture developing in the myocardial muscle[88]. Such a scheme is indicated in Figure 5.5. In my opinion the hypothesis that myocardial infarction is due to thrombosis in the coronary artery is overstated at the present time. The mechanism is

Table 5.5 Possible initiating and exacerbating factors in myocardial infarction

Rupture, fissure or haemorrhage into plaque of atheroma

Thrombosis

Coronary constriction (spasm)

Compression of capillaries by contracted and non-relaxing myocardium

Platelet aggregation

Emboli

Viscosity

Coronary steal

Others: trauma, arteritis, aortic dissection etc.

Table 5.6 A metabolic mechanism for myocardial infarction

Atheroma
+
Increased ATP consumption (caused by ↑ cardiac work)
or reduction of blood flow (leading to ↓ ATP production, retention of metabolites)
↓
Ischaemia
                    → intracellular acidosis (↓ contractility)
                    → extracellular accumulation of K^+ (ECG changes, pain)
                    → needs 1/52 for complete recovery
Recurrent episodes
↓
Prolonged episodes
↓
Contracture of myocardium around capillaries
Contraction of smooth muscle
↓
Further reduction of blood flow
↓
Myocardial infarction

---

likely to be multifactorial and the contribution of each factor will vary in individual patients. The important considerations appear to be the severity of coronary stenosis, the ability of platelets to adhere to the wall of the atheromatous plaque (rupture), contraction of the smooth muscle in the wall of the artery, pre-existing anatomy of the atheromatous plaque allowing shortening of the smooth muscle, the presence of collaterals, the degree of activity of the natural thrombolytic system and finally the degree of compression of the capillaries in the distal coronary bed by contracting myocardium.

CLINICAL RELEVANCE

Angina pectoris and angioplasty

A major puzzle in cardiology is the precise cause of the symptom, angina pectoris. The presence of angina is poor testimony to the presence of ischaemia, since as many as 25% of myocardial infarctions may be silent and numerous episodes of myocardial ischaemia are not associated with chest pain[89,90]. Since pain is a late manifestation (60 seconds) of myocardial ischaemia it may be that the initiating factor for pain is the rise in the extracellular potassium concentration. When a threshold is reached, sufficient nerve fibres may be activated to give rise to the sensations that the clinicians call *angina*. The perception of pain by the patient will depend on many other factors.

The word angina was initially used to describe a feeling of tightness in the throat and lower neck. Part of this symptom may occur because of a rise in the left arterial pressure associated with a reduction in cardiac contraction. The sensation in the chest would then have some of the features in common with acute heart failure.

A large proportion of patients with coronary artery disease die suddenly without evidence of acute myocardial infarctions. The presumption is that they die of an arrhythmia. The arrhythmia may occur either in the presence of an acute event in the coronary arteries (an unstable plaque) or merely in the presence of severe atheromatous coronary artery disease. Many factors are known to contribute to arrhythmias including stimulation of the autonomic nervous system and alterations in the concentration of many substances in the blood and within the cell. Examples are the extracellular potassium concentration, the extracellular magnesium concentration and the intracellular accumulation of lipids. A major factor may be the extracellular accumulation of potassium in the ischaemic myocardium. The edge of a myocardial infarct is now known to be sharp, so that normal myocardial cells being perfused at a potassium concentration of 4.5 mmol l^{-1} will be adjacent to cells with an extracellular potassium concentration of up to 10 mmol l^{-1}. There will be a gradient between the high extracellular potassium concentration in the middle of the infarcted area and the normal tissues. Such electrical inhomogeneity within the heart can provide the electrical basis for arrhythmias. The trigger factor may be stimulation of the sympathetic nervous system or sudden alterations in the extracellular potassium concentration of the normal tissue. Recent work shows that the plasma potassium concentration alters from minute to minute, particularly with exercise.

The recent introduction of angioplasty has provided a model whereby the early effects of ischaemia can be studied in man. It is apparent that the monophasic action potential shortens after about the 16th heart beat[19] and at the same time contraction falls[20], potassium is lost from the myocardium[38] and there is the development of an intracellular acidosis[26]. Thus, angioplasty has allowed the demonstration of many phenomena known to occur in animals also occur in man. Arrhythmias in general are fortunately rare during angioplasty but can occur on reperfusion after a more prolonged period of ischaemia. The alterations of ionic haemostasis outlined above provide a reasonable basis for the genesis of these arrhythmias. Most currently available antiarrhythmic drugs are aimed at the interruption of established arrhythmias, or at preventing those electrical phenomena within single cells, that may initiate arrhythmias. A more effective therapy may be to prevent ischaemia or to influence those mechanisms responsible for the early loss of potassium from the ischaemic myocardium.

Sudden death

Sudden death should not be equated or confused with acute myocardial infarction. The circumstances in which these occur and the underlying mechanisms may be very different. Reports vary greatly in the incidence of coronary thrombosis in patients with sudden death[84,85,87]. This almost certainly reflects the different definitions of sudden death, the exclusion of selected groups of patients and different techniques for pathological examination of the post mortem specimen. If sudden death is defined as death in a person who has been well 24 hours previously in one study and a person who has been well 6 hours previously in another study, then the proportion of patients with myocardial infarction in the populations studied will differ. Even six hours is a long time in terms of the development of an infarction, but post mortem techniques cannot easily detect myocardial infarction if it has been present for less than about three hours. Studies on patients who have survived cardiac resuscitation indicate that only a small proportion (17%) develop a myocardial infarct.

A common feature of most patients dying suddenly is that they do have severe coronary artery disease[84,85,87]. It seems likely therefore, that many of these deaths are due to an arrhythmia and this may have been induced by the ionic events described above, which accompany a short period of myocardial ischaemia. One report indicates a high incidence of unstable atheromatous plaques and thrombosis in patients with coronary artery disease[85]. This could indicate that in this study there was a greater proportion of patients with early myocardial infarction compared to other studies. The clinical implication is that agents known to prevent or interfere with the alleged mechanisms of myocardial infarction may not necessarily be effective in the prevention of sudden death. Agents which terminate arrhythmias or interfere with the early mechanisms of ischaemia likewise may not be effective in preventing myocardial infarction.

Infarct size

In the 1970s the belief was that a myocardial infarct was surrounded by myocardium, which had a marginal blood flow and could be regarded as 'jeopardized' or 'threatened'. Experiments were undertaken with a variety of drugs and interventions which appeared to indicate that 'infarct size' could be reduced[91]. Subsequently, clinical trials were undertaken with drugs and certainly in the case of beta-blockers it has been shown that when used in patients after myocardial infarction there is a reduction in subsequent death and reinfarction[1]. The original experiments in animals and isolated tissue that demonstrated the supposed reduction of infarct size have been challenged[92,93]. The challenge has been based largely on the question of whether the experiments showed a reduction of infarct size or merely a delay in the development of the infarct[7]. The issue is complicated by the criticism of techniques used to demonstrate the amount of muscle at risk of infarcting when a vessel is occluded and the actual final size of an infarct. Further, there is the important question of whether animals that die during an experiment are excluded from the final analysis of results. If this is done and were those animals to have the larger infarcts, only animals with smaller infarcts will survive and an apparent reduction of infarct size would be observed. More recent experiments have not confirmed early enthusiasm[50] and indeed now there is strong reason to believe that the whole concept of infarct size reduction is flawed[7].

There are large species differences in the anatomical arrangement of the coronary arteries[51]. In the guinea pig there is an extensive collateral flow so that it is almost impossible to induce an infarct by occlusion of a coronary artery. In the pig most of the coronary arteries are end arteries. The dog has extensive collateral circulation on the endocardium. Man, in general, appears to have end arteries in his coronary system but in the presence of coronary artery disease collaterals develop over the years, in which case the anatomy is somewhat similar to that which exists in the dog. These observations are crucial in attempting to interpret animal data. In the pig without collaterals and the dog, where there is no collateral circulation in the epicardium, occlusion of a coronary artery leads to a clearly demarcated infarct on the endocardial surface of the heart. With time the infarct spreads from the endocardial surface to the epicardial surface until a full thickness infarct develops[92-94]. The edge of the infarct does not alter. The reason why the endocardium appears to be more vulnerable than the epicardium is not clear but may relate to different wall tension, metabolic rate or distribution of blood vessels. Necrosis begins in the subendocardium independent of collateral flow and wall tension[95]. Detailed investigation of the nature of the edge of the infarct shows that there is no border zone (or certainly it is less than one cell thick) and that the capillary beds supplied by the normal tissue and ischaemic tissue interdigitate and are immediately adjacent.

These observations have an important clinical significance since it is unlikely that infarct size will be altered in any way unless coronary blood flow is restored. Blood flow might be increased: by reopening of the natural occluded coronary artery; by opening of pre-existing collaterals; by the development of new collaterals (this process requires a minimum of 48 hours); or by redistribution of the collateral flow between the epicardium and the endocardium[7]. The factors determining infarct size are shown in Table 5.7.

An important issue is the use of enzyme release of the myocardium to measure the size of an infarct. Simple consideration of this method suggests that it should not work. In a severe infarct there will be little blood flow to the centre of the infarct and the enzymes will not be

Table 5.7 Factors determining infarct size in man

Duration of ischaemia

Underlying anatomy ('area at risk')

Residual flow or reperfusion
  (a) collaterals
  (b) 'stuttering ischaemia'

Myocardial oxygen consumption at onset of ischaemia

reduced from that area of muscle. In a small infarct, a small residual coronary flow will be present and the enzymes will be released. Thus the amount of enzyme release is not precisely related to the size of the myocardial infarct. A further important problem arises from consideration of the mechanism by which enzyme leaves cells[54]. Certainly if the cell membrane is disrupted enzymes pass out of the myocardial cell. It is also clear that early in ischaemia and on reperfusion after short periods of ischaemia enzymes can leave the myocardial cell without gross disruption of the cell membrane. Thus small increases in blood enzymes in the presence of chest pain may not necessarily mean that cell necrosis has occurred.

'Stuttering ischaemia'

If myocardial infarction is caused by the sudden and total occlusion of a coronary artery then, in the absence of collateral flow, the myocardium will only survive for approximately 40 minutes. It is unlikely that interventions can be applied to patients so quickly. However, if the occlusion were not sudden or if there is a collateral blood flow to supply a small quantity of blood, then the time course over which cell necrosis develops will be greatly extended. Studies on patients very early in the development of infarction indicate that the ST segments on the surface electrocardiogram may change from moment to moment[96]. This can be interpreted as representing so called 'stuttering ischaemia'. That is, the processes limiting blood flow are varying from moment to moment allowing blood to pass to the muscle perhaps by the mechanisms outlined in Table 5.5. This may be partly because of the washout of ions so altering the degree of vasoconstriction of the smooth muscle, or due to natural lysis of a thrombus by the body's normal thrombolytic mechanisms. If stuttering ischaemia is a reality and common in the context of myocardial infarction it becomes an important concept, because it greatly lengthens the time which is available to the physician to introduce an intervention, with the intention of increasing blood flow, or delivering drugs to delay myocardial necrosis until blood flow can be restored.

'Stunned myocardium'

As indicated above, following acute myocardial ischaemia the function of the myocardium and many metabolic changes do not recover instantly but can persist for several weeks. Chest pain has clearly been shown to be a poor indicator of myocardial ischaemia. Patients with angina have frequent episodes of changes in the ST segment on the surface electrocardiogram and only a proportion of these are associated with chest pain[89,90]. If coronary arteries are occluded frequently and regularly, then it is possible that the myocardium remains stunned on an almost continuous basis. This would give rise to a reduction in contraction and a picture indistinguishable from that referred to by the older concept of 'chronic ischaemia'. Repeated episodes of ischaemia might initiate processes leading to myocardial infarction. The accumulative effect of repeated episodes of ischaemia is contested[97–101].

Thrombolysis

The availability of a variety of new thrombolytic agents and recent evidence that thrombosis is an important cause of myocardial infarction have given rise to great interest in the clinical application of these substances. Initial results appear to indicate that occluded coronary arteries can be opened and that provided patients are treated early, the opening of the coronary artery is accompanied by an improvement of left ventricular function. These findings are entirely compatible with the results of earlier animal experiments. Reocclusion of the coronary artery in man appears to be a problem and will need to be overcome. However, the expectations of thrombolytic therapy should not be set too high. Only about 70% of patients with myocardial infarction have an occluded coronary artery at one hour. Of these only 70% can be opened by thrombolytic therapy. Up to 50% may reocclude in the following days. In a proportion of patients (say 40%) the thrombotic processes may not be the key mechanism for the occurrence of myocardial infarction and may be a secondary event. Considering these figures in total thrombolytic therapy would be expected to be of some benefit but not a panacea for the treatment of a complex and a multifactorial entity such as myocardial infarction. Newer drugs may delay the onset of tissue necrosis and prevent damaging metabolic events at the time of reperfusion. In the next few years many drugs will be tested as adjuncts to thrombolytic therapy.

References

1. Yusuf, S., Peto, R., Lewis, J. Collins, R. and Sleight, P. (1985). Beta-blockade during and after myocardial infarction: an overview of the randomised trials. *Prog. Cardiovascular Dis.*, 27, 335–71
2. Yusuf, S., Collins, R., Peto, R., Furberg, C., Stampfer, M. L., Goldhaber, S. Z. and Hennekens, C. H. (1985). Intravenous and intracoronary fibrinolytic therapy in acute myocardial infarction: overview of results on mortality, reinfarction and side-effects from 33 randomised controlled trials. *Eur. Heart J.*, 6, 556–83
3. Harker, L. A. (1986). Clinical trials evaluating platelet-modifying drugs in patients with atherosclerotic cardiovascular disease and thrombosis. *Circulation*, 73, 206–23
4. GISSI Study (1986). Effectiveness of intravenous thrombolytic treatment in acute myocardial infarction. *Lancet*, 1, 397–401
5. Yellon, D. M., Hearse, D. J., Crome, R. and Wyse, R. K. H. (1983). Temporal and spatial characteristics of evolving cell injury during regional myocardial ischemia in the dog: the "border zone" controversy. *J. Am. Coll. Cardiol.*, 2, 661–70
6. Factor, S. M., Okun, E. M., Takashi, M. and Kirk, E. S. (1982). The microcirculation of the human heart: end-capillary loops with discrete perfusion fields. *Circulation*, 66, 1241–8

7. Hearse, D. H. and Yellon, D. M. (eds.) (1984). In *Therapeutic Approaches to Myocardial Infarct Size Limitation*. (New York: Raven Press)
8. Marcus, M. L. (1983). *The Coronary Circulation in Health and Disease*. (New York: McGraw-Hill)
9. Shaper, W. (1979). *The Pathophysiology of Myocardial Perfusion* (Amsterdam and New York: Elsevier/North Holland Biomedical Press)
10. Neely, J. R., Whitmer, J. T. and Rovetto, M. J. (1975). Effect of coronary blood flow on glycolytic flux and intracellular pH in isolated rat hearts. *Circ. Res.*, 37, 733–41
11. Neely, J. R., Morgan, H. E. (1974). Relation between carbohydrate and lipid metabolism and the energy balance of the heart. *Ann. Rev. Physiol.*, 36, 413–59
12. Neely, J. R., Rovetto, M. J., Whitmer, J. T. and Morgan, H. E. (1973). Effects of ischemia on function and metabolism of the isolated working rat heart. *Am. J. Physiol.*, 226, 651
13. Sayen, J. J., Sheldon, W. F., Pierce, G. and Kuo, P. T. (1958). Polarographic oxygen, the epicardial electrocardiogram and muscle contraction in experimental acute regional ischaemia of the left ventricle. *Circ. Res.*, 6, 779–98
14. Braasch, W., Gudbjarnason, S., Puri, P. S., Ravens, K. G. and Bing, R. J. (1968). Early changes in energy metabolism in the myocardium following acute coronary artery occlusion in anaesthetized dogs. *Circ. Res.*, 23, 429–38
15. Gudbjarnason, S., Mathes, P. and Ravens, K. G. (1970). Functional compartmentalisation of ATP and creatine phosphate in heart muscle. *J. Mol. Cell. Cardiol.*, 1, 325–39
16. Wollenberger, A. and Krause, E. G. (1968). Metabolic control characteristics of the acutely ischemic myocardium. *Am. J. Cardiol.*, 22, 349–59
17. Tennant, R. and Wiggers, C. J. (1935). The effect of coronary occlusion on myocardial contraction. *Am. J. Physiol.*, 112, 351–61
18. Tennant, R. (1935). Factors concerned in the arrest of contraction in an ischaemic myocardial area. *Am. J. Physiol.*, 113, 677–82
19. Donaldson, R. M., Taggart, P., Bennett, J. G. and Rickards, A. F. (1984). Study of electrophysiological ischemic events during coronary angioplasty. *Texas Heart Inst. J.*, 11, 23–30
20. Serruys, P. W., Wijns, W., Van den Brond, M., Meij, S., Slager, C., Schuubiers, J. C. H., Hugenholtz, P. G. and Brower, R. W. (1984). Left ventricular performance, regional blood flow, wall motion and lactate metabolism during transluminal angioplasty. *Circulation*, 70, 25–36
21. Poole-Wilson, P. A., Fleetwood, G. and Cobbe, S. M. (1983). Early contractile failure in myocardial ischaemia – role of acidosis. In Refsum, H., Jynge, P. and Mjos, O. D. (eds.) *Myocardial Ischaemia and Protection*. pp. 9–17 (Edinburgh: Churchill Livingstone)
22. Apstein, C. S., Mueller, M. and Hood, W. B. (1977). Ventricular contracture and compliance changes with global ischaemia and reperfusion, and their effect on coronary resistance changes in the rat. *Circ. Res.*, 41, 206–17
23. Arnold, G., Kosche, F., Meissner, E., Neitzert, A., Lochner, W. (1968). The importance of the perfusion pressure in the coronary arteries for the contractility and the oxygen consumption of the heart. *Pfluegers Arch.*, 299, 339–56
24. Jacobus, W. E., Pores, I. H., Lucas, S. K., Clayton, H. K., Weisfeldt, M. L. and Flaherty, J. T. (1983). The role of intracellular pH in the control of normal and ischaemic myocardial contractility: a 31P nuclear magnetic resonance and mass spectrometry study. In Nuccitelli, R. and Deamer, D. W. (eds.) *Intracellular pH: Its Limitation, Regulation and Utilization in Cellular Functions*. pp. 537–65 (New York: Alan Liss)
25. Cobbe, S. M. and Poole-Wilson, P. A. (1980). The time of onset and severity of acidosis in myocardial ischaemia. *J. Mol. Cell. Cardiol.*, 12, 745–60
26. Cobbe, S. M., Parker, D. J. and Poole-Wilson, P. A. (1982). Tissue and coronary venous pH in ischemic canine myocardium. *Clin. Cardiol.*, 5, 153–6
27. Allen, D. G. and Orchard, C. H. (1983). The effect of pH on intracellular calcium transients in mammalian cardiac muscle. *J. Physiol*, 335, 555–67

28. Kubler, W. and Katz, A. M. (1977). Mechanism of early "pump" failure of the ischemic heart: possible role of adenosine triphosphate depletion and inorganic phosphate accumulation. *Am. J. Cardiol.*, **40**, 467–71
29. Kentish, J. C. (1985). The effect of inorganic phosphate and creatine phosphate on force production in skinned muscle from rat ventricle. *J. Physiol.*, **370**, 585–604
30. Bricknell, O. L., Daries, P. S. and Opie, L. H. (1981). A relationship between adenosine triphosphate, glycolysis and ischaemic contracture in the isolated rat heart. *J. Mol. Cell. Cardiol.*, **13**, 941–5
31. Higgins, T. J. C., Allsopp, D., Bailey, P. J. and D'Souza, E. D. A. (1981). The relationship between glycolysis, fatty acid metabolism and membrane integrity in neonatal myocytes. *J. Mol. Cell. Cardiol.*, **13**, 599–615
32. Weiss, J. and Shine, K. I. (1981). Extracellular K^+ accumulation during early myocardial ischemia. Implications for arrhythmogenesis. *J. Mol. Cell. Cardiol.*, **13**, 699–704
33. Hirche, H. J., Franz, C., Bos, L., Bissig, R., Lang, R. and Schramm, M. (1980). Myocardial extracellular K^+ and H^+ increase and noradrenaline release as possible cause of early arrhythmias following acute coronary artery occlusion in pigs. *J. Mol. Cell. Cardiol.*, **12**, 579–94
34. Hill, J. L. and Gettes, L. S. (1980). Effect of acute coronary artery occlusion on local myocardial extracellular K^+ activity in swine. *Circulation*, **61**, 68–78
35. Wiegand, V., Guggi, M., Meesmann, W., Kessler, M. and Greitschus, F. (1979). Extracellular potassium activity changes in the canine myocardium. *Cardiovasc. Res.*, **13**, 297–302
36. Weiss, J. and Shine, K. I. (1982). Extracellular K^+ accumulation during myocardial ischaemia in isolated rabbit heart. *Am. J. Physiol.*, **242**, H619–H628
37. Webb, S. C., Fleetwood, G. G., Montgomery, R. A. P. and Poole-Wilson, P. A. (1984). Absence of a relationship between extracellular potassium accumulation and contractile failure in the ischemic or hypoxic rabbit heart. In Dhalla, N. S. and Hearse, D. J. (eds.) *Advances in Myocardiology*. Vol. 6, pp. 405–15 (New York: Plenum Press)
38. Webb, S. C., Rickards, A. F. and Poole-Wilson, P. A. (1983). Coronary sinus potassium concentration recorded during coronary angioplasty. *Br. Heart J.*, **50**, 146–8
39. Weiss, J. and Shine, K. I. (1982). $(K^+)o$ accumulation and electrophysiological alterations during early myocardial ischaemia. *Am. J. Physiol.*, **243**, H318–27
40. Gaspardone, A., Shine, K. I., Seabrooke, S. R. and Poole-Wilson, P. A. (1986). Potassium loss from rabbit myocardium during hypoxia; evidence for passive efflux linked to anion extrusion. *J. Mol. Cell. Cardiol.*, **18**, 389–99
41. Kleber, A. G. (1984). Extracellular potassium accumulation in acute myocardial ischemia. *J. Mol. Cell. Cardiol.*, **16**(5), 389–94
42. Kleber, A. G. (1983). Resting membrane potential, extracellular potassium activity and intracellular sodium activity during acute global ischaemia in isolated perfused guinea pig hearts. *Circ. Res.*, **52**, 442–50
43. Jennings, R. B., Hawkins, H. K., Lowe, J. E., Hill, M. C., Klotman, S. and Reimer, K. A. (1978). Relation between high energy phosphate and lethal injury in myocardial ischemia in the dog. *Am. J. Pathol.*, **92**, 187–214
44. Jennings, R. B., Ganote, C. E. and Reimer, K. A. (1975). Ischaemic tissue injury. *Am. J. Pathol.*, **81**, 179–98
45. Poole-Wilson, P. A. (1984). What causes cell death? In Hearse, D. J. and Yellon, D. M. (eds.) *Therapeutic Approaches to Myocardial Infarct Size Limitation.* pp. 43–60. (New York: Raven Press)
46. Jolly, S. R., Kane, W. J., Bailie, M. B., Abrams, G. D. and Lucchesi, B. R. (1984). Canine myocardial reperfusion injury: its reduction by the combined administration of superoxide dismutase and catalase. *Circ. Res.*, **54**, 227–85
47. Shine, K. I., Douglas, A. M. and Ricchiuti, N. V. (1978). Calcium, strontium, and barium movements during ischemia and reperfusion in rabbit ventricle. Implications for myocardial preservation. *Circ. Res.*, **43**, 712–20

48. Allen, D. G. and Orchard C. H. (1983). Intracellular calcium concentration during hypoxia and metabolic inhibition in mammalian ventricular muscle. *J. Physiol.*, **339**, 107–22
49. Steenbergen, C. and Jennings, R. B. (1984). Relationship between lysophospholipid accumulation and plasma membrane injury during total in vitro ischaemia in dog heart. *J. Mol. Cell. Cardiol.*, **16**, 605–21
50. Reimer, K. A., Jennings R. B., Cobb, F. R., Murdock, R. H. *et al.* (1985). Animal models for protecting ischaemic myocardium: results of the NHLBI cooperative study. Comparison of unconscious and conscious dog models. *Circ. Res.*, **56**, 651–65
51. Schaper, W. (1984). Experimental infarcts and the microcirculation. In Hearse, D. H. and Yellon, D. M. (eds.) *Therapeutic Approaches to Myocardial Infarct Size Limitation*. pp. 79–90. (New York: Raven Press)
52. Hearse, D. J. (1977). Reperfusion of the ischemic myocardium. *J. Mol. Cell. Cardiol.*, **9**, 605–16
53. Poole-Wilson, P. A. (1983). The mechanism of cell death in heart muscle after hypoxia or ischaemia. In Refsum, H., Jynge, P. and Mjos, O. D. (eds.) *Myocardial Ischaemia and Protection*. pp. 123–30. (Edinburgh and New York: Churchill Livingstone)
54. Poole-Wilson, P. A. (1984). Enzyme loss and calcium exchange in ischemic or hypoxic myocardium. In Opie, L. H. (ed.) *Calcium Antagonists and Cardiovascular Disease*. pp. 97–104. (New York: Raven Press)
55. Poole-Wilson, P. A. (1985). The nature of myocardial damage following reoxygenation. In Parratt, J. R. (ed.) *Control and Manipulation of Calcium Movement*. pp. 325–40. (New York: Raven Press)
56. Shen, A. C. and Jennings, R. B. (1972). Myocardial calcium and magnesium in acute ischemic injury. *Am. J. Pathol.*, **67**, 417–40
57. Bourdillon, P. D. and Poole-Wilson, P. A. (1982). The effects of verapamil guiescence and cardioplegia on calcium exchange and mechanical function in ischemic rabbit myocardium. *Circ. Res.*, **50**, 360–8
58. Hearse, D. J., Humphrey, S. M. and Bullock, G. R. (1978). The oxygen paradox and the calcium paradox: two facets of the same problem? *Cardiology*, **10**, 641–68
59. Fleetwood, G. and Poole-Wilson, P. A. (1986). Diastolic coronary resistance after ischaemia in the isolated rabbit heart: effect of nifedipine. *J. Mol. Cell. Cardiol.*, **18**, 139–47
60. Humphrey, S. M., Gavin, J. B. and Herdson, P. B. (1980). The relationship of ischemic contracture to vascular reperfusion in the isolated rat heart. *J. Mol. Cell. Cardiol.*, **12**, 1397–406
61. Kloner, R. A., Reimer, K. A., Willerson, J. T. and Jennings, R. B. (1974). The "no-reflow" phenomenon after temporary coronary occlusion in the dog. *J. Clin. Invest.*, **54**, 1496–508
62. Powers, E. R., DiBona, D. R. and Powell, W. J. Jr. (1984). Myocardial cell volume and coronary resistance during diminished coronary perfusion. *Am. J. Physiol.*, **247**, H467–77
63. Yamazaki, S., Fujibayashi, Y., Rajogopalan, R. E., Meerbaum, S. and Corday, E. (1986). Effects of staged versus sudden reperfusion after acute coronary occlusion in the dog. *J. Am. Coll. Cardiol*, **7**, 564–72
64. Jennings, R. B. and Reimer, K. A. (1981). Lethal myocardial ischemic injury. *Am. J. Pathol.*, **102**, 241–55
65. Ganote, C. E. and Kaltenbach, J. P. (1979). Oxygen-induced enzyme release: early events and a proposed mechanism. *J. Mol. Cell. Cardiol.*, **11**, 389–406
66. Poole-Wilson, P. A., Harding, D. P., Bourdillon, P. D. V. and Tones, M. A. (1984). Calcium out of control. *J. Mol. Cell. Cardiol.*, **16**, 175–87
67. Steenbergen, C., Hill, M. L. and Jennings, R. B. (1985). Volume regulation and plasma membrane injury in aerobic, anaerobic and ischemic myocardium in vitro: effects of osmotic cell swelling on plasma membrane integrity. *Circ. Res.*, **57**(6), 864

68. Fleckenstein, A., Janke, J., Doring, H. J. and Leder, O. (1984). Myocardial fibre necrosis due to intracellular Ca overload – a new principle in cardiac pathophysiology. In Dhalla, N. S. (ed.) *Recent Advances in Studies on Cardiac Structure and Metabolism*. pp. 563–580. (Baltimore: University Park Press)
69. Nayler, W. G., Poole-Wilson, P. A. and Williams, A. (1979). Hypoxia and calcium. *J. Mol. Cell. Cardiol.*, **11**, 683–706
70. Denton, R. M. and McCormack, J. G. (1981). Calcium ions, hormones and mitochondrial metabolism. *Clin. Sci.*, **61**, 135–40
71. Parr, D. R., Wimhurst, J. M. and Harris, E. F. (1975). Calcium-induced damage of rat heart mitochondria. *Cardiovasc. Res.*, **9**, 366–72
72. Wrogeman, K. and Pena, S. D. J. (1976). Mitochondrial calcium overload: a general mechanism for cell necrosis in muscle diseases. *Lancet*, **1**, 672–4
73. Lazdunski, M., Frelin, C. and Vigne, P. (1985). The sodium/hydrogen exchange system in cardiac cells: its biochemical and pharmacological properties and its role in regulating internal concentrations of sodium and internal pH. *J. Mol. Cell. Cardiol.*, **17**, 1029
74. Werns, S. W., Shea, M. J., Driscoll, E. M., Cohen, C. *et al.* (1985). The independent effects of oxygen radical scavengers on canine infarct size: reduction by superoxide dismutase but not catalase. *Circ. Res.*, **56(6)**, 895
75. McCord, J. M. and Roy, R. S. (1982). The pathophysiology of superoxide: roles in inflammation and ischaemia. *Can. J. Physiol. Pharmacol.*, **60**, 1346–52
76. Guarnieri, C., Flamigni, F. and Calderera, C. M. (1980). Role of oxygen in the cellular damage induced by re-oxygenation of hypoxic heart. *J. Mol. Cell. Cardiol.*, **12(8)**, 797–808
77. Werns, S. W., Shea, M. J., Mitsos, S. E., Dysko, R. C., Fantone, J. C., Schork, M. A., Abrams, G. D., Pitt, B., Lucchesi, B. R. (1986). Reduction of the size of infarction by allupurinol in the ischemic-reperfused canine heart. *Circulation*, **73**, 518–24
78. Bush, L. R., Buja, L. M., Samowitz, W., Rude, R. E. *et al.* (1983). Recovery of left ventricular segmental function after long-term reperfusion following temporary coronary occlusion in conscious dogs. Comparison of 2 and 4 hour occlusions. *Circ. Res.*, **53**, 248–63
79. Jennings, R. B., Reimer, K. A., Hill, M. L. and Mayer, S. E. (1981). Total ischemia, in dog hearts, in vitro. I. Comparison of high energy phosphate production, utilization and depletion and of adenine nucleotide catabolism in total ischemia in vitro vs. severe ischemia in vivo. *Circ. Res.*, **49**, 892–900
80. Swain, J. L., Hines, J. J., Sabina, R. L. and Holmes, E. W. (1982). Accelerated repletion of ATP and GTP pools in postischemic canine myocardium using a precursor of purine de novo synthesis. *Circ. Res.*, **51**, 102–5
81. Braunwald, E. and Kloner, R. A. (1982). The stunned myocardium: prolonged, postischemic ventricular dysfunction. *Circulation*, **66**, 1146–9
82. Herrick, J. B. (1912). Clinical features of sudden obstruction of the coronary arteries. *J. Am. Med. Assoc.*, **59**, 2015–20
83. Davies, M. J. and Thomas, T. (1981). The pathological basis and microanatomy of occlusive thrombus formation in human coronary arteries. *Phil. Trans. R. Soc. Lond. B*, **294**, 225–9
84. Davies, M. J. and Thomas, A. C. (1985). Plaque fissuring – the cause of acute myocardial infarction, sudden ischaemic death, and crescendo angina (review 60-refs). *Br. Heart J.*, **53**, 363–73
85. Davies, M. J. and Thomas, A. (1984). Thrombosis and acute coronary-artery lesions in sudden cardiac death. *N. Engl. J. Med.*, **310**, 1137–40
86. DeWood, M. A., Spores, J., Notske, R., Mouser, L. T. *et al.* (1980). Prevalence of total coronary occlusion during the early hours of transmural myocardial infarction. *N. Engl. J. Med.*, **303**, 897–902
87. Warnes, C. A. and Roberts, W. C. (1984). Sudden coronary death: comparison of patients with to those without coronary thrombus at necropsy. *Am. J. Cardiol.*, **54(10)**, 1206–11

88. Harris, P. (1975). A theory concerning the course of events in angina and myocardial infarction. *Eur. J. Cardiol.*, **3**, 157–63
89. Schang, S. J. and Pepine, C. J. (1977). Transient asymptomatic S-T segment depression during daily activity. *Am. J. Cardiol.*, **39**, 396–402
90. Selwyn, A. P., Fox, K., Oakley, D., Dargie, H. and Shillingford, J. (1978). Myocardial ischaemia in patients with frequent angina pectoris. *Br. Med. J.*, **2**, 1594–6
91. Maroko, P. R., Kjekshus, J. K., Sobel, B. E., Watanabe, T. *et al.* (1971). Factors influencing infarct size following experimental coronary artery occlusions. *Circulation*, **43**, 67–82
92. Hearse, D. J. and Yellon, D. M. (1981). The "border zone" in evolving myocardial infarction: controversy or confusion? *Am. J. Cardiol.*, **49(6)**, 1321–34
93. Yellon, D. M., Hearse, D. J., Crome, R. and Wyse, R. K. H. (1983). Temporal and spatial characteristics of evolving cell injury during regional myocardial ischemia in the dog: the "border zone" controversy. *J. Am. Coll. Cardiol.*, **2**, 661–70
94. Reimer, K. A., Lowe, J. E., Rasmussen, M. M. and Jennings, R. B. (1977). The wavefront phenomenon of ischaemic cell death. 1. Myocardial infarct size vs duration of coronary occlusion in dogs. *Circulation*, **56**, 786–94
95. Lowe, J. E., Cummings, R. G., Adams, D. H. and Hull-Ryde, E. A. (1983). Evidence that ischemic cell death begins in the subendocardium independent of variations in collateral flow or wall tension. *Circulation*, **68**, 190–202
96. Davies, G. J., Cherchia, S. and Maseri, A. (1984). Prevention of myocardial infarction by very early treatment with intracoronary streptokinase. *N. Engl. J. Med.*, **311**, 1488–92
97. Lange, R., Ware, J. and Kloner, R. A. (1984). Absence of cumulative deterioration of regional function during three repeated 5 or 15 minute coronary occlusions. *Circulation*, **69**, 400–8
98. Liedtke, A. J. and Nellis, S. H. (1980). Effects of coronary washout on cardiac function during brief periods of ischemia and hypoxia. *Am. J. Physiol*, **8**, H371–9
99. Nicklas, J. M., Becker, L. C. and Bulkley, B. H. (1982). Repeated brief coronary occlusion: Effects on regional shape, function and ultrastructure. *Cardiovasc. Res.*, **30**, 209A
100. Theroux, P., Ross, J. Jr., Fanklin, D., Kemper, W. S. and Sasayama, S. (1976). Regional myocardial function in the conscious dog during acute coronary occlusion and responses to morphine, propranolol, nitroglycerine and lidocaine. *Circulation*, **53**, 302–14
101. Weiner, J. M., Apstein, C. S., Arthur, J. H., Pirzada, F. H. and Hood, W. B. (1976). Persistence of myocardial injury following brief periods of coronary occlusion. *Cardiovasc. Res.*, **10**, 678–86

6
Investigation and management of chronic stable angina

H. J. DARGIE

INTRODUCTION

Like many ancient terms in medicine, angina pectoris is not a diagnosis but a symptom. The term implies the occurrence of myocardial ischaemia, the usual mechanism of which is an increase in myocardial oxygen demand that cannot be met by an appropriate increase in coronary blood flow because of the physical obstruction imposed by atheromatous coronary heart disease. Thus, as noted by Heberden in 1772, angina is precipitated mainly by effort and disappears with rest[1]. Several non-cardiac mechanisms, including anaemia or polycythaemia, can also cause angina; as can a number of other cardiac or vascular mechanisms independently of or in association with atheroma – including coronary vasoconstriction, ventricular hypertrophy with or without associated valve disease and platelet aggregation or thrombosis.

In this chapter we will concentrate on the investigation and management of those patients in whom angina due to coronary heart disease is suspected and in whom the pattern of symptoms is stable, in that angina usually is induced by exercise (albeit variably) and relieved by rest. It is in these patients that clinical investigation has reached the stage where it allows the cardiologist to formulate a therapeutic strategy based not only on the symptoms but also on the prognostic information provided by non-invasive and invasive assessment.

But, equally, the availability of such an array of powerful diagnostic tests as computer assisted exercise electrocardiography, radionuclide ventriculography, thallium perfusion scintigraphy and coronary arteriography poses some of the most crucial and controversial questions in cardiology today:

(1) Which patients should be investigated?
(2) When and how far?
(3) Who should have surgery or angioplasty?
(4) Who may safely continue on medical treatment?

Basically three related questions arise at the outset. *Firstly,* are the symptoms definitely due to coronary heart disease? *Secondly,* do they significantly limit exercise capacity and detract from the quality of life? And *thirdly,* irrespective of symptoms, does the underlying coronary heart disease pose a threat to life or well being in the short or medium term? The inevitable paradox of the practice of medicine is that in most diseases, including coronary heart disease, the need for investigation is usually signalled by the onset of a symptom such as chest pain. But since sudden death, unheralded by any symptom, is a common presentation of coronary heart disease[2] and since in certain categories of patients with angina, coronary bypass surgery may improve prognosis[3], it is important not to depend entirely on the perceived severity of the symptoms when considering further investigation. Moreover, personality factors may be such that symptoms might be minimized by some patients and exaggerated by others. Modern non-invasive methods enable us to quantify the severity of the underlying coronary heart disease thus providing information on prognosis that, regardless of the symptoms, may be very important in management.

Another stimulus to careful investigation is that often it may exclude a cardiac cause for chest pain in a very symptomatic patient, thereby allowing the withdrawal of a complex drug regimen and removal of the fear of heart disease that could be contributing significantly to the symptoms. Also a negative cardiac investigation may lead to a change in the diagnostic direction towards the correct identification of, for example, oesophageal or other upper alimentary pathology[4].

THE APPROACH TO INVESTIGATION

At the outset it is very important to make a working clinical diagnosis by means of a detailed history supplemented by a careful clinical examination – to exclude other forms of heart disease or serious pathology, especially concomitant vascular disease, to detect hypertension and to identify any other attendant coronary risk factors. Strong pointers to the presence of coronary heart disease are a characteristic history of effort related retrosternal or epigastric pain that builds up gradually, radiates to the throat, jaw, back, shoulders or arms and which passes off gradually but promptly with cessation of activity (or, subsequently, with the use of nitrates). Dyspnoea commonly accompanies the chest discomfort and may be the main or, indeed, the only complaint in some patients – the pathophysiological basis for which could be one or other or a combination of reversible myocardial ischaemia and poor left ventricular function, although associated airways disease may be a factor in smokers. Often the presence of one or more coronary risk factors is a persuasive factor, especially when the symptoms are atypical. The differential diagnosis and investigation of chest pain that is not typical for coronary heart disease is beyond the scope of this chapter, but caution must be observed in ascribing such symptoms to anxiety or to other non-cardiac sites (such as the oesophagus) when the underlying problem might indeed be coronary spasm.

It is helpful to categorize patients into those with a strong clinical probability of having coronary heart disease and those who do not; because interpretation of any diagnostic test is highly dependent on the prevalence of the disease in the population from which the patient comes[5]. Inevitably some patients with chest pain will be difficult to classify but most will fall into one of three groups – those with typical symptoms, those with atypical but suggestive symptoms and those in whom coronary heart disease is thought unlikely. The prevalence of coronary heart disease in these groups has been reported to be approximately 90%, 50% and 5–10% respectively[6-8]. Thus a good history, in itself, is a reasonable clinical indicator for coronary heart disease. Its further investigation can be considered in three stages – primary, secondary and tertiary.

PRIMARY INVESTIGATION

In the absence of clinical pointers to the presence of non-cardiac or non-coronary causes, a number of routine tests form the primary investigation of the patient with chest pain:

Urinalysis for glucose

This is essential and, although a full biochemical screen is not required, the serum cholesterol level is important because this may influence management. Fasting is unnecessary and if a random sample were to be normal, no further lipid tests would be needed; but if the serum cholesterol were to be elevated, a fasting sample to evaluate triglycerides would be advisable. Height and weight should be recorded so that a reducing diet can be instituted, if appropriate.

Chest X-ray

A chest X-ray may provide diagnostic information that is not already available from clinical examination – the heart size is important and there may be other intrathoracic pathology especially in smokers. Rarely a hiatus hernia may be seen.

Electrocardiogram

In the patient with chest pain, a resting ECG is of most help when it is abnormal because a normal ECG does not exclude coronary heart disease. The spectrum of abnormalities that confirm or suggest that chest pain is due to myocardial ischaemia is wide, but evidence of previous myocardial infarction (that may have been silent)[9] is most predictive; while other abnormalities, such as left bundle branch block and ventricular hypertrophy, raise the suspicion that the chest pain might be due to a cardiomyopathy or any cause of secondary hypertrophy including systemic or, rarely, pulmonary hypertension. Since the relationship between the height of the blood pressure and left ventricular mass is not close[10] moderate or even mild essential hypertension could be important. In the context of chest pain the importance of establishing the presence of coronary heart disease is such that minor abnormalities, such as non-specific repolarization changes, should be taken seriously and may provide the stimulus for further investigation.

SECONDARY INVESTIGATION (NON-INVASIVE)

Though more sophisticated and perhaps more accurate methods of detecting and quantifying ischaemia are under development, those that most commonly are applied in clinical practice are exercise electrocardiography, radionuclide ventriculography, myocardial perfusion scintigraphy and echocardiography. Exercise is an integral part of each test, when a change in pattern due to myocardial ischaemia may occur that is reversible with rest. Each of the tests provides different information from which the presence and severity of myocardial ischaemia can be inferred and an estimate made of the area of myocardium likely to be involved and therefore in jeopardy. In selected patients, ambulatory monitoring of the ST segment can also provide valuable and clinically relevant information.

Since a good history of angina is probably as good as any non-invasive test in diagnosing coronary heart disease, the aims of secondary investigation are:

(1) To quantify the severity of the ischaemia
(2) To estimate the prognosis
(3) To define the most appropriate treatment, be it medical, angioplasty or surgical.

However, in a significant proportion of patients the history, though suggestive, is less than typical for coronary heart disease. Similarly, many patients give a history of chest pain that is thought unlikely to be anginal. It is in these categories of patients that the diagnostic ability of these tests is most commonly sought. That is, to confirm the clinical suspicion of coronary heart disease in patients whose symptoms nonetheless are atypical, and firmly to exclude it in patients with chest pain who, on clinical grounds, are thought not to have it. Probably, these patients comprise the majority of out-patient referrals, so that the accuracy with which this information can be obtained is of considerable importance in management.

A number of definitions are used to describe the diagnostic reliability of these tests:

(1) *The sensitivity* is the intrinsic ability of the test to detect the

disease and is defined as the percentage of all the patients in a population with coronary heart disease (CHD) that the test will identify.

> Sensitivity = true positives (i.e. all patients with CHD ÷ all positives)

(2) *The specificity* refers to the percentage of those who do not have coronary heart disease, whom the test will correctly identify and is influenced by the number of falsely positive tests.

> Specificity = true negatives (i.e. all patients without CHD ÷ all negatives)

A perfect test would be both completely sensitive and specific – always detecting coronary heart disease when it existed and never diagnosing it when it was absent. But the disease in question and the technology involved do not allow such diagnostic utopia, so that present techniques will miss some with the disease and falsely diagnose it in others. Thus from a clinical point of view how confident can we be that the result of the test is accurate – be it positive or negative?

(3) *The predictive accuracy* is the percentage of those who have a positive or negative result that is truly positive or negative.

> Predictive accuracy = true positives or negatives ÷ all positives or negatives

In accordance with Bayesian theory[11] this is highly dependent on the prevalence of coronary heart disease in the population under study. For example, if we apply a test that is 90% sensitive and specific to an asymptomatic population in whom the disease prevalence is low, say 5%, there will be a few positive tests and many negative tests. Thus false positives and negatives will form small and large proportions of their respective totals; therefore the predictive accuracy of a positive test will be relatively low, while that of a negative test will be very high.

In a group of patients with atypical symptoms in whom the prevalence of coronary heart disease is, say, 50% the predictive accuracies of both positive and negative tests will be high. In a population with typical symptoms in which the prevalence of coronary heart disease approaches 90%, the impact of a falsely negative test will be considerable since the total number of negative tests will be small; thus the reliability of a negative test in excluding it will be low because the high proportion of false negatives relative to true negatives reduces the predictive value of a negative test to just over 50%[5].

The effect of the prevalence of coronary heart disease in the population on the predictive accuracy of a diagnostic test is best illustrated with respect to sex differences. The poorer reliability of ST segment depression during exercise as a marker for coronary heart disease in women can be accounted for by the lower prevalence of the disease. In the Coronary Artery Surgery Study, in which exercise tests and coronary arteriography were performed on over 3000 patients, the rate of false positive and negative results were similar in men and women, when allowance was made for the disease prevalence[12].

Exercise electrocardiography

Commonly referred to as exercise testing, the rationale for its use is that clinical and ECG evidence of coronary heart disease often are present only during or after exercise. Supervised exercise was first employed as a provocative test for angina by Masters and Oppenheim in 1929[13]; but it was not until 1941 that ST segment depression, the hallmark of myocardial ischaemia, was described after exercise[14]. Since then many modifications both of the form of exercise and of the method of recording the electrocardiogram have been made, such that several different techniques are now used in routine clinical practice – though the information sought and obtained is broadly similar.

Mode of exercise

Both supine and upright bicycle exercise can be used, though the latter is more common. The workload can be accurately determined and is usually increased in stages by some form of brake. Less distortion of the ECG tracing occurs than with treadmill exercise, though the maximum heart rate and oxygen consumption during bicycle ergometry is slightly lower[15].

Treadmills are more expensive than bicycles, but probably are more popular. Many eponymous protocols have been described, the best known of which is the Bruce protocol (full or modified)[16-18]. For clinical purposes, exercise capacity is usually described in terms of the stage of the exercise protocol that the patient achieves or the time at which pain or >1 mm ST segment depression occurs.

Performance of the test

Whatever mode of exercise is chosen a variety of end-points may be used to terminate the test, the most common of which are the attainment of a certain heart rate say (1) either 150 beats per minute, or (2) 90% of the age-predicted maximum, which could be described as submaximal. But it is more usual in the clinical setting of chronic stable angina to ask the patient to exercise to a symptom limited maximum level, the end-points being intolerable fatigue, dyspnoea or pain. In more sophisticated exercise laboratories, continuous recording of the oxygen consumption by direct measurement enables the maximum aerobic capacity to be identified, though in clinical practice this information has so far not been regarded as essential.

During any protocol safety demands that the test be terminated if any event occurs that renders continuation of the test hazardous – such markers are an important arrhythmia, marked planar ST segment depression (>2 mm) or a sustained fall in blood pressure (>10 mmHg).

Detection of myocardial ischaemia

Myocardial ischaemia may be diagnosed electrocardiographically, clinically or by both criteria.

(1) *Electrocardiographic*

Several groups of ECG leads have been recommended for recording the exercise ECG[19-21] though generally the most popular has been the conventional 12 lead system using a three channel recorder. Single bipolar lead systems utilizing the V5 monitoring position and different sites on the chest as the reference position (e.g. CM5 meaning V5 and the manubrium sterni) can be used with a single channel recorder but the yield relative to the 12 lead system is highly variable[22].

Use of sites on the torso for limb leads makes a 12 lead recording relatively simple and free of the distortion caused by leg and arm movement. This is the preferred and most widely adopted method at the present time.

(a) *ST segment shift.* The association between ST segment depression and clinical episodes of angina pectoris was described many years ago[23] and such ECG changes are now regarded as sensitive, though not entirely specific indicators of myocardial ischaemia. For clinical purposes, ST segment depression of $> 1\,mm$ $(0.1\,mV)$ that is downsloping or planar and occurs during or after exercise is regarded as indicating myocardial ischaemia. ST segment elevation occurring during exercise usually reflects underlying dyskinesia due to scarring from previous myocardial infarction but occasionally, and especially if it is very marked $(> 3\,mm)$, ST elevation may be due to severe reversible transmural ischaemia, when it is often accompanied by widening of the QRS complex[24-26].

(b) *Other ECG criteria.* Other reversible changes in the ECG affecting the QRS amplitude, the QT interval and the T-wave have been studied but in the absence of ST segment shift they are probably less reliable[27].

Ventricular arrhythmias occurring during exercise may be an indication for termination of the test, but in the absence of ST segment change they are poor indicators of the presence of coronary heart disease; however, the probability of developing clinical features of it in the future is enhanced and moreover the occurrence of ventricular arrhythmias in association with ST depression carries a poorer prognosis than ST depression alone[28,29].

(2) *Clinical*

(a) *Chest discomfort.* Although the patient's usual symtoms develop in only about half the tests in which significant ST shift occurs, when they do so, the likelihood of coronary heart disease is enhanced[30].

(b) *Exercise capacity.* The inability to sustain a normal peak level of cardiac work in the absence of other forms of disability also is suggestive[31]. This may be due to irreversible left ventricular dysfunction consequent upon previous myocardial infarction, or the development of reversible left ventricular dysfunction due to exercise induced myocardial ischaemia.

Other indicators of ischaemic left ventricular dysfunction are an inadequate blood pressure response (<10 mmHg), or a sustained fall in blood pressure (>10 mmHg); and such signs usually indicate severe underlying coronary heart disease[32].

Obfuscating factors

(1) Drugs

(a) Resting ST depression on the ECG, induced by *digoxin* may increase during exercise and even if the resting ECG is normal, significant ST depression may occur during exercise in the absence of coronary heart disease. However, very severe (>4 mm) ST depression is unlikely to be due simply to digoxin therapy.

(b) *Certain antidepressant drugs* and the phenothiazines can cause resting repolarization changes that are aggravated by exercise.

(c) *Diuretic* induced hypokalaemia may cause non-ischaemic ST depression during exercise.

(d) *Antianginal drugs.* Nitrates, calcium antagonists and beta-blockers all permit a higher workload before ischaemia develops, though less commonly will nitrates abolish ST depression in a progressive exercise test. If the exercise test is negative on drug therapy, while the clinical suspicion remains high, gradual discontinution of medication should be advised – the patient continuing only on nitrates as required and the test repeated.

(2) Pre-existing ECG abnormalities

Left bundle branch block and Wolff–Parkinson–White Syndrome render interpretation of the ST segment response during exercise invalid, though in right bundle branch block ischaemia of the left ventricle may be inferred from ST segment depression affecting the lateral ECG leads[33,34].

Left ventricular hypertrophy may predispose to subendocardial ischaemia during exercise and since left ventricular hypertrophy can occur with a normal ECG, especially in systemic hypertension, the latter may cause a false positive response.

Recent advances

More recently three new methods of recording or interpreting the ECG during exercise testing have been described.

(1) Precordial mapping

Introduced by Fox *et al.*, this test utilized 16 chest leads that were recorded almost simultaneously after maximal upright bicycle exercise.

Sensitivity was 96% and specificity 90%[35,36]. The site of ST segment depression also enabled information to be adduced about the likelihood of single or multivessel disease and some indication of which vessels were involved. The disadvantages of the test were the number of leads and the problem of obtaining satisfactory recording during exercise. Nonetheless it is an extremely accurate test that has been useful in assessing the effect of antianginal therapies, including drugs and surgery.

(2) Computer assisted exercise testing
Distortion of the ECG by artifact has always been a major problem in the interpretation of an exercise test. Computer averaging of the complexes represents a major advance with the abolition or marked reduction of muscle or movement artifact, thus facilitating the production of high quality recordings during exercise in multiple leads (Figure 6.1). This

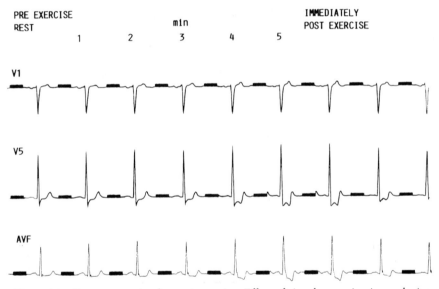

Figure 6.1 Computer assisted exercise testing. Effect of signal averaging in producing high quality distortion free complexes: summary of each minute of the test

enables continuous assessment to be made during exercise as well as giving computer derived measurements of several variables[37–40]. These innovations make it easier to apply exercise electrocardiography not only in the diagnosis and initial assessment of each patient but also in the evaluation of therapy.

Using a computer assisted 12 lead system and treadmill exercise a sensitivity and specificity of about 85% and 98% respectively can be expected[41].

(3) *ST segment/heart rate slope*

In 1982 a new test based on maximal treadmill exercise and utilizing the rate of development and extent of ST segment depression was claimed to be 100% reliable, not only detecting coronary heart disease but also in separating patients with one, two and three vessel disease. This would represent a significant advance but these results await confirmation at other centres – at present the analysis is very time consuming[42,43].

Prognostic implications of exercise testing (ETT)

The occurrence of significant ST segment depression during exercise is an important determinant of future coronary events and survival. Using

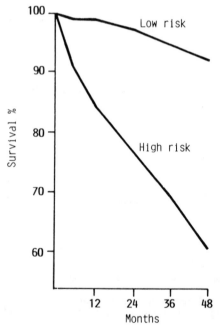

Figure 6.2 Risk stratification by exercise testing. Prediction of survival on basis of exercise test: 'low risk' patients had normal response, while 'high risk' patients did not. Modified from McNeer *et al.* (1978)

the exercise duration, ST segment response and the achieved heart rate, the exercise test can classify patients with chest pain into high and low risk groups (Figure 6.2).

Even in the presence of significant ST segment depression, if the exercise capacity is good then the prognosis is favourable (Figure 6.3).

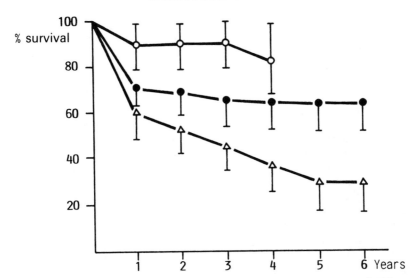

Figure 6.3 ST depression and exercise duration. In the presence of ST segment depression > 2 mm, progression of coronary disease is directly related to exercise duration. Modified from Ellestad (1975) △ = 3 min; ● = 5 min; ○ = 7 min

Value of the ETT in management

An exercise test is useful, partly because it strengthens the clinical diagnosis of coronary heart disease, but mainly because it provides information about certain objective variables from which the severity of the underlying coronary heart disease may be inferred. Assessment of exercise capacity is often helpful in assessing the symptoms and establishing a baseline with which future progress can be compared after either medical or surgical therapy. Population studies claim a fair correlation between symptoms and the severity of coronary heart disease[44,45], but the disparity between symptoms and pathology can be considerable in the individual patient[46]. Thus, importantly, the ETT can provide an objective index of the severity of ischaemia in those patients whose symptoms, though typical, are mild in that they do not preclude a 'normal' lifestyle.

Therefore the information that is useful in management is:

(1) The stage of exercise, or the heart rate/blood pressure product (double product), at which ST segment depression, or the patient's usual pain develops
(2) The maximum depression of the ST segment and its distribution in the 12 lead ECG
(3) The blood pressure response
(4) The total duration of exercise
(5) The occurrence of an important arrhythmia.

These variables illustrate the impact of the underlying coronary heart disease on cardiac function and thus are helpful in deciding whether medical treatment is appropriate, or whether coronary arteriography is warranted to assess the suitability for coronary bypass surgery.

Who should have an exercise test?

If, as the accumulating evidence suggests, the exercise test can be a powerful predictor of prognosis and can guide the therapeutic strategy[31,47-49], then the question is not 'who should have an exercise test?' but what reasons are there for not performing one in all patients with a history of chest pain that is at least suggestive of a cardiac origin? In some it is impracticable, including those who are physically incapable of exercising, because of severe claudication or other physical disability. In some it is unsafe – for example those in whom a non-coronary but serious cardiac cause, such as aortic stenosis or hypertrophic cardiomyopathy, may be obvious from clinical examination, and those in whom the symptoms are unstable.

In general, since the safety of maximal or submaximal exercise tests is extremely high[50] when carried out by properly trained staff according to safe guidelines, an exercise test ought to be regarded as a routine part of the clinical management in all other patients.

Non-invasive imaging techniques

Three techniques have evolved as non-invasive methods of studying cardiac function and structure and myocardial perfusion. In the management of coronary heart disease the two most commonly used are radionuclide ventriculography and thallium perfusion scintigraphy[51], though echocardiography also has a place.

Radionuclide ventriculography

This technique aims to provide and extend in a non-invasive way the information on ventricular structure and function that formerly was obtainable only by a contrast injection directly into the ventricle at the time of cardiac catheterization. In addition to studies carried out at rest, exercise is usually performed to provoke ischaemia so that its distribution and its effect on cardiac function can be studied. Thus the technique is useful in assessing the degree of irreversible dysfunction caused by previous myocardial infarction, the extent of reversible ischaemia induced by exercise, and the effect of the latter on global, regional and ventricular function. Most attention has been paid to the left ventricle, though recently there has been renewed interest in right ventricular function and structure. There are two methods by which this information may be obtained, first pass and multiple gated acquisition, or MUGA, scanning[52].

The left ventricular ejection fraction is a most important prognostic indicator in patients with coronary heart disease and with good technique, radionuclide ventriculography reliably provides this information non-invasively[60,61].

During exercise in normals, the ejection fraction rises by at least 5 units; while in patients with coronary heart disease the ejection fraction fails to rise normally, or falls revealing the effect of exercise induced ischaemia on global left ventricular function[62].

(b) Regional wall motion. With either technique wall motion abnormalities can be detected. When present at rest they may indicate the presence of an old myocardial infarction and when induced by exercise an assessment of the area of myocardium in jeopardy can be made.

(c) Ventricular volumes. The area length formula applied to contrast angiography has been widely applied also to radionuclide ventriculography. Accurate in normal ventricles, there are problems inherent in these calculations with asymmetric diseased ventricles and so non-geometric methods utilizing the relationship between ventricular activity and blood activity may be more reliable[63].

(d) Filling phase indices. Although ejection phase indices have received most attention, of considerable interest also is that portion of the time activity curve representing relaxation or diastole. This is because an early marker of ischaemia is delayed filling that may be detectable in the absence of abnormal systolic function[64].

(5) *Value of radionuclide ventriculography in management* – There is now good evidence that the most important prognostic factor in patients with coronary heart disease, not only after myocardial infarction but also in patients with chronic stable angina is the degree of left ventricular functional impairment. Evidence for this comes from several sources including the Coronary Artery Surgery Study (CASS) and the Veterans Administration Study (VA) of surgery for angina and from the CASS registry of patients suitable for randomization but who were not randomized (*vide infra*)[65-67]. The normal response to exercise is a rise in ejection fraction of 5% or more and failure to do so, or a fall, is a useful and graphic demonstration not only of the reversible effects of ischaemia but also the potential irreversible effect on left ventricular function of subsequent myocardial infarction. The fall in ejection fraction may be accompanied by a wall motion abnormality in the territory of the diseased vessel, whose size and effect on global LV function are useful clinical indices of the area of myocardium in jeopardy. As would be expected, the prognosis of patients with exercise induced ischaemia leading to left ventricular dysfunction is poorer compared to those with normal exercise responses despite the presence of anatomical evidence of coronary heart disease[48].

Thus not only is a radionuclide ventriculogram an accurate reflection of resting left ventricular function, it also demonstrates the degree of ventricular dysfunction caused by exercise induced myocardial ischaemia. These two items of information provide powerful prognostic information and are now being used with increasing frequency in the decision to proceed to coronary arteriography in patients with chronic stable angina and to complement the anatomical information gained by defining the effect of the coronary stenoses on left ventricular function.

In a severely symptomatic patient with an unequivocally strongly positive exercise test, there may be no compelling need to perform radionuclide ventriculography prior to coronary arteriography – though it would be of great value in a mildly symptomatic patient when, if strongly positive, it might persuade the physician to recommend coronary arteriography with a view to surgery. If, on the other hand, rest and exercise left ventricular function were found to be normal, then a conservative approach would be indicated.

Clearly it is of value in patients with ECG abnormalities such as left ventricular hypertrophy, resting ST segment changes, conduction disturbances, digoxin effect and evidence of previous myocardial infarction all of which preclude a precise diagnosis of ischaemia by exercise testing.

It is of value also in the very symptomatic patient, whose exercise test surprisingly is normal. The normal scan might suggest a change or direction in investigation and certainly question the need for coronary arteriography. In patients whose coronary arteriogram shows triple vessel disease and whose left ventricular function at rest is normal, a positive exercise scan might tip the scales in favour of surgery.

The functional significance of coronary stenoses that anatomically seem less than critical is also facilitated.

Myocardial perfusion scintigraphy

It is almost 25 years since the first attempts at myocardial perfusion scintigraphy were made using rubidium-86, followed by the potassium analogue caesium-131 and potassium-43[68–70]. The modern invasive techniques involve the direct intracoronary injection of radioactive inert gases, such as xenon or krypton-81m, and primarily are used in research studies.

(1) *Thallium* – For non-invasive assessment of myocardial perfusion, the most widely used agent is thallium-201 introduced in 1975 by Lebowitz et al.[71]. Thallium substitutes for potassium in the ATPase dependent sodium–potassium pump and when injected intravenously is widely distributed in the body. Although only 4% of the dose accumulates in the heart, the myocardial uptake is rapid – 80% being extracted during the first passage through the coronary circulation[72–74].

Like most non-invasive tests for coronary heart disease, thallium scanning usually incorporates both rest and exercise studies. This is because the distribution of thallium in the myocardium may change as a function of time following administration during exercise. Areas of reversible ischaemia induced by exercise are seen as cold spots when the heart is imaged immediately after exercise. These disappear when scanning is repeated four hours later, while defects due to infarction do not resolve. This redistribution phenomenon is due to continuous exchange with thallium circulating in the blood pool, resulting in wash-out from normal tissues and accumulation into previously underperfused areas (Figure 6.5).

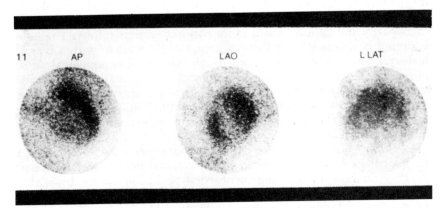

Figure 6.5 Thallium perfusion scintigraphy. Exercise thallium image showing infero-apical reversible defect indicating ischaemia.

(2) *Technique* – Routinely, thallium is injected at peak exercise on either a treadmill or bicycle ergometer system and, to maximize myo-cardial bloodflow, the patient is encouraged to continue exercising for a further minute. Fasting for 6 hours prior to the test will minimize splanchnic bloodflow, though this could adversely affect exercise per-formance. The heart is imaged immediately after exercise in several views (usually AP, LAO 30° and 60° and left lateral) and again four hours after injection.

(3) *Information obtained* – Although abnormalities of thallium dis-tribution are not specific for coronary heart disease, simplistically (in the context of the patient with chronic stable angina) a fixed thallium defect indicates previous infarction, while a reversible defect implies myocardial ischaemia. Thallium images may be analysed visually with or without computer processing, though many processing techniques have been applied to thallium images to improve their diagnostic accu-racy including tomography and statistical analysis.

(4) *Value of thallium scintigraphy in management* – The sensitivity and specificity of thallium scintigraphy in detecting coronary heart disease is between 80–90% and 85–95% respectively[75]. Since this is similar to a good history of angina, as with all non-invasive tests for ischaemia, it is not recommended for the diagnosis of coronary heart disease in the patient with typical symptoms. Thus an important clinical

use of thallium perfusion scintigraphy is in the diagnosis and assessment of coronary heart disease in patients in whom the history is atypical, or when the exercise ECG is positive in an asymptomatic patient – for example, after myocardial infarction or when an exercise test carried out for screening purposes is positive. In the patient with chronic stable angina its main use is to indicate the severity of underlying ischaemia when the symptoms are mild and the exercise ECG is strongly positive, or if the ECG cannot be interpreted because of pre-existing abnormalities. Large or multiple defects might suggest a sizeable area of myocardium in jeopardy and indicate the need for coronary arteriography. Thallium scanning is also helpful in the evaluation of the patient with a typical history when the exercise test surprisingly is negative or equivocal. Also, in patients in whom coronary arteriography has revealed a borderline stenosis in an important vessel, a thallium study may contribute to the assessment of its functional significance. But thallium scanning often underestimates the severity of disease and may not reliably identify multivessel disease[76].

(5) *Other non-invasive tests of myocardial perfusion* – The use of radiolabelled substrates utilized in myocardial energy metabolism is another method of assessing myocardial perfusion on the basis that absolute or relative reduction in perfusion leads to metabolic abnormalities and a failure of uptake of substrate. Much research work has been carried out using positron emitting substances, such as [^{11}C]palmitate or [^{13}N]amino acids, but as this requires the nearby presence of a cyclotron to produce this short-lived isotope (half-life 20 minutes) and a special camera to image it, the technique of positron emission tomography is likely to remain a research tool at least in the present economic climate. However, certain fatty acids, notably hexa- and hepta-decanoic acid, may be conveniently labelled with ^{123}I and, following intravenous injection, are rapidly taken up by the myocardium the distribution being proportional to bloodflow[77,78]. In ischaemia β-oxidation is impaired and uptake of the fatty acid is reduced. Early studies are promising but much more work is required before this technique will be available for the clinical evaluation of patients with chronic stable angina.

Echocardiography

This may be the simplest and most 'non-invasive' way of investigating global LV function and would be very useful in centres without a gamma camera. Moreover studies with exercise can indicate areas of reversible ischaemia, but for technical reasons this is unlikely to be preferable to radionuclide ventriculography, though it could substitute for it in its absence.

Ambulatory monitoring

Ambulatory electrocardiography is a routine investigation in cardiac units and in many general hospitals where it is usually employed for the detection of arrhythmias. More recently, ambulatory electro-cardiographic monitoring has been used to detect and record shifts in the position of the ST segment as a method of detecting the presence and measuring the frequency of myocardial ischaemia in patients with chest pain[79,80]. This has been facilitated by the introduction into clinical use of recorders with a frequency response low enough to record and faithfully reproduce episodes of ST segment depression. While there is debate concerning the meaning and cause of ST segment depression or elevation in asymptomatic normal individuals[81,82] there is now abundant evidence available to conclude that episodes of ST segment depression, or elevation > 1 mV, in patients with coronary heart disease do represent myocardial ischaemia[83–85]. Much useful and interesting information has been gained from ambulatory monitoring in such patients.

(1) Ambulatory episodes of ischaemia often occur at a significantly lower heart rate than during a standardized treadmill test.

(2) They are more frequent in patients with the most severe coronary heart disease, especially those with left main disease and triple vessel disease, though there is considerable overlap between individual patients.

(3) There are many more episodes of silent ischaemia than of angina and in some studies the frequency of painless ischaemia has been 70% of all episodes. Some patients, however, have only painful and some only painless ischaemia (Figure 6.6).

There is debate about the mechanism of these episodes of ST segment change which occur at a relatively low workload at rest or during the night[84,86]. Do they result from a reduction in coronary blood flow due to vasoconstriction adjacent to a coronary stenosis, or indeed spasm in a normal coronary artery; or do they simply represent increases in myocardial oxygen demand? Platelet aggregation, analogous to that responsible for cerebral transient ischaemia attacks, also could be a factor. It may be that any of these three mechanisms could be responsible in different patients, for it is now accepted that several different mechanisms may be responsible for myocardial ischaemia.

In carefully conducted studies with ECG and haemodynamic monitoring, Maseri and his colleagues found that no change in heart rate and blood pressure preceded the ischaemic episodes, which were characterized by ST depression, ST elevation or pseudonormalization of the T wave[87]. Pain was a late feature and this may explain the finding of others of an increase in the heart rate and blood pressure preceding attacks of angina. The earliest sign of ischaemia was a decrease in left ventricular function[88] and a reduction in oxygen saturation in the

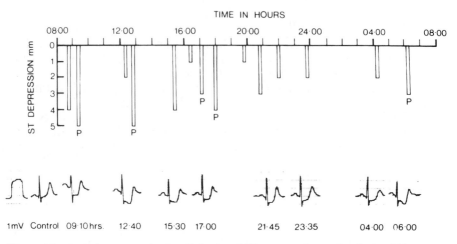

Figure 6.6 Ambulatory monitoring. Episodes of ST segment depression during 24 hour ambulatory monitoring. Note episodes denoted (P) were painful but that the majority were silent

coronary venous blood indicated that a fall in myocardial perfusion had occurred – indeed, angiographic confirmation of coronary spasm was demonstrated in some patients[89]. In contrast, other workers using ambulatory ECG recordings in a large consecutive series of patients undergoing diagnostic coronary arteriography noted that a significant increase in heart rate did precede episodes of ischaemia, though the magnitude of this change varied considerably between patients and for a given severity of coronary heart disease[84]. In their studies, nocturnal angina usually occurred in the context of severe triple vessel disease or left main stem disease and also was preceded by an increase in myocardial oxygen consumption[90]. Their conclusion was that coronary spasm need not necessarily be the cause of these episodes, since myocardial oxygen demand had increased. In only one patient out of 26 with normal coronary arteries could spasm be demonstrated as the cause of myocardial ischaemia.

It seems likely that a different spectrum of patients was studied by each group but that the latter study may be more representative of that seen by most physicians investigating chest pain. The greatest value of the studies of Maseri *et al.* is that they have shown beyond all reasonable doubt that mechanisms other than increased myocardial oxygen demand can cause ischaemia, which in many cases can be attributed to a dynamic obstruction to coronary flow either with or without pre-existing disease. Pathological studies have revealed the heterogeneity of atheroma from rigid calcific lesions to softer and more fibrous lesions that may or may not completely encircle the artery[91] – such eccentricity suggests that the unaffected segment of the media could be susceptible to vasomotor stimuli leading to vasoconstriction (Figure 6.7).

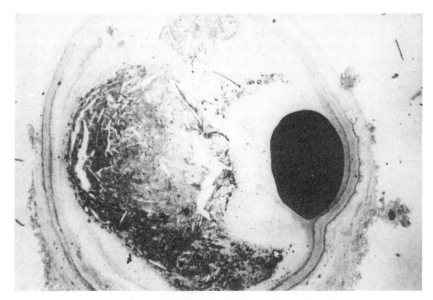

Figure 6.7 Eccentric coronary arterial stenoses. Note area of unaffected vessel wall on which the action of vasomotor stimuli could significantly influence the luminal diameter

Value of ambulatory monitoring in management

It is clear from ambulatory studies of ST segment changes that the total number of episodes of myocardial ischaemia in the patient with chronic stable angina is considerably greater than the frequency of angina itself would suggest. Thus, only by using a technique like ambulatory monitoring can episodes of silent ischaemia be detected and the magnitude of the 'total ischaemic burden' determined.

Ambulatory monitoring of the ST segment has been used most commonly in the investigation of patients with chest pain that occurs primarily or exclusively at rest in whom exercise testing may have been negative and not in the patient with chronic stable (usually effort related) angina pectoris.

In the context of chronic stable angina it may be of greatest value in the patient whose symptoms are mild but whose exercise test or nuclear studies suggest severe myocardial ischaemia – frequent episodes of ischaemia would support the consideration of surgery.

It has perhaps been of the greatest value in the assessment of the treatment of angina both medical and surgical[84]. Whether this application of the technique should move from the research area to clinical practice is debatable. There is always a case for obtaining maximum information about patients before embarking on medical treatment that may be lifelong and to ensure that that regimen has abolished or reduced the frequency of silent ischaemia as well as episodes of angina. There may not yet be sufficient evidence concerning the prognostic importance of silent ischaemia to justify this on a routine basis[92]. But in certain categories of patients, for example those who have declined or are unsuitable for surgery or in whom it has been unsuccessful, ambulatory monitoring could help by ensuring that medical treatment was indeed optimal.

Also in those with chest pain and less than critical coronary arterial lesions, in whom exercise testing and nuclear studies have been negative, the demonstration of episodes of ST depression at a low heart rate could suggest a dynamic component to the lesion and indicate that the most appropriate therapeutic approach would be to reduce coronary arterial tone rather than to reduce myocardial oxygen consumption. Ambulatory monitoring for ischaemia is a technique that awaits definition of its place in management. The demonstration of the frequency of silent ischaemia ensures that its role will increase.

TERTIARY (INVASIVE) INVESTIGATION

Invasive techniques

Coronary arteriography is the most expensive of all the routine inves-tigations of coronary heart disease because it requires several types of personnel: including an operator, who is usually a cardiologist (but may be a radiologist); an assistant; a nurse, who may double as the assistant; a radiographer; and a physiological measurement technician. In addition, overnight accommodation is usually required for at least the night of the procedure. However, if a brachial arteriotomy is used, coronary arteriography may be carried out as a day case and several centres using Judkins femoral approach also use the day case approach, especially when smaller catheters are used.

Primarily, coronary arteriography and left ventriculography are car-ried out to define the suitability for bypass surgery in patients with angina that is not adequately controlled on medical therapy, or in those whose symptoms may be mild but whom non-invasive investigation has classed as 'high risk'. Occasionally it may be performed in very symptomatic patients in whom non-invasive tests have been normal or equivocal and in whom doubt has arisen concerning the diagnosis of coronary heart disease. This indication ought to be diminishing in frequency as confidence in the results of these tests grows; but, presently, the 'normal coronary arteriogram' rate is about 20% in most centres.

In expert hands it is a painless procedure, complications are rare and the information gained is usually extremely valuable in management. Left ventricular function is assessed visually for the presence of areas of reduced or absent contractility consistent with previous myocardial infarction and for an 'eyeball' estimate of the ejection fraction. Left ventricular volumes can be estimated from the area length formula and the ejection fraction then may be calculated. Coronary stenosis are considered 'surgical' if there is a reduction in luminal diameter of >70% in two planes. Multiple views are usually taken to assist accuracy.

In all patients in whom the site and severity of the proximal lesions indicate that surgery should be considered great attention must be paid to the distal vessels and the likely adequacy of the 'run off' following bypass grafting.

INTEGRATED APPROACH TO INVESTIGATION

At the present time, the exercise ECG has become so widely and routinely used that the term exercise test is synonymous with it, even though exercise is a standard part of radionuclide ventriculography and thallium perfusion scintigraphy.

None of these tests is 100% sensitive or specific for diagnosing coronary heart disease nor is any diagnostic test ever likely to be. While the debate will continue, at the present time the nuclear tests probably are slightly more sensitive (though radionuclide ventriculography may be slightly less specific) in detecting coronary heart disease[5]. Exercise testing is simple to perform, involves no injections and employs a monitoring modality with which most clinicians are familiar (that is, the ECG). Thus it is the most acceptable of the non-invasive tests both to patients and physicians; and with the added sensitivity (without loss of specificity) that computer assistance confers, it is likely to remain as the initial step in the investigation of the patient with chronic stable angina. The choice of the mode of exercise will inevitably vary but as most patients still walk more often than cycle, treadmill exercise seems preferable and usually generates a greater maximal oxygen uptake than bicycle ergometry. The use of standard protocols enables the results of exercise tests to be widely interpreted, applied and understood; moreover, prognostic groupings are facilitated by referral to results obtained using standard protocols.

The patient with typical symptoms

Although the exercise test is likely to confirm the diagnosis, of greater interest are those variables that may be used to describe the test as strongly positive (Table 6.1). Patients in this category have a poorer prognosis that can be improved by surgery[93], so that such a result is an unequivocal indication for coronary arteriography. Although further information on myocardial perfusion or function using the nuclear techniques would be of value in any patient with a good history of angina, these tests are of greatest help in assessing those patients who have a good history but in whom, surprisingly, the exercise test is negative or equivocal. The predictive accuracy of the latter is sufficiently low to justify applying a further test, which if strongly positive might indicate coronary arteriography and if negative should obviate it. While the combination of a negative ETT and thallium or RNVG does not

Table 6.1   A 'strongly positive' exercise test

Those variables that define an exercise test as strongly positive and confer a poorer prognosis

(1) Exercise capacity:
    (a) Failure to complete Stage 2 of Bruce protocol (of equivalent)
    (b) Failure to achieve 70% maximum predicted heart rate

(2) Systolic blood pressure (SBP):
    (a) SBP rise of < 10 mmHg over 2 stages
    (b) Fall in SBP > 10 mmHg

(3) ST segment:
    (a) Depression (planar or downsloping) of > 2 mm
    (b) Post exercise persistence of ST depression for > 5 minutes

exclude coronary heart disease it does place such patients in a very low risk category and other factors, especially the severity of the symptoms, would be the deciding factors in proceeding to coronary arteriography.

The patient with atypical symptoms

In a male patient, a positive ETT would be regarded similarly as that in a patient with typical symptoms. In a female patient, the specificity and predictive accuracy are not sufficiently high to warrant coronary arteriography but if the thallium study or radionuclide ventriculography also were to be positive then coronary arteriography would be indicated.

Paradoxically, a negative exercise test in this population carries a high predictive accuracy of sufficient clinical importance to justify terminating the investigative process in most patients; though on an individual basis, persistent symptoms often lead to further investigation despite the fact that the diagnostic return often is little greater.

The mildly symptomatic patient

Decisions about further investigation in this group of patients are, presently, difficult and controversial. The knowledge that episodes of silent ischaemia usually outnumber episodes of angina means that the history does not give an accurate assessment of the total ischaemic burden in all patients. Moreover, sudden cardiac death and myocardial infarction unheralded by severe symptoms (or in many cases, by any symptoms) means that uncertainty must surround a management strategy based purely on the history. However, if an ETT is carried out on such a patient it may allow classification into a high or low risk category. If strongly positive, further confirmation of the severity of ischaemia should be sought by thallium scanning or radionuclide ventriculography. The latter may be more helpful, since it also provides a measurement of left ventricular function that could be of prognostic importance. This information is extremely useful in deciding whether to proceed to coronary arteriography and will be helpful in the discussions with the surgeons at a later stage, since more evidence of severe ischaemia may be required before operation is advised in a patient with mild symptoms that do not limit his lifestyle or prevent him from working (Figure 6.8).

The move towards better risk stratification in patients with chronic stable angina has been stimulated by the findings of the randomized trials of coronary artery bypass surgery. The European Study showed that a strongly positive exercise test was an important determinant of an improved prognosis after surgery[93]. But it may not be sensitive enough to identify all the patients who would benefit from surgery. The main determinant of prognosis apart from the distribution of coronary artery stenosis is left ventricular function so that its non-invasive assessment by radionuclide ventriculography could be justified in many patients. An important problem as far as exercise testing is concerned is that exercise capacity, one of the important variables in an exercise test, is poorly related to the ejection fraction and a 'normal' exercise capacity in association with a normal blood pressure response is quite feasible in the presence of mildly or moderately impaired left ventricular function. Thus assessment of left ventricular function should be practised more widely; for example, in those with impairment of exercise capacity or a poor blood pressure response that is not thought to be due to drug therapy, such as beta-blockade. Significant impairment of left ventricular function, especially when associated with reversible ischaemia, is a valid indication for coronary arteriography.

Many studies, of which the Cleveland Clinic series was the most comprehensive, have attested to the prognostic importance of the number and severity of coronary stenoses identified by coronary arteriography[46]. More recently the randomized trials of medical and surgical treatment have provided more information[66,67,93,94]. In addition to the CASS study, the CASS registry of patients with angina who have undergone coronary arteriography has yielded even more data on a much larger population.

Although the modern data suggest a more favourable prognosis than was suggested by the original studies, essentially the message is similar and fairly obvious: those with the most severe manifestations of coronary heart disease have a poorer prognosis, this being related to the number and site of the lesions. Left main stem lesions[93,95] and triple vessel disease (especially when the proximal left anterior descending artery is involved)[93] carry the worst prognosis. The more recent studies have also drawn attention to the importance of left ventricular function and if left ventricular function is impaired the prognosis is worse still[65,66]; even in patients with single vessel disease, the prognosis is poorer than those with triple vessel disease and good left ventricular function[65]. Among other factors, the ability to maintain good myocardial function in the presence of apparently extensive coronary disease will depend on the development of a collateral circulation. This can also be assessed to some extent by coronary arteriography, when the larger collaterals may be visible, and may be important in deciding about future treatment.

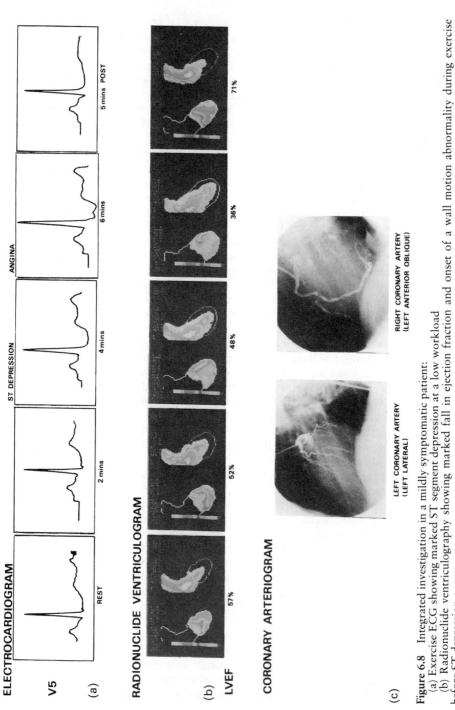

Figure 6.8 Integrated investigation in a mildly symptomatic patient:

(a) Exercise ECG showing marked ST segment depression at a low workload

(b) Radionuclide ventriculography showing marked fall in ejection fraction and onset of a wall motion abnormality during exercise before ST depression occurs

(c) Coronary arteriogram showing tight proximal stenosis of left anterior descending and right coronary arteries

However, the limitations of purely anatomical information is recognized and indeed highlighted by the results of non-invasive investigation, which can demonstrate the functional importance of those lesions identified by coronary arteriography. These factors indicate the need for an integrated approach to the investigation of the patient with chronic stable angina. Non-invasive testing should not be seen as being in competition with coronary arteriography, but rather as an indicator for and a complement to it in those who require it and as a means of avoiding it in those who do not.

MEDICAL TREATMENT OF ANGINA

Introduction

Before embarking on drug therapy for angina that is likely to be lifelong, it is important to make a general assessment of the patient to identify those adverse features of lifestyle that can be improved if necessary. These include cigarette smoking, hyperlipidaemia, obesity, lack of exercise and employment that is unsuitable either physically or mentally. Primarily medical antianginal treatment aims to relieve symptoms or episodes of myocardial ischaemia but also it seems prudent to reduce the coronary risk profile in the hope of influencing the progression of the disease and preventing future coronary events[96,97]. Some of these measures may be important in complementing the action of drugs. For example, reversal of obesity will reduce myocardial oxygen demand during exercise and stopping smoking is mandatory for it is now clear that in addition to imposing an increased coronary risk[97] cigarette smoking decreases the efficacy of certain antianginal drugs – notably the beta-blockers and calcium antagonists[98].

Dietary advice may be helpful not only to control obesity but also to lower the serum cholesterol level. The simplest message for those whose cholesterol is moderately high (>6 mmol l^{-1}) is to reduce the intake of saturated fat by 25%. Often this may be accomplished by reducing the consumption of dairy produce and red meat with replacement by fibre rich carbohydrates, white meat and fish. For those in whom the cholesterol is >7 mmol l^{-1}, the data from the lipid research clinics provides a sound base for prescribing a cholesterol lowering agent, such as cholestyramine, if dietary measures are insufficient[99]. More complex hyperlipidaemias will require more specific dietary and pharmacological treatment, consideration of which is outwith the scope of this chapter.

There is little doubt that the majority of middle-aged people are physically unfit. Equally, there is no doubt that physical conditioning and the acquiral of a 'training effect' leads to a markedly decreased double product during exercise, thus reducing the myocardial oxygen requirement of any given level of exercise[100]. A significant training effect can be achieved by moderate exercise for 30 minutes three times a week and the intensity of exercise likely to produce this can be ascertained by an exercise test. However, since exercise is the main stimulus to the development of myocardial ischaemia, it must be advised with caution. Strenuous sports[101] should be avoided, while more gentle but regular exercise such as walking, swimming, cycling and in selected low risk cases jogging should be encouraged. Dynamic exercise of this kind can lead to a modest training effect that favourably influences the anginal threshold, well being, effort capacity and body weight.

Antianginal therapy

Physiological considerations

Ideally the prescription of an antianginal regimen for an individual patient should be guided by the mechanism of ischaemia presumed most likely to be predominant. Broadly speaking the 'medical' approach is

(1) To reduce myocardial oxygen requirements, which can be accomplished in most patients
(2) To improve myocardial perfusion, which may be possible in some
(3) Most frequently, to use a combined strategy.

Angina pectoris occurs when there is an imbalance between myocardial oxygen supply and demand, and traditional teaching emphasizes the relationship between physical effort and the production of chest pain that first was described by Heberden in 1792[1]. Although Osler in 1920 suggested that coronary arterial spasm might be the cause of angina[102], until fairly recently, conventional wisdom had it that artheromatous coronary arteries were incapable of alterations in tone. But it is now more widely appreciated that areas of unaffected vessel wall adjacent to atheromatous plaques are susceptible to vasoconstrictor (and vasodilator) influences that can dramatically affect the residual cross sectional area (Figure 6.7). Indeed this was the mechanism postulated by Prinzmetal in 1959[24] when he described ST segment elevation in a group of patients with angina occurring at rest that was relieved by glyceryl trinitrate. Moreover in 1976[103] Maseri and his colleagues elegantly demonstrated large areas of reversible transmural myocardial ischaemia associated with documented coronary aterial spasm in patients with angiographically normal coronary arteries. This concept of dynamic variation in coronary tone with or without coronary artery stenosis provides a useful working hypothesis to explain the various clinical presentations of angina pectoris. It helps to account for the occurrence of angina, albeit rarely, in patients with normal coronary arteries, the variation in exercise threshold (such as the early morning 'walk-through' phenomenon) and the effect of cold in patients with effort related angina pectoris. Increased coronary arterial tone also could explain the episodes of angina at rest and of nocturnal angina reported by some patients with predominantly angina of effort. However, in such patients coronary arterial disease is usually very severe and other mechanisms, such as platelet aggregation, also have been suggested. Nonetheless this concept of 'mixed angina' provides a basis for the rational use of the various antianginal agents now at our disposal for the medical treatment of angina pectoris.

Presently, the three main groups of drugs available for the treatment of angina are the nitrates, beta-blockers and calcium antagonists; associated drug therapy may include lipid lowering drugs, anti-hypertensive agents (other than those used for angina), digoxin, diuretics and anti-arrhythmic agents. The clinical pharmacology of these agents is dealt with in detail in a companion volume[104] so only a brief summary of the main points that are relevant to the overall management of the patient is given here.

Nitrates

In 1857 Lauder Brunton described the dramatic clinical effect of amyl nitrate and in 1879 William Murrell demonstrated that glyceryl trinitrate had similar effects[105,106]. This profound relief of symptoms is the product of a series of events resulting from the basic pharmacologic action of nitrates, which is relaxation of vascular (especially venous) smooth muscle[107]; pooling of blood peripherally diminishes the heart volume and the associated fall in left ventricular systolic pressure reduces wall stress and myocardial oxygen consumption, while the fall in left ventricular end diastolic pressure facilitates greater capillary bloodflow to the ischaemic area. Although dilatation of collateral vessels also enhances perfusion, dilatation of the large coronary arteries (as suggested by Sir Thomas Lewis) probably is important only in unstable angina and those rare cases of 'variant' angina, when severe coronary vasoconstriction is important[108]. In patients with chronic stable angina, glyceryl trinitrate failed to alleviate pacing induced angina despite evidence of increased coronary bloodflow[109]. There is also a small reduction in left ventricular afterload due to arteriolar dilatation, though the reflex tachycardia induced by these effects may limit the oxygen sparing effect somewhat.

(1) *Glyceryl trinitrate (GTN)* – Sublingual GTN has stood the test of time as an effective and rapid treatment for the acute attack of angina and for its immediate prophylaxis. Its onset of action is usually within one to three minutes, though its short duration of action of about 20 minutes limits its usefulness for chronic prophylaxis.

(2) *Isosorbide dinitrate (ISDN)* – ISDN was introduced for oral therapy and if given in large enough doses therapeutic blood levels are attained[110]. Numerous studies have addressed the questions of effectiveness or otherwise of the oral nitrates and of tolerance[111–115]. Results are conflicting and, formerly, negative results were attributed to inadequate dosing; but subsequent double blind placebo controlled studies with large doses also have not been encouraging. After 4 weeks, treatment with ISDN in a dose of 160 mg per day was found to be no better than

placebo in reducing attacks of angina and during exercise testing there was no improvement in the time to angina or exercise induced ST segment depression[116]. Benefit has been reported in a number of other studies, however, and in one of these a further increase in exercise duration was found after sublingual glyceryl trinitrate indicating that tolerance to the effects of glyceryl trinitrate had not occurred, as had been previously suggested[117].

In an investigation of tolerance the effects of acute single and multiple doses varying fom 15 to 120 mg were compared[118]. Acutely time to angina and total exercise time were prolonged to the same extent by each dose, an effect that persisted for 8 hours and was unrelated to plasma levels. During chronic therapy, improvement in these variables was evident only at 2 hours despite higher plasma levels than in the acute study; again these effects were not dose related. This suggests that during chronic therapy a high rapidly rising plasma concentration of ISDN is required to produce significant effects. Thus sustained release preparations may not be ideal and some studies have been discouraging.

Thus, although the general clinical impression is that oral nitrates may confer some benefit, their true place in chronic therapy is not established and this may be related to inappropriate dosing regimens and the development of tolerance.

(3) *Alternative nitrate delivery systems* – Nitroglycerin ointment was the first attempt to deliver nitroglycerin in a non-oral form and a number of studies have demonstrated adequate blood levels for up to 8 hours[119]. Major disadvantages are the need for application up to three times a day and practical difficulties with clothing particularly during warm weather making it a less than ideal route of administration in the active patient.

(a) *Transdermal nitrates.* Transdermal glyceryl trinitrate patches have become available and are designed to deliver a steady supply of glyceryl trinitrate through the skin for 24 hours. The rate of absorption is reported to be constant and related to the impregnated dose. Several studies have now been reported and the data are conflicting regarding both efficacy and duration of action. There have been several negative studies but some have been promising, however, especially when a nitrate free interval has been used between dosing[120-122].

(b) *Buccal GTN.* The buccal mucosa provides a site of rapid absorption avoiding first pass hepatic metabolism. The acute anti-anginal action appears to be as effective as sublingual glyceryl trinitrate and a prolonged action has been documented; a double blind study has reported no decrease in anti-anginal effect on chronic dosing[123]. Clinical experience, however, remains limited though the preparation appears well tolerated and side effects are comparable to those obtained with sublingual glyceryl trinitrate.

(c) *Nitrate aerosols.* Also available now are metered dose aerosols of GTN; the spray is directed to the buccal mucosa and absorption is rapid. This is more expensive than ordinary glyceryl trinitrate but its rapid absorption is particularly beneficial in patients who have difficulty in dissolving the tablets and the formulation is not subject to loss of activity on storage.

(4) *Mononitrates* – Oral ISDN is extensively metabolized in its first pass through the liver and its bioavailability is about 25%. The drug has two pharmacologically active mononitrate metabolites, 5-mononitrate and 2-mononitrate. The plasma half-life of the 5-mononitrate is 4.2 hours and it undergoes no significant first pass metabolism[124]. This compound is now available in a variety of proprietary preparations and appears to offer predictable systemic bioavailability. It remains to be determined whether it is more effective clinically than ISDN. In summary, glyceryl trinitrate sublingually remains the drug of choice for acute attacks of angina pectoris and even today the long term efficacy of ISDN or glyceryl trinitrate remains in doubt. Tolerance probably does develop despite the maintenance of adequate plasma levels and it may be that peak levels are more important, thus necessitating more frequent dosing intervals and possibly lower doses than are used at present.

Beta-blockers

Acute decreases in myocardial perfusion and oxygen supply may be an important mechanism of ischaemia in some patients with chronic stable angina, but increased myocardial oxygen demand caused by exercise or emotion is the usual reason for an attack of angina pectoris in most. Beta-blockers reduce myocardial oxygen demand by lowering heart rate, blood pressure and contractility especially during exercise; the increased oxygen requirements caused by the attendant increase in left venticular end diastolic volume detracts from this effect only slightly.

That beta-blockers have remained so prominent in the treatment of myocardial ischaemia during two decades is testimony to the original

Table 6.2 Beta-blockers. Ancillary properties of several commonly used beta-blockers

	Beta 1 selectivity	Partial agonist activity	Membrane stabilizing activity	Half-life (Hours)
Acebutolol	?	+	+	3
Atenolol	+	—	—	6–9
Metoprolol	+	—	+	3–4
Nadolol	—	—	—	14–24
Oxprenolol	—	+	+	1–4
Pindolol	—	+ +	—	2–5
Propranolol	—	—	+	3–5
Sotalol	—	—	—	7–18
Timolol	—	—	—	2–5

+ = Present
— = Absent

hypothesis of Sir James Black[125] that reduction in sympathetic stimulation would reduce myocardial oxygen demand and to the importance of the latter in the provocation of myocardial ischaemia. The first beta-blocker to be used in routine clinical practice, propranolol, has been followed by more than 20 others and still more are undergoing clinical trails. Since their efficacy is related to beta-blockade, equivalent doses of all beta-blockers ought to be equally good in the treatment of exercise induced angina pectoris. However, certain ancillary properties are of clinical importance and should be considered when choosing a beta-blocker – these include lipid solubility, cardioselectivity, partial agonist activity and membrane stabilizing activity (Table 6.2).

(1) *Solubility* – Lipophilic beta-blockers, for example propranolol and metoprolol, are well absorbed but are subject to first pass hepatic metabolism and show marked variability in plasma levels[126]. Hydrophilic beta-blockers are poorly absorbed from the gut, but plasma levels after single and multiple dosing (for example with atenolol) are relatively uniform. They are excreted essentially unchanged by the kidney. These factors may be of more than a pharmacokinetic curiosity, since with lipophilic drugs the potential exists for a pharmacokinetic interaction with other agents that undergo similar biotransformation, such as cimetidine, the plasma levels of which are enhanced by propranolol[127]. The plasma levels of verapamil, however, seem not to be significantly affected by propranolol[128].

Also of clinical importance is the influence of cigarette smoking, which has been shown to reduce the anti-ischaemic efficacy of nifedipine, propranolol and atenolol[98]. Plasma levels of propranolol and nifedipine are significantly lower during smoking, possibly due to induction of hepatic metabolism by nicotine. This observation may have important implications not only for the management of patients with angina for in the recently published MRC trial in mild hypertension, only the non-smokers in the propranolol treated group showed a reduction in cardiovascular events[129].

The narrow effective dose range and long half-life of the hydrophilic beta-blockers may be an advantage in that once daily dosage is possible without resort to special formulations, as are often required with the lipophilic beta-blockers. Hydrophilic beta-blockers cross the blood–brain barrier poorly, in contrast to the lipophilic beta-blockers and this may be associated with a lower incidence of CNS side effects. With increasing age hepatic and renal function deteriorate and hepatic blood flow may fall by 50%, thereby reducing the first pass hepatic metabolism and clearance of lipophilic drugs leading to higher plasma levels. Thus the hydrophilic beta-blockers also may be preferable in the elderly, since renal excretion is not a problem until glomerular filtration rate falls below 35 ml min^{-1}.

(2) *Cardioselectivity* – This term denotes those agents that preferentially and reversibly bind to beta-1 receptors and it should be emphasized that since the heart is not unique in possessing beta-1

receptors a better term is beta-1 selectivity. Also it should be remembered that selectivity is not synonymous with specificity and increasing dosage leads to beta-2 receptor blockade. Although much commercial import-ance is attached to this property, all beta-blockers will effectively anta-gonize cardiac beta-1 receptors; but in the treatment of angina not only is beta-2 receptor blockade unnecessary, in some patients (notably those with reversible airways disease) it could be deleterious. Others in whom non-selective beta-blockade potentially is disadvantageous are diabetics and patients with peripheral vascular disease. Since the use of a beta-1 selective agent allows access to and stimulation of the beta-2 receptors in bronchial smooth muscle by inhaled beta-2 stimulants, beta-1 selective drugs might be preferred in patients with reversible airways obstruc-tion[126,130]. But all beta-blockers are best avoided if suitable alternatives, for example, calcium antagonists can be used.

The metabolic response to hypoglycaemia is mediated not only by glycolysis but also by gluconeogenesis resulting from beta-2 stimulation of hepatocytes; thus hypoglycaemia affecting insulin dependent diabetics may be prolonged by non-selective beta-blockade. The adrenergic ner-vous response to hypoglycaemia, which alerts the patient, also may be limited especially by non-selective drugs[130]. In peripheral vascular disease sparing of beta-2 receptors, theoretically, may be beneficial for cutaneous blood flow but the reduced cardiac output that occurs to some extent with all beta-blockers at rest and more importantly during exercise reduces limb blood flow and potentially could aggravate symptoms.

(3) *Partial agonist activity (PAA)* – The possible advantages of this property previously termed intrinsic sympathomimetic activity have always been debated. Beta-adrenoceptor stimulation occurs when sym-pathetic tone is low, for example at rest or during sleep, while during exercise these drugs display their status as beta-blockers. The degree of PAA for each such agent is expressed as that percentage of the maximum beta-adrenoceptor stimulating effect attainable with isoprenaline (usu-ally on heart rate) and is 10% for oxprenolol, 20% for practolol and 35% for pindolol. Mild stimulation of beta-2 receptors may relax smooth muscle in the peripheral vasculature, the bronchi and the cor-onary tree. However, during exercise access to the beta adrenoceptors by the increased levels of circulating catecholamines is competitively antagonized. The net result of treatment with these drugs is little or no reduction of resting heart rate but reduction of exercise induced tachycardia that is slightly less than with a full beta-blocker[131].

Clinical situations in which PAA has been claimed to be important include angina in patients with poor left ventricular function, reversible airways disease, or peripheral vascular disease. No clinically significant advantage in patients with impaired left ventricular function has been documented over beta-blockers devoid of PAA, although drugs with even greater degrees of PAA are being developed that may be especially useful in this context.

In reversible airways obstruction beta-1 selectivity may be preferable to PAA, since non-selective beta-blockers with or without PAA impair the response to inhaled beta-2 stimulants.

PAA may be an advantage in patients with peripheral vascular disease, though the reduced exercise cardiac output may offset any local effects of beta-2 stimulation. Some studies suggest that cold hands and feet are less frequent with beta-blockers with PAA. In the absence of a consensus, the same care that should apply to the prescription of any beta-blocker should be observed with these dugs. When pindolol and atenolol were compared in a double blind clinical trial in patients with both effort related and nocturnal angina pectoris the frequency of ST segment depression on 24 hour ambulatory ECG monitoring was lower both during the day and night on atenolol[132]. Day and night time heart rates were lower on atenolol, suggesting that in patients with severe angina a reduction of heart rate even at rest appears to be beneficial, whether the underlying mechanism of ischaemia is reduced myocardial perfusion or increased oxygen demand.

With the possible exception of a significant degree of PAA these pharmacological differences do not affect the peak degree of beta-blockade conferred by equivalent doses of the currently available beta-blockers. Many would agree that since beta-2 blockade is non-contributory to the antianginal effect, a beta-1 selective agent seems preferable. The choice would then depend on duration of action with a convenient dosing interval, physician experience and individual patient acceptability.

(4) *Value in management* – Beta-blockers have remained the standard therapy for chronic stable angina pectoris since their introduction to clinical practice 20 years ago; indeed they have become the treatment against which novel agents must be compared.

Although there are several reasons for this, the most important is that they are very effective in relieving symptoms and evidence of ischaemia in patients with effort related angina pectoris[83,133]. Yet they do not treat the underlying problem, which is restriction of coronary blood flow, and quite simply reduce the increased myocardial oxygen requirements that exercise (or emotion) imposes by limiting the associated rise in heart rate, blood pressure and contractility, thus restoring the imbalance between oxygen delivery and demand.

Another reason for their popularity among the prescribing medical public is the notion that beta-blockade may prevent myocardial infarction or sudden death in patients with coronary heart disease or hypertension. This seems plausible given the known arrhythmogenic inotropic and chronotropic effects of catecholamines, which beta-blockade competitively antagonizes. That they also lower the blood pressure facilitates the treatment of that sizeable minority of patients with angina who also are hypertensive. The efforts of the pharmaceutical industry were at their most apposite with the coining of the term 'cardioprotective', a label which has stuck. The greatest stimulus to this image was the demonstration that certain beta-blockers reduced mortality and recurrent myocardial infarction in patients with proven myocardial infarction[134-136]. These factors have influenced cardiological thinking profoundly especially in the United Kingdom where the idea of beta-blockers was conceived and where they were first used. But now that the beneficial effects after myocardial infarction are being seen in perspective and since a primary protective effect in hypertension is not apparent[129] there may be a time for reappraisal. This is particularly so in view of the symptom side effects of beta-blockers and the growing appreciation of the effect of these on the quality of life. But these must be kept in perspective since neither has any drug been shown to be superior to beta-blockade in relieving effort related ischaemia, nor is any drug ever likely to be free from side effects. Moreover it is probable that in a symptomatic disease, such as angina, the importance of mild side effects is much less than in an asymptomatic condition, such as hypertension.

However, a significant proportion of patients do not respond adequately to beta-blockers or experience intolerable side effects with them and in some patients they are contraindicated.

Recently calcium antagonists have been introduced in the treatment of angina and have been claimed by some to be an effective alternative to beta-blockade.

Calcium antagonists

(1) *General considerations* – More than twenty years ago the name 'calcium antagonist' was given by Fleckenstein to those compounds, of which verapamil was the first, that inhibited the slow influx of calcium necessary for the contraction of myocardial and vascular smooth muscle cells[137]. From their coronary and peripheral vasodilatory properties together with their negative inotropic effect he recognized their potential in the treatment both of hypertension and angina pectoris[138,139]. At that time beta-blockers were becoming established as the first line treatment for angina and, in general, they have proved to be effective and safe in long term use. Recently, new concepts about the pathophysiology of angina have resulted in a reappraisal of traditional therapeutic strategies, such that calcium antagonists are now being used with increasing frequency in the treatment of angina. It could be argued that calcium antagonists would be a more appropriate treatment for angina, since they have the potential to increase coronary blood flow[140]. Indeed it was the recognition of the importance of increased coronary vascular tone in some patients with myocardial ischaemia that facilitated the emergence of calcium antagonists as important agents in the treatment of coronary heart disease[141-143].

As expected, they are particularly useful in the treatment of ischaemia caused by coronary spasm, as in Prinzmetal or variant angina[144-146]. Also in many patients with unstable angina there is evidence for coronary vasoconstriction as an important component on a basis of coronary heart disease and improvement has followed treatment with calcium antagonists[147-149].

The calcium antagonists have also been advocated in the treatment of patients with chronic stable angina, since variation in coronary arterial tone may influence myocardial perfusion and therefore the pattern of symptoms in such patients. In these patients the mechanisms of action of calcium antagonists could include improvement in coronary blood flow due to coronary vasodilatation, a reduction in myocardial oxygen demands due to peripheral vasodilatation, a small negative inotropic effect and a metabolic effect involving more efficient energy utilization[150-153].

Three calcium antagonists are in routine clinical use. These are, in order of discovery, verapamil, nifedipine and diltiazem. Unlike the beta-blockers, structurally the calcium antagonists are a heterogeneous group of compounds with important differences in pharmacological action (Table 6.3). For example, the negative inotropic effect is most pronounced with verapamil, an effect that is energy sparing and which

Table 6.3 Calcium antagonists. Main pharmacological effects of the three clinically available calcium antagonists

	Heart rate	Arteriolar tone	Cardiac pacemaker tissue	Cardiac contractility
Nifedipine	0/↑	↓↓↓	0	0/↓
Verapamil	0/↓	↓↓	0/↓	0/↓↓
Diltiazem	0/↓	↓↓	0/↓	0/↓

0 = no effect
↓ = decrease
↑ = increase

contributes to its antianginal action. Though the peripheral vaso-dilatory effect leads to a reduction in left ventricular systolic stress it may be accompanied by a reflex tachycardia, which is more pronounced with nifedipine than verapamil or diltiazem – perhaps because of their weak depressant effects on the sinoatrial node. In groups of patients with coronary heart disease, there is no increase in mean heart rate with nifedipine during chronic therapy but a mild increase in heart rate persists in some patients[154].

Many studies have shown that calcium antagonists can increase coronary blood flow in man and increase the luminal diameter of coronary arterial lesions. Increased post-stenotic myocardial blood flow has also been demonstrated following nifedipine[140]. While increased coronary vascular resistance may not be an important mechanism in effort related angina due to concentric coronary stenoses, many lesions may be eccentric and thus remain susceptible to vasoactive influences including the vasodilatory effect of calcium antagonists. Thus the mechanisms of action of the calcium antagonists in chronic stable angina are complex but it seems likely that an increase in coronary blood flow to the ischaemic area, either directly or through the collateral circulation, could be important.

(a) Efficacy in chronic stable angina. Preliminary open data suggested that nifedipine decreased angina frequency by 70% but in placebo controlled studies it reduced episodes of angina and glyceryl trinitrate consumption by 40–50% – studies of exercise induced ischaemia and exercise duration have given similar results[83,155,156]. The variable therapeutic response to nifedipine may be due partly to marked differences in plasma levels, as a result of first pass metabolism, but it has also been suggested that coronary anatomical factors that might favour a 'steal' phenomonen could be important[157].

Early studies with verapamil in angina were equivocal due to inadequate dosage, but recent studies using higher doses (360–480 mg daily) show significant reductions in anginal frequency and glyceryl trinitrate consumption of at least 50% together with improvements in exercise induced ischaemia and exercise duration of similar magnitude as can be obtained by beta-blockade[158–160]. Diltiazem was the third calcium antagonist to be available for clinical use. Like verapamil, its spectrum of effects include delay in conduction through the atrioventricular node together with a mild negative chronotropic effect. In common with both verapamil and nifedipine, peripheral arteriolar vasodilatation is the major effect in man together with the potential to dilate large coronary arteries. In double blind clinical studies, diltiazem has been shown to improve both subjective and objective indices of myocardial ischaemia[161,162].

(2) *Combination therapy with beta-blockers* – The potential for coronary vasodilation by the calcium antagonists – either in promoting better myocardial perfusion during exercise or preventing vasoconstriction – together with the favourable effects of peripheral arteriolar dilation in reducing left ventricular afterload, suggest a beneficial drug interaction with β-adrenoceptor blockers whose action is to reduce myocardial oxygen demands mainly by reducing heart rate.

(a) Nifedipine. Of the few double-blind placebo controlled trials in which the combined effect of nifedipine and beta-blockers have been studied, three illustrate some general points about antianginal trials in addition to defining the role of nifedipine in management of angina[163–165]. In the first[163], recording of angina frequency and nitrate consumption showed that although combination therapy was more effective than placebo or nifedipine alone, it was only slightly better than propranolol alone. In the second study, a small improvement in symptoms occurred on the combination compared with beta-blockers alone and exercise tolerance increased[164]. In the third study[165], the objective indices used (24 hour ambulatory monitoring of the ST segment and exercise testing using precordial ST segment mapping) allowed clear separation of individual drug effects and identification of the added effects of the combination. These data showed conclusively that the combination, which reduced exercise ischaemia and episodes of ischaemia on ambulatory monitoring (many of which are painless) by 90 and 95%, respectively, was better than either drug alone. Propranolol was better than nifedipine and there was no difference in the two doses of propranolol, which were 240 and 480 mg daily (Figure 6.9(a)). By contrast, the subjective indices of chest pain and nitrate consumption were only slightly improved on the combination than on propranolol alone, which in turn was superior to nifedipine alone. These studies emphasize the difficulty in demonstrating an improvement when combination therapy is compared

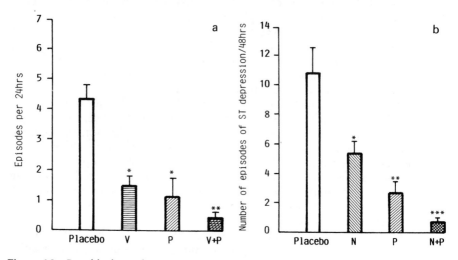

Figure 6.9 Beta blocker/calcium antagonist combinations.

(a) Effects of verapamil 360 mg/day, atenolol 100 mg/day and that combination on episodes of ischaemia during ambulatory monitoring

(b) Effects of nifedipine 60 mg/day, propranolol 480 mg/day and that combination on episodes of ischaemia during ambulatory monitoring

with an effective treatment like beta-adrenoceptor blockade alone in effort related angina pectoris; and the importance of using objective techniques, which detect ischaemia electrocardiographically rather than depending solely on the subjective data. Moreover it is important to record the severity of ischaemia during exercise as well as the exercise time or work done, which could be influenced by factors other than ischaemia such as tiredness of the legs on beta-blockers. Also these studies suggest that rather than being prescribed as a single agent in chronic stable angina nifedipine may be used to best advantage in combination with a beta-adrenoceptor blocker.

(b) Verapamil. Five placebo controlled studies of verapamil and propranolol have shown that the combination is superior to either drug alone; the doses of verapamil ranged from 320 to 480 mg daily, which is much higher than recommended initially[159,166–169]. In three of these studies the combination was used when monotherapy had failed to control the symptoms. All these studies confirmed that combination therapy had additive effects and was superior to either drug alone, using both subjective and objective criteria of efficacy. In one study[159] verapamil, atenolol and that combination were compared in a double-blind placebo controlled study of identical design to that with nifedipine already described. The objective indices confirmed the superiority of the combination and also agreed with earlier studies showing that verapamil was as effective as a beta-adrenoceptor blocker in reducing exercise induced ischaemia (Figure 6.9(b)).

(c) Diltiazem. In keeping with the beneficial effects noted with the combination of beta-blockers and either nifedipine or verapamil, that with diltiazem has also been shown to be superior to beta-blockade alone when objective criteria were assessed in double blind placebo controlled studies[162].

(3) *Potential adverse effects of combination therapy* – Since calcium influx is important in the generation of normal pacemaker activity in the sinus node and in the conduction of these impulses through the atrioventricular node and since sympathetic activity also facilitates these mechanisms and promotes myocardial contractility the possibility of adverse cardiac interactions with beta-blockers arises. But the structural heterogeneity of the calcium antagonists is reflected in their different properties with respect to contractility, cardiac conduction and automaticity and arterial tone in man[137–139,170].

(a) Myocardial depression. While all the currently available calcium antagonists share vasodilatation as their main property, nifedipine is the most potent both experimentally and clinically. In patients with normal left ventricular function, this causes a rise in cardiac output when nifedipine is given alone. By contrast, the acute administration of verapamil usually does not increase cardiac output, despite peripheral vasodilatation, thus implying a negative inotropic effect – indeed, a fall in left ventricular contractility occurs transiently after intravenous injection[171]. These haemodynamic differences probably reflect both the more potent arteriolar dilating effects of nifedipine and the greater intrinsic negative inotropic effect of verapamil. They assume greater importance if calcium antagonists are combined with beta-blockers, when a small increase in cardiac output occurs with nifedipine despite a fall in LV dp/dt, while indices of contractility decrease with verapamil[171,172]. The potential for myocardial depression during long term oral therapy may be greater with verapamil than with nifedipine or diltiazem but this complication is unlikely to occur in patients with normal left ventricular function prior to treatment in whom ejection fraction responses have been shown to remain unchanged[166,167]. In such patients, an increase in echocardiographic dimensions or diastolic volume has been demonstrated in double blind placebo controlled studies but the bradycardic effect of combination treatment may have been partly responsible for this[174,175].

While there are anecdotal reports of cardiac failure with the combination of calcium antagonists and beta-blockers[176–180], careful studies with nifedipine in patients with good left ventricular function have been reassuring[133,173]. There is little information about this combination in patients with impaired left ventricular function in whom removal of the sympathetic drive by beta-blockade could be disadvantageous. Nor is there any definite evidence that the vasodilating effect of nifedipine improves cardiac function in patients with poor left ventricular function who are already receiving a beta-blocker.

(b) Heart rate and conduction. *In vitro*, sinoatrial automaticity and atrioventricular nodal conduction are depressed by nifedipine, verapamil and diltiazem but only nifedipine is devoid of these effects in man[137–139,170,173,176]. Since sympathetic activity enhances both functions the combination of beta-blockers and verapamil or diltiazem could depress sinoatrial and AV nodal function further. This has been documented in patients with ischaemic heart disease in some studies with either verapamil or diltiazem but not in others[159,167,181]. In a double blind study in hypertensive patients, the combination of verapamil and propranolol significantly prolonged the PR interval though ambulatory monitoring revealed no important bradyarrhythmias[174].

In most reported studies maximal doses of beta-blockers and calcium antagonists have been used, while in clinical practice the addition of low doses of one drug to another would be more usual and probably safer. Combination therapy with beta-blockers and calcium antagonists is very effective in angina and double blind controlled studies confirm that this is more effective than beta-blockers alone. When safety aspects only are considered the obvious combination is that with nifedipine and a beta-blocker, though in patients with good left ventricular function and normal sinoatrial and atrioventricular nodal function serious clinical problems related to combination therapy with beta-blockers and either nifedipine, verapamil or diltiazem are likely to be few. In those patients in whom left ventricular function is impaired great caution is required with any beta-blocker/calcium antagonist combination and especially with verapamil.

In general the results of clinical studies with calcium antagonists alone are consistent with the predictions made from the original observations on their basic pharmacology. The recent and increasing use of these drugs in combination with beta-blockers has posed a new set of problems that will be answered only by further clinical experience which, thus far, is promising[182]. Perhaps surprisingly, there have been few serious problems.

Drug treatment strategy

Despite the growing appreciation of the effect of coronary vasomotion on coronary bloodflow, myocardial ischaemia and angina usually occur in the setting of coronary atheroma that is severe enough to significantly limit the coronary reserve. The most successful therapeutic strategy, therefore, is likely to be that aimed at reducing myocardial oxygen demands for any given external workload – either to facilitate routine activities or to counter the effects of situations when myocardial oxygen demands increase suddenly or unexpectedly, as in daily life.

In the patient who experiences exertional angina at least once a day, most physicians would still recommend a beta-blocker as their first line drug in chronic prophylaxis. Apart from efficacy, the convenient dosing intervals (especially for the hydrophilic drugs) is attractive and side effects are usually not a major problem in comparison with the relief of symptoms that beta-blockade usually affords. At the present time although there is no definite proof that beta-blockers are protective against the subsequent development of myocardial infarction, the evidence of benefit when given early or late after myocardial infarction demonstrates some 'cardioprotective effect'[134–136] – in contrast to the studies with calcium antagonists, which have been disappointing in this context[183–185].

Since a significantly better effect on objective evidence of myocardial ischaemia (including silent ischaemia) is achieved with concomitant treatment with a calcium antagonist there is a good case for introducing this at an early stage rather than simply increasing the dose of the beta-blocker, which will probably not help and will almost certainly increase side effects. This approach may be particularly valuable in those patients whose symptoms, though basically effort related, may be variable or aggravated by factors thought to increase coronary vasomotor tone such as cold or emotion. The calcium antagonist of choice in this context is nifedipine, on account of proven efficacy and for safety considerations with respect to left ventricular function, heart rate and conduction. Combination treatment with beta-blockers and verapamil or diltiazem may be cautiously tried in selected patients with good left ventricular function and no evidence of sinoatrial or atrionodal dysfunction, if the addition of nifedipine is ineffective or contraindicated or if it causes side effects.

In the presence of a contraindication to a beta-blocker, or when beta-blockade has been ineffective, verapamil seems the most appropriate alternative in view of its proven efficacy, which is similar to that of a beta-blocker.

In patients with impaired left ventricular function, the calcium antagonists seem a better option than the beta-blockers and the less prominent negatively inotropic effects of nifedipine or diltiazem may be more reassuring compared with the possibility of myocardial depression with verapamil, though this is likely to be important only in those with severe left (or right) ventricular functional impairment.

The use of 'long acting' oral nitrates alone or in combination with beta-blockers or calcium antagonists remains controversial, as does the use of alternative nitrate delivery systems. Undoubtedly the superior bioavailability of the mononitrates as compared with di- or trinitrates has been a step forward in oral therapy, but the development of tolerance to any form of chronic nitrate therapy still requires to be understood and overcome.

The flexibility of modern drug therapy means that the majority of patients with chronic stable angina can be significantly improved by medical therapy. Perhaps more attention ought to be paid to finding the optimum regimen for individual patients who seem difficult to control medically, especially if non-invasive or even invasive investigation has shown them to be a relatively low risk.

(1) *Infrequent angina* – The decision whether to treat patients with infrequent angina in a similar fashion to their more symptomatic peers can be difficult. It seems logical to base the decision on the results of non-invasive evaluation – if the risk is low, then GTN as required seems appropriate, since the frequency or severity of the symptoms does not justify chronic (and therefore expensive) treatment with a beta-blocker or other drugs. On the other hand, if non-invasive testing indicates a high risk, then coronary angiography is indicated to define the suitability for surgery. Patients whose symptoms are mild but whose investigative profile suggests an intermediate risk should probably be advised to receive medical therapy with a beta-blocker or, where appropriate, a calcium antagonist.

In all patients GTN sublingually (or as a spray) remains, as it has done for over a century, the best treatment for the acute episode; though sublingual nifedipine is also useful when the episodes are more severe or unresponsive to the nitrate. Despite classical medical teaching, patients still seem resistant to or unaware of the practice of using GTN as an acute prophylactic when anticipating some activity that usually results in angina – reaffirming this advice is often helpful.

CORONARY BYPASS SURGERY

Introduced by Favorolo in 1967[186], coronary artery bypass surgery soon will come of age. The operation now is commonplace, especially in the United States of America, and in experienced centres the mortality is comparable with other types of major surgery. Even in higher risk patients with compromised ventricular function the risk is acceptable and not of paramount importance in deciding about surgery when other factors indicate its value.

The two main reasons for considering surgery in the patient with angina are to relieve symptoms and to prolong life and, although many studies have addressed these issues, most have not been controlled. Fortunately three randomized controlled trials, the European Coronary

Surgery Study (ECSS)[93], the Veterans Administration Study (VA)[66] and the Coronary Artery Surgery Study (CASS)[94] have been carried out. When considering the management of the patient with chronic stable angina it must be remembered that the results of these trials are, strictly, applicable only to the specific population concerned; their respective strengths and weaknesses have been extensively reviewed recently[187–189]. Nevertheless they do provide the best available information concerning the efficacy of surgery in achieving its main goals – the improvement of the quality and the length of life.

A brief description of the trials is necessary to place the role of coronary bypass surgery in the context of everyday cardiological practice.

Veterans Administration Study

This was the first randomized trial of medical and surgical treatment and initially comprised 1015 male patients recruited over a five year period at 13 centres. Because the surgical mortality was so high at certain less experienced centres, the results now quoted refer to the 686 patients randomized between 1972 and 1974.

Patients with all grades of severity of chronic stable angina and with >50% stenosis of at least one major coronary artery were included; most were in NYHA Classes II and III with the latter having a slight preponderance. Thus the study comprised a relatively symptomatic spectrum of patients more representative of that seen in referral centres than in the primary care or general medical sectors. The patients had a relatively severe degree of coronary heart disease with a high frequency of previous myocardial infarction (61%), multi-vessel disease (85%), resting ST segment abnormalities and impaired left ventricular function (70%).

The baseline characteristics of the medical and surgical group were similar apart from the serum cholesterol levels which were significantly higher in the medical group[190].

Crossover of patients to the alternate group was small (20 allocated to surgery were not operated on and 42 allocated to medical treatment were eventually operated on).

European Coronary Surgery Study

This comprised men under 65 years of age in whom surgery was not deemed essential on account of symptoms but who had angina and angiographic evidence of >50% stenosis in 2 or 3 major coronary arteries and who had a resting left ventricular ejection fraction >50%. Although the European population comprised symptomatically less severe patients than the VA study, 57% being in functional classes II and III, 40% of patients had moderately severe symptoms. Moreover, although patients with impaired global left ventricular function were excluded, more than half had regional wall motion abnormalities on angiography. A total of 768 patients were randomized either to medical or surgical treatment – of the 373 assigned to medical treatment, 83 subsequently underwent surgery; while 27 of the 395 surgical patients did not undergo surgery.

Coronary Artery Surgery Study

As it had been shown previously that surgery reduced mortality in left main stem disease, such patients were excluded from this study, as were those whose symptoms were severe enough to justify surgery in their own right. Thus the study comprised patients with mild angina pectoris (79% were in NYHA Classes I and II) together with patients who were asymptomatic following a myocardial infarction. Angiographic criteria were the presence of >70% stenosis in at least one major vessel excluding the left main stem artery. Impairment of left ventricular function was not a contraindication provided heart failure was not present and the ejection fraction was at least 0.35, ejection fraction was less than 0.5 in 20% of the patients.

In this study 2095 patients were considered randomizable, though only 780 were randomized equally to medical or surgical treatment.

Effect on symptoms, exercise capacity and drug treatment

Chest pain

In the European Study 46% of patients treated surgically were free of symptoms at 5 years, as compared with 28% of those treated medically; most of the apparent change in the medical group could be attributed to surgery in those subsequently crossing over from medical treatment. The figures from the CASS study are similar for medically treated patients, while a slightly higher proportion (55%) of surgical patients were free of symptoms at 5 years. It should be remembered that patients with severe symptoms were excluded from these studies but the VA study on the other hand, which was symptomatically selective for more severely affected patients, produced broadly similar results. Thus, after 5 years about half of the patients treated surgically will be free of symptoms, while surgery can be expected to improve symptoms in about three-quarters of the patients.

Exercise capacity

In the CASS study after 5 years, exercise time was greater by about a minute and a half in the surgical group from a similar baseline; but the percentage of those with exercise induced ST segment depression >1 mm, which was dramatically reduced after one year, was only slightly though significantly less than medically treated patients. The trend in the European study was similar and the difference in exercise performance between the two groups was no longer significant after 5 years.

Drug treatment

In all the trials there is a striking decrease in both beta-blocker and nitrate therapy in the surgical group; approximately 30% of surgical patients were receiving a beta-blocker after 5 years compared with 70% in the medical group, with a similar trend in nitrate therapy.

Employment status

Employment status after surgery is very dependent on that prior to surgery. In the CASS study there was no difference eventually in employment status between medically and surgically treated patients, which was approximately 70% before and after the study[191].

Effect on mortality

Veterans Administration Study

The initial report was the first from a randomized controlled study to confirm earlier uncontrolled reports of a highly significant difference in mortality for patients with left main stem disease. At 4 years this was 33% for medically treated patients and 7% for surgically treated patients (Figure 6.10(a)).

Excluding left main stem disease, there was no significant difference in mortality between the two groups. At first there appeared to be a trend towards a better surgical mortality but this disappeared between 7 and 11 years – due, it is widely believed, to progressive occlusion of the vein grafts.

Scrutiny of the survival characteristics of the medically treated group produced interesting data concerning high and low risk groups. Apart from left main stem disease, the variable most associated with decreased survival was impaired left ventricular function as defined by a left ventricular ejection fraction <35%. In those patients with three vessel disease who had impaired left ventricular function, survival in medically treated patients was 52% as compared with 76% in surgically treated patients after 7 years.

In a clinically defined high risk subgroup who had two of the following, resting ST segment depression, history of myocardial infarction or history of hypertension, survival in the medical group was 52% as compared with 72% in the surgical group.

Thus it was concluded that among patients with stable ischaemic heart disease surgery increased longevity only in those with a high risk of dying as defined by certain angiographic or clinical criteria. The

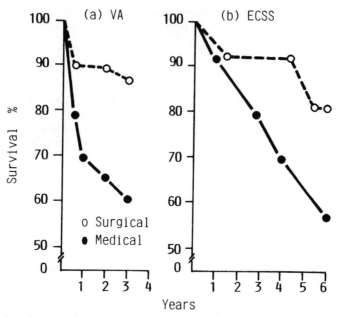

Figure 6.10 Coronary bypass surgery – left main stem disease. The Veterans Administration study (a) VA and the European coronary surgery study, (b) ECSS both showed a dramatic reduction in mortality in the surgical groups

subsequent analysis at 11 years showed that the survival benefit appeared to diminish after 7 years.

European Coronary Surgery Study

In patients with left main stem disease survival was 85.7% and 81.7% for surgical patients and 67.9% and 63.6% for medical patients at 5 and 8 years respectively. Although this was the largest difference between the groups the small numbers precluded statistical significance (Figure 6.10(b)).

Excluding left main stem disease, survival in surgically treated patients was significantly better in the group as a whole largely due to benefit in patients with triple vessel disease in whom survival at 5 and 8 years was 94% and 91.8% respectively compared with 82.4% and 76.7% for medical patients[192] (Figure 6.11(a)).

The study emphasizes the importance of disease in the proximal left anterior descending coronary artery in that while surgically treated patients with two vessel disease but without a proximal LAD stenosis fared no better than medically treated patients, those with proximal LAD disease did. Since few patients with triple vessel disease did not have a proximal LAD lesion the influence of the latter in this group was less obvious.

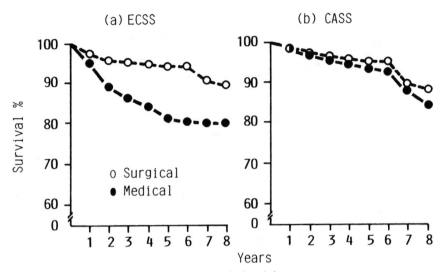

Figure 6.11 Coronary bypass surgery – excluding left main.
(a) The European Coronary Surgery Study (ECSS) and (b) the Coronary Artery Surgery Study (CASS). The ECSS showed a significant reduction in mortality, while the CASS study did not – note the excellent survival in the medically treated group in the CASS study, suggesting less severe coronary heart disease

Importantly, the study identified a number of other non-angiographic variables that were predictive of a better result following surgery, including the presence of ST segment depression of greater or equal to 1.5 mm on a standard bicycle exercise test. Even in the presence of proximal LAD stenosis, if ST segment depression of this magnitude was not present then the prognosis remained equally good in medically and surgically treated patients with respect to both double and triple vessel disease (Figure 6.13).

Another clinical indicator of benefit from surgery was the presence of peripheral vascular disease.

Coronary Artery Surgery Study

Analysis at 5 years showed that there was no difference in survival between medically and surgically treated patients being 92% and 95% respectively (Figure 6.11(b))[94].

It was anticipated at the outset that there might be differences within subgroups and a recent analysis demonstrated that those with three vessel disease and impaired left ventricular function had a better prognosis when treated surgically. Of 160 patients with an ejection fraction between 35 and 50%, 82 were randomized to medical therapy and 78 to surgery. After 7 years 30% of those treated medically were dead as compared with 16% of those who had had surgery (Figure 6.12)[65]. Moreover, when those who had a reduced ejection fraction, together

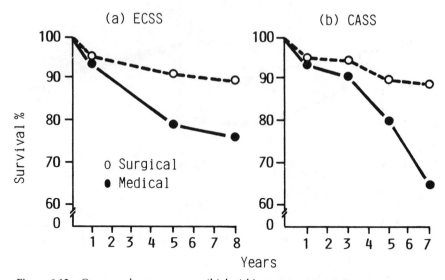

Figure 6.12 Coronary bypass surgery: 'high risk' groups.
(a) The ECSS study and (b) the CASS study. The presence of exercise induced ST segment depression > 1.5 mm in the ECSS and an impaired ejection fraction in patients with triple vessel disease in the CASS study conferred a poorer prognosis on medically treated patients

with triple vessel disease (who comprised about half of this subset) are considered, 35% of those treated medically were dead after 7 years compared with only 12% of those treated surgically.

While the CASS and VA studies are in agreement concerning the survival advantage of surgery in patients with triple vessel disease and impaired left ventricular function, the improved survival of surgically treated patients with triple vessel disease and preserved left ventricular function noted in the ECSS was not confirmed by the CASS study. Interestingly the survival of surgically treated patients of this type in both studies was identical, while the survival of medically treated patients in the ECSS was poorer. It has been argued that this reflects the greater severity of coronary heart disease in the ECSS patients, since the survival of a much larger group of medically treated patients in the CASS registry is very similar to the ECSS.

Summary of the trials

Bearing in mind that these studies are neither perfect in design or execution, nor are they strictly comparable, a number of clinical conclusions that bear on the management of patients with chronic stable angina reasonably may be drawn.

(1) When treated medically patients who have > 50% stenosis of the

    left main stem coronary artery have a poor prognosis that can be improved by surgery

(2) Those with impaired left ventricular function in the presence of triple vessel disease also live longer after surgery. The benefit in these patients is very similar when the Veterans Administration and the CASS studies are compared with the mortality being halved by surgery

(3) Stenosis of the proximal LAD in patients with multivessel disease confers a poor prognosis for those treated medically, even when left ventricular function is unimpaired

(4) Certain patients with clinical variables suggesting a high risk also fare better after surgery including those with a previous myocardial infarction, a history of hypertension or resting ST segment depression on the electrocardiogram

(5) Surgery also improves survival in patients with ST segment depression of 1.5 mm appearing early in exercise and indeed in patients with negative or less positive exercise tests. There is no difference in survival between medically and surgically treated patients

(6) The incidence of subsequent myocardial infarction is not reduced by surgery though the outcome may be more preferable.

Coronary bypass surgery in the elderly

No randomized trial has been carried out in patients aged 65 or over but in a non-randomized subset from the CASS registry the results were similar to those in younger patients – in 'low risk' patients with mild symptoms preserved left ventricular function and absence of left main stem disease there was no difference in survival after 6 years; and in 'high risk' patients, defined preoperatively, there appeared to be a survival benefit from surgery[193]. Although these data are from a non-randomized study, they are in keeping with the results of randomized studies in that the prognosis of those patients with the most severe coronary heart disease can be improved by surgery.

Serious complications of coronary surgery

Operative mortality

Modern cardiopulmonary bypass techniques and methods of myocardial preservation have evolved and improved with the passage of time such that the mortality associated with cardiac surgery of any kind has decreased markedly, especially with coronary artery surgery. In the most experienced centres, the operative mortality is now reputed to be < 1% having been 3% more than a decade ago. As would be expected mortality increases with age and the complexity of the underlying coronary disease and when left ventricular function is impaired. In the CASS study operative mortality was 1.4%, 2.1% and 2.8% in one, two and three vessel disease respectively and ranged from 1.9% to 6.7% in patients with normal and those with severe impairment of left ventricular function (EF <19%)[194].

Thus there is a range of operative mortality that reflects surgical skill and experience on the one hand and severity of coronary heart disease on the other. Such factors must not be forgotten when considering the individual patient in his own environment.

Perioperative myocardial infarction

The major factor in the decrease in perioperative myocardial infarction has been the use of cold cardioplegia. Despite the quoted figures of 1–3%, the true incidence of myocardial infarction may be higher and will vary according to the sensitivity of the techniques used to diagnose it[195]. In the CASS registry of 9777 bypass operations, myocardial infarction occurred in 561 (5.7%) and, importantly, long term survival was reduced in these patients[196].

Cerebral dysfunction

The reduction in cerebral blood flow that, inevitably, accompanies cardiopulmonary bypass has always been a source of concern. Brain death, cerebrovascular accidents and visual disturbances are the recognized serious cerebral complications of cardiopulmonary bypass the frequency of which has been variably reported.

In a prospective study of 312 elective coronary bypass procedures evidence of some early neurological deficit can be detected in approximately 60% of patients[197]. Fatal brain damage was rare (0.3–0.7%) but definite stroke occurred in about 5% and ophthalmological defects in 25% of patients, though in only 3% were significant field defects present. Moreover, peripheral nerve lesions (12%) and especially brachial plexopathy (7%) were not uncommon.

In another prospective study in which a control group undergoing other forms of surgery was included, although new neurological signs could be elicited in 64% of bypass patients and in none of the controls at 24 hours, there was no significant difference between the groups at 8 weeks. Interestingly, minor neuropsychological abnormalities were common in both groups and were still identifiable in about one third of patients at 8 weeks[198].

Although most patients with detectable neurological damage have no important residual functional disability, other aspects of cerebral dysfunction (such as subtle intellectual impairment or personality change) await full evaluation. Much more information on this aspect is needed but sufficient evidence exists to demand that at least extracranial carotid arterial disease be excluded routinely in all older patients and all smokers; and to suggest that more attention be paid to the cerebral reserve before submitting the brain to the inevitable reduction in cerebral bloodflow imposed by cardiopulmonary bypass.

Who should have surgery?

While no rigid set of criteria can cater completely for patient individuality, a number of guidelines may be constructed based on the symptoms and on the premise that surgery does improve the prognosis in certain categories of patients. Few would argue that those patients who are genuinely incapacitated by angina and whose vessels are suitable for grafting should be offered surgery when optimum medical treatment has failed to allow a reasonable quality of life. Value judgements enter the equation in patients who would like to be more active than their peers and who find the side effects of medical treatment intolerable even though it has improved their angina. But the accumulating information on risk stratification in coronary heart disease together with the results of the randomized trials indicate that the perceived severity of symptoms should not be the sole or indeed always the major criteria in deciding about surgery. A summary of recommendations is given in Table 6.4.

Table 6.4 Who should have surgery? Indications based on symptoms, risk stratification and randomized trials

---

(1) *Based on symptoms*
   (a) Unacceptable limitation of lifestyle because of symptoms despite optimum medical treatment
   (b) Inability to tolerate drug therapy because of side effects

(2) *Regardless of symptoms*
   (a) Significant stenosis (> 50%) of left main coronary artery
   (b) Triple vessel disease when:
      (i) Proximal left anterior descending coronary artery is stenosed.
      (ii) Left ventricular function is impaired.

(3) *Clinical variables suggesting 'high risk'*
   (a) Strongly positive exercise test
   (b) Myocardium in jeopardy:
      – fall in ejection fraction > 5% on exercise
      – large exercise induced wall motion abnormality
      – large or multiple thallium perfusion defects

Can surgery be improved?

It seems certain that there will be no further large scale randomized trials of coronary artery surgery compared with medical therapy. Equally certain is that surgery itself will continue to evolve as it has already done during and since the trials. The improved prognosis in certain subsets of patients following surgery is impressive and of considerable clinical significance; and it is matched by marked relief of symptoms and improved functional capacity, at least in the short and medium term. But the recurrence of symptoms, even at a late stage, after such a

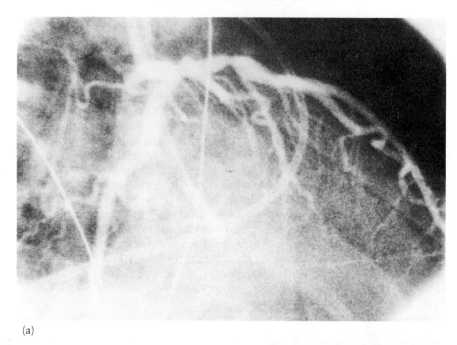

(a)

(b)

Figure 6.13 Percutaneous transluminal coronary angioplasty (PTCA). (a) Before angioplasty, (b) inflation of balloon

Figure 6.13 (cont.)

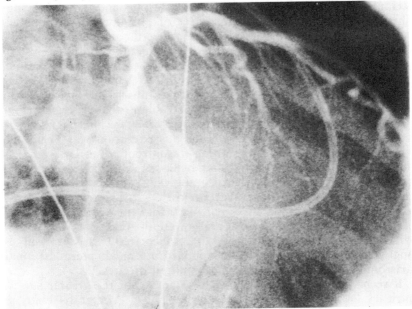

(c) Final result

major procedure is disappointing and demands continued research into the development of new procedures or techniques that will improve long term graft patency. Two innovations, antiplatelet therapy and internal mammary artery grafting, are promising in this respect.

Antiplatelet therapy

In a recent large double blind placebo controlled study in which dipyridamole was started before and aspirin a few hours after surgery, the rate of early and late graft occlusion was more than halved[199]. Previous trials suggested that, to be effective, dipyridamole had to be started before surgery and since there is no reason to suppose that aspirin need be withheld until after surgery, it seems more logical and convenient to start combined antiplatelet therapy one day prior to surgery. Experimental data from other forms of vascular surgery support this strategy[200].

Internal mammary artery grafting

It seems likely that even in the very best centres for cardiac surgery, at least one third of coronary vein grafts will have occluded in the first decade after operation[201]; indeed the average patency rate may well be lower, conducive with the frequency of recurrent symptoms that has been reported in the randomized trials of medical and surgical therapy. The recently reported beneficial effect of peri-operative antiplatelet therapy may well improve the symptomatic result and the prognosis but the search continues for novel and hopefully better conduits.

The internal mammary artery (IMA) has been used in the surgical treatment of coronary artery disease for more than 30 years. Vineberg implanted it into a tunnel of left ventricular muscle with an apparently impressive relief of symptoms that was supported by experimental evidence of partial re-vascularization[202]; certainly, the internal mammary seemed to maintain its patency[203] but this operation was abandoned when coronary artery bypass grafting was introduced in 1967.

The IMA was first used in man as a bypass graft in 1968[204], but despite its reputation for patency, it was employed by few cardiac surgeons until the report by the Montreal group in 1984[205]. They described a 95% patency over 10 years compared with 30% for vein grafts inserted in the same institution – moreover the grafts were in good condition with no evidence of atheroma. Use of the IMA has increased greatly, not only for single anastomoses but also for sequential grafts and bilateral mammary anastomoses are now being used for multiple arteries.

It seems clear that despite the disadvantage of the greater surgical intricacy and complexity involved in their use, IMA grafts enjoy the advantage of relative immunity from atheroma, in contrast to radial arteries for example.

The largest series and longest follow up was reported from the Cleveland Clinic in which 2306 IMA grafts were compared with 3625 vein grafts to the LAD over a 7 year period in a non-randomized study[206]. The actuarial curves show a significant difference in survival in all grades of severity of coronary artery disease, a difference that is widened when decreased LV function is added into the equation. In one, two and three vessel disease twice as many died in the vein graft group as in the IMA group. The survival rates at 10 years were 93.4% v. 88.0%, 90% v. 79.5%, 82.6% v. 71% for one two and three vessel disease respectively. This was associated with a significant reduction in non fatal myocardial infarction, cardiac reoperation and all cardiac events. There was no effect on hospitalization for arrhythmia (which may be due to fibrosis pre-existing pre-operatively) or on the recurrence of angina. This may be consistent with the theory that late angina is related to associated vein graft closure and that improved survival is related to continued perfusion of the LAD. Objective assessment of exercise capacity is greater following IMA both in single and multivessel disease. Sequential flow studies suggest that at least initially vein graft flow is greater but that IMA grafts enlarge with time such that the relief of angina even in the short term is equally good with either conduit.

There is little doubt that the use of IMA grafting will increase further.

PERCUTANEOUS TRANSLUMINAL CORONARY ANGIOPLASTY

In 1977, when Andreas Gruentzig first demonstrated his new technique of percutaneous transcoronary angioplasty (PTCA) to a gathering of distinguished but somewhat incredulous European cardiologists he was given a standing ovation. Although angioplasty had already been performed by Dotter in 1964 on peripheral arteries using coaxial dilating catheters[207] it was obvious that the innovative Gruentzig with PTCA had steered the treatment of coronary heart disease into a new era[208].

'Like a footprint in the snow' was Gruentzig's description of his belief that the atheroma was being squashed by the inflation of the balloon at the tip of the catheter. There is now good evidence that compression and longitudinal redistribution of atheroma is indeed one mechanism of dilatation, but a common result of PTCA is tearing of the intima with overstretching or frank dissection of the media. The integrity of the vessel is maintained by the adventitia but desquamation of the endothelium occurs with exposure of subendothelial microfibrils and subsequent deposition of platelets and fibrin[209]. Dilatation of vessels with eccentric plaques is associated with separation of the plaque from the media which stretches, thins and sometimes ruptures. When stenoses are concentric, frequently there is rupture of the plaque with the formation of clefts between the plaque and the media[210]. The artery heals by scarring with the formation of a fibrous neointima within the lumen.

Technique

The coronary artery is catheterized selectively by a guiding catheter and, with the help of a soft flexible and steerable guide wire, a small balloon tipped catheter is manoeuvred across the lesion. The balloon is then inflated several times to a pressure of 600–1000 kPa (6–10 atmospheres). The inflation time is variable and may be as long as 60 seconds, though 10–20 seconds is more typical (Figure 6.13).

Results

Successful angioplasty is associated with marked relief of symptoms together with a significant reduction or indeed abolition of objective evidence of exercise induced ischaemia either on electrocardiography, thallium perfusion scintigraphy or radionuclide ventriculography[211–213].

The most comprehensive information about PTCA is available from the NHLBI registry on 3248 patients who had 3567 angioplasties between 1979 and 1982[214–216].

In 25% the catheter could not be passed across the lesion and in a further 8% dilatation could not be achieved. Taking an improvement of luminal diameter of 20% as the minimal criteria for success this was achieved in 70%.

Complications

Acute coronary occlusion, occurring as a result of dissection, spasm or thrombosis is the most important and commonest of the serious angioplastic complications. This may supervene at any point following passage of the balloon catheter across the lesion until about 30–60 minutes after the end of the procedure – thereafter occlusion is unlikely. If acute occlusion persists despite intracoronary nitrates, calcium antagonists or repeat dilatation, emergency coronary bypass grafting is usually performed[217].

The serious complication rate (death, myocardial infarction or emergency bypass) in the NHLBI registry was 9%, surgery being performed in 6.6%. Death occurred in 0.9%; mortality in those suffering myocardial infarction was 8.4% and in those requiring surgery 4.4%. Of 1418 patients followed for one year by the NHLBI registry – 2.7% had died, 8.5% had had repeat PTCA and 33.3% had undergone bypass surgery. Of those who were not operated on, only 36.5% were symptom free and had not suffered a myocardial infarction. Restenosis occurred in 34% within six months.

Although 62.7% were symptom free at one year and had not sustained a myocardial infarction, only 36.5% of those not operated on enjoyed a similar status. In the small numbers followed for up to three years approximately one third remain symptom free. Interestingly, 7% of those whose angioplasties were unsuccessful but who had not had surgery also were symptom free at this time.

As with any manual skill there is a definite learning curve and the early success rates of 65–75% have risen to around 90% in the most experienced hands. Increasing expertise is not the only factor responsible for the improved results; better design of the catheter, guidewire and balloon has contributed greatly, while more appropriate patient selection will also have played a part. Death is perhaps surprisingly uncommon, even in inexperienced hands, with a prevalence of about 1%. Myocardial infarction occurs in about 3% and usually in those who require emergency surgery.

Even in the best centres, recurrence or restenosis occurs in about one third of all patients between one and nine months after angioplasty. Typically, symptoms reappear at about four months and restenosis is rather rare after nine months. These lesions may be treated by repeat angioplasty, which is successful in 80% and carries a very low risk. Clearly this is the biggest single problem with angioplasty because apart from being traumatic to the patient it reduces the margin of difference between the cost of angioplasty and surgery. Nonetheless, repeat angioplasty carries a high probability of initial success, though the tendency to restenosis is not removed.

Who should have angioplasty?

The principal indication remains a single discrete proximal lesion in a patient whose symptoms or non-invasive evaluation justify surgery. It is salutory that despite the burgeoning experience with balloon angioplasty, there is no evidence of a decline in the numbers undergoing bypass surgery. It seems that despite the accepted and overriding indication for angioplasty, that the patient is indeed a 'surgical option', many patients must be undergoing angioplasty as an alternative to medical therapy[218]. The degree of stenoses being dilated also may be less than critical if a pre-dilatation mean stenosis of 71%, as in the NHLBI Registry, is typical. There seems therefore to be an urgent need to compare modern medical therapy with angioplasty in similarly experienced hands. Safety issues must be paramount since the mortality rate of angioplasty itself is around 1%, while there is a further significant mortality in those who require emergency surgery. Moreover, myocardial infarction occurs in about 3–5% of patients with its resultant effect on left ventricular function and ultimately on prognosis. These issues can only be addressed properly in large well designed clinical trials. Newly occluded vessels may also be dilated having been reopened with a guidewire. Distal anastomoses of coronary vein grafts also are amenable to angioplasty and some surgeons have used the technique intraoperatively. Lesions near large branching vessels are less suitable as are those lesions that are longer than the balloon itself. In experienced centres, multiple lesions and those of the main stem are now being tackled with a success rate of 60–70%, though no long term data are available.

With the passage of time, the proportion of patients who would be candidates for surgery and who now may be considered for angioplasty is increasing – estimates vary widely from 10–50%.

Much has been made of the financial savings of angioplasty as compared with surgery. It must be remembered, however, that repeat angioplasty may be necessary in about a third and coronary bypass surgery in a significant minority.

Coronary angioplasty undoubtedly is here to stay but its true place remains to be defined. It should not be simply seen as a competitor to surgery, rather as an alternative or indeed complementary treatment for a progressive disease[218]. Possibly surgery may only be postponed in many patients but it seems probable that procedures at selected sites over a period of time, chosen on the basis of non-invasive evaluation, may become a routine treatment. Never since the advent of coronary artery bypass surgery has there been a more pressing need for careful evaluation against surgery and indeed medical therapy. It should not be regarded as a morale booster for jaded cardiologists but as a powerful new treatment modality that has not yet come of age.

The success of angioplasty is reflected not only in the rapidly growing population of treated patients but also in the stimulus it has given to the development of different percutaneous catheter-based techniques designed to remove or reduce atheromatous coronary obstruction. The most widely studied, experimentally and now clinically, is laser angioplasty; though the use of a device that shaves the plaque with a protected blade has been described recently.

CONCLUSIONS

The choice of a management strategy in chronic stable angina will depend on the severity of symptoms and the risk stratification group in which the overall clinical picture together with clinical investigation places the patient.

The randomized trials of medical and surgical therapy have answered some questions and posed others, but one byproduct of this research and of the registries set up in non-operated patients has been to stratify risk more accurately. To many general physicians and cardiologists the favourable prognosis of many patients with angina, even those with apparently severe coronary heart disease based on anatomical features but in whom functional assessments have been reassuring, has been illuminating.

While the prognostic differences between medical treatment and surgery many now be clearer, much remains to be answered concerning the overall quality of life. Both medical and surgical treatment have improved since the trials were carried out – the advent of the calcium antagonists together with novel nitrate delivery systems have rendered medical therapy much more flexible; while the use of perioperative antiplatelet drugs and of the internal mammary artery as a conduit have made striking improvements in graft patency in the short and long term. Clarification of the cerebral complications of cardiopulmonary bypass is urgently required as are better techniques for monitoring and ensuring the adequacy of intraoperative cerebral perfusion. Percutaneous revascularization by its very nature will remain an attractive option and it seems that with practice safety for balloon angioplasty at least is perhaps surprisingly high. Thus in appropriately selected patients, this is a reasonable alternative to surgery and there seems no reason why angioplasty cannot be repeated over a period of years – perhaps until the surgical option becomes more favourable, as the odds on requiring a second operation shorten with the increasing age of the patient and the improving surgical techniques.

Unfortunately, as was abundantly clear at the first Consensus Development Conference on Coronary bypass surgery, many patients in this country are denied this option because of lack of facilities for both investigation and operation[219]. Doubtless, the decisions made on the basis of the recommendations of this conference will be political and financial rather than medical. Research has made it clearer what we ought to do but whether it can be done is another matter.

It may be of more than passing interest that beta-blockers and bypass surgery arrived on the clinical scene almost simultaneously and began the revolution in the treatment of coronary heart disease that continues today with the introduction of rival therapeutic options – on the one hand, calcium antagonists and, on the other, coronary angioplasty. To some extent effective treatments preceded the accurate patient evaluation that is possible now through an integrated approach to non-invasive and invasive investigation. Only now are the true roles of beta-blockers and surgery becoming clearer, while the place of new medicines and new physical techniques, such as angioplasty, remain to be established.

Some revolutions lead to progress while others cause confusion as the more powerful (or superficially more attractive) factions begin to dictate policy. Never has there been a greater need for continuing evaluation of these treatment modalities in well designed clinical trials.

ACKNOWLEDGEMENTS

I am extremely grateful to Miss Esther Henderson and to Dr Iain Findlay for their help in preparing this manuscript.

References

1. Heberden, W. (1772). Some accounts of a disorder of the breast. *Med. Trans. R. Coll. Physicians* (London) **2**, 59
2. Kannel, W. B., Doyle, J. T., MacNamara, P. M., Quickanton, P. and Gordon, T. (1975). Precursors of sudden coronary death. Factors related to incidence of sudden death. *Circulation*, **51**, 608
3. Julian, D. G. (1985). The practical implications of the coronary artery surgery trials. *Br. Heart J.*, **54**, 343
4. Ockene, I. S., Shay, M. J., Alpert, J. S. *et al.* (1980). Unexplained chest pain in patients with normal coronary arteriograms. *N. Engl. J. Med.*, **303**, 1249
5. Gibson, R. S. and Beller, G. A. (1983). Should exercise electrocardiographic testing be replaced by radioisotope methods? In Rahimtoola, S. H. and Brest, A. N. (eds.) *Controversies in Coronary Artery Disease.* Vol. 1 (Philadelphia: F.A. Davis Co.)
6. Proudfit, W. L., Shirey, E. K. and Sones, F. M. (1966). Selective cine coronary angiography; correlation with clinical findings in 1,000 patients. *Circulation*, **33**, 901
7. Campeau, L., Bourassa, M. G., Bois, M. A. *et al.* (1968). Clinical significance of selective coronary cine arteriography. *Can. Med. Assoc. J.*, **99**, 1063
8. Weiner, D. A., Ryan, T. J., McCabe, C. H. *et al.* (1979). Exercise stress testing. Correlations among history of angina, ST segment response and prevalence of coronary artery disease in the Coronary Artery Surgery Study (CASS). *N. Engl. J. Med.*, **301**, 230
9. Bayliss, R. I. S. (1985). The silent coronary. *Br. Med. J.*, **290**, 1093
10. Messerli, F. H. (1983). In Hedj ter Keurs and Shipperheyn, J. J. (eds.) *Determinants and Modulators of Left Ventricular Structure in Cardiac Left Ventricular Hypertrophy*, p. 38 (Boston: Martinus Nijhoff)
11. Bayes, T. (1763). An essay towards solving problems in the doctrine of chance. *Philos. Trans. R. Soc. London*, **53**, 570
12. Weiner, D. A., McCabe, C. H., Fisher, L. D., Chaitman, B. R. and Ryan, T. J. (1978). Similar rates of false positive and false negative exercise tests in matched males and females (CASS). *Circulation*, **58**, (Suppl. II), 11–140

13. Master, A. M., Jaffe, H. L. and Oppenheimer, E. T. (1929). *Am. J. Med. Sci.*, **177**, 223

14. Wilson, F. N. and Johnston, F. D. (1941). The occurrence in angina pectoris of electrocardiographic changes similar in magnitude and kind to those produced by myocardial infarction. *Am. Heart J.*, **22**, 64

15. Bruce, R. A. (1971). Exercise testing of patients with coronary heart disease. *Ann. Clin. Res.*, **3**, 323

16. Bruce, R. A. and Hornsten, T. R. (1969). Exercise stress testing in evaluation of patients with ischemic heart disease. *Prog. Cardiovasc. Dis.*, **11**, 371

17. Patterson, J. A., Naughton, J., Pietras, R. J. and Gunnar, R. M. (1972). Treadmill exercise in assessment of the functional capacity of patients with cardiac disease. *Am. J. Cardiol.*, **30**, 757

18. Sheffield, L. T. (1972). Graded exercise text (GXT) for ischemic heart disease. A submaximal test to a target heart rate. In *Exercise Testing and Training of Apparently Healthy Individuals: A Handbook for Physicians*. American Heart Association Committee on Exercise, pp. 35–38 (Bethesda: American Heart Association)

19. Chaitman, B. R., Bourassa, M. G., Wagnairt, P., Corbara, F. and Ferguson, R. J. (1978). Improved efficiency of treadmill exercise testing using a multiple lead ECG system and basic hemodynamic exercise response. *Circulation*, **57**, 71

20. Froelicher, V. F. Jr, Wolthius, R., Keiser, N. *et al.* (1976). A comparison of two bipolar exercise electrocardiographic leads to lead V5. *Chest*, **70**, 611

21. Simoons, M. L., Boom, H. B. K. and Smallenburg, E. (1975). On-line processing of orthogonal exercise electrocardiogram. *Comput. Biomed. Res.*, **8**, 105

22. Sheffield, L. T. (1980). Exercise stress testing in heart disease. In Braunwalde, E. (ed.) *A Textbook of Cardiovascular Medicine*. p. 253 (Philadelphia: W. B. Saunders)

23. Feil, H. and Siegel, M. L. (1928). Electrocardiographic changes during attacks of angina pectoris. *Am. J. Med. Sci.*, **175**, 225

24. Prinzmetal, M., Kennamer, R., Merliss, R., Wada, T. and Bor, N. (1959). Angina pectoris. I. A variant form of angina pectoris. *Am. J. Med.*, **27**, 375

25. Chahine, R. A., Raizner, A. E. and Ishmori, T. (1976). The clinical significance of exercise-induced ST-segment elevation. *Circulation*, **54**, 209

26. Fortuin, N. J. and Friesinger, G. C. (1970). Exercise-induced S-T segment elevation. Clinical electrocardiographic and arteriographic studies in twelve patients. *Am. J. Med.*, **49**, 459

27. Lekven, J., Chatterjee, K., Tyberg, J. V., Stowe, D. F., Mathey, D. G. and Parmley, W. W. (1978) Pronounced dependence of ventricular endocardial QRS potentials on ventricular volume. *Br. Heart J.*, **40**, 891

28. Koppes, G., McKiernan, T., Bassan, M. and Froelicher, V. F. (1977). Treadmill exercise testing. Part II. *Curr. Probl. Cardiol.*, **7**, 1

29. Udall, J. A. and Ellestad, M. H. (1977). Predictive implications of ventricular premature contractions associated with treadmill stress testing. *Circulation*, **56**, 985

30. Cole, J. P. and Ellestad, M. H. (1978). Significance of chest pain during treadmill exercise. Correlation with coronary events. *Am. J. Cardiol.*, **41**, 227

31. McNeer, J. F., Margolis, J. R., Lee, K. L. *et al.* (1978). The role of the exercise test in the evaluation of patients for ischaemic heart disease. *Circulation*, **57**, 64

32. Thomson, P. D. and Kelleman, K. H. (1975). Hypotension accompanying the onset of exertional angina. *Circulation*, **52**, 28

33. Whinnery, J. E., Froelicher, V. F. Jr., Stewart, A. J., Longo, M. R. Jr. and Triebwasser, J. H. (1977). The electrocardiographic response to maximal treadmill exercise of asymptomatic men with right bundle branch block. *Chest*, **71**, 335

34. Johnson, S., O'Connel, J., Becker, P., Moran, J. F. and Gunar, R. (1975). The diagnostic accuracy of exercise ECG testing in the presence of complete right bundle branch block. *Circulation*, **52** (Suppl. II) 11–48

35. Fox, K. M., Selwyn, A. P. and Shillingford, J. P. (1978). A method for praecordial surface mapping of the exercise electrocardiogram. *Br. Heart J.*, **40**, 1339

36. Fox, K. M., Selwyn, A., Oakley, K. and Shillingford, J. P. (1979). Relation between the precordial projection of S-T segment changes after exercise and coronary angiographic findings. *Am. J. Cardiol.*, **44**, 1068

37. Simoons, M. and Hugenholtz, P. G. (1977). Estimation of the probability of exercise-induced ischaemia by quantitative ECG analysis. *Circulation*, **56**, 552

38. McHenry, P. L., Phillips, J. F. and Knoebel, S. B. (1972). Correlation of computer-quantitated treadmill exercise electrocardiogram with arteriographic location of coronary artery disease. *Am. J. Cardiol.*, **30**, 747

39. Sheffield, L. T. and Roitman, D. (1976). Stress testing methodology. *Prog. Cardiovasc. Dis.*, **19**, 33

40. Hollenberg, M., Zoltick, J. M., Mateo, G., Yaney, S. F., Daniels, W., Davis, R. C. and Bedynek, J. L. (1985). Comparison of a quantative treadmill exercise score with standard electrocardiographic criteria in screening asymptomatic young men for coronary artery disease. *N. Engl. J. Med.*, **313**, 600

41. Hollenberg, M., Budge, W. R., Wisneski, J. A. and Gertz, E. W. (1980). Treadmill score quantifies electrocardiographic response to exercise and improves test accuracy and reproducability. *Circulation*, **61 No. 2.**, 276

42. Elamin, M. S., Mary, D. A. S. G., Smith, D. R. and Linden, R. J. (1980). Prediction of severity of coronary artery disease using slope of submaximal ST segment/heart rate relationship. *Cardiovasc. Res.*, **14**, 681

43. Elamin, M. S., Kardash, M. M., Smith, D. R. *et al.* (1982). Accurate detection of coronary heart disease by new exercise test. *Br. Heart J.*, **48**, 311

44. Webster, J. S., Moberg, C. and Rincon, C. (1974). Natural history of severe proximal coronary artery disease as documented by coronary cine angiography. *Am. J. Cardiol.*, **33**, 195

45. Cohn, D. F., Harris, P., Barry, W. H., Rosati, R. A., Rosenbaum, P. and Waternaux, C. (1981). Prognostic importance of anginal symptoms in angiographically defined coronary artery disease. *Am. J. Cardiol.*, **47**, 233

46. Bruschke, A. V. G., Proudfit, W. L. and Sones, F. M. (1973). Progress study of 590 consecutive non surgical cases of coronary disease followed 5–9 years. Ventriculographic and other correlation. *Circulation*, **47**, 1154

47. Ellestad, M. H., Wan, M. K. C. (1975). Predictive implications of stress testing. Follow-up of 2700 subjects after maximum treadmill stress testing. *Circulation*, **51**, 363

48. Bonow, R. O., Kent, K. M., Rosing, D. R. (1984). Exercise-induced ischaemia in mildly symptomatic patients with coronary-artery disease and preserved left ventricular function. *N. Engl. J. Med.*, **311**, 1339

49. Gohlke, H., Samek, L., Betz, P. and Roskamm, H. (1983). Exercise testing provides additional prognostic information in angiographically defined subgroups of patients with coronary artery disease. *Circulation*, **68 No. 5**, 979

50. Rochmis, P., Blackburn, H. (1971). Exercise Tests. A survey of procedures, safety and litigation experience in approximately 170000 tests. *J. Am. Med. Assoc.*, **217**, 1061

51. Elliott, A. T. (1982). Radionuclides in cardiology: An overview. In Short, M. D., Pay, D. A., Leeman, S. and Harrison, R. M. (eds.) *Physical Techniques in Cardiological Imaging.* pp. 65–75

52. Dymond, D. S. (1982). First pass and equilibrium measurements of ventricular function. In Short, M. D., Pay, D. A., Leeman, S., Harrison, R. M. (eds.) *Physical Techniques in Cardiological Imaging*, pp. 87–98. (Bristol: Adam Hilger)

53. Marshall, R. C., Berger, H. J. and Costin, J. C. (1977). Assessment of cardiac performance with quantative radionuclide angiocardiography. Sequential left ventricular ejection fraction, normalised left ventricular ejection rate, regional wall motion. *Circulation*, **56**, 820

54. Dymond, D. S., Elliott, A., Stone, D., Hendricks, G. and Spurrell, R. (1982). Factors that affect the reproducibility of measurements of left ventricular function from first pass radionuclide ventriculograms. *Circulation*, **65**, 311

55. Jordan, L. J., Jeffrey, B. S., Borer, S. *et al.* (1983). Exercise versus cold temperature

stimulation during radionuclide cine angiography: diagnostic accuracy in coronary artery disease. *Am. J. Cardiol.,* **51,** 1091

56. Wainwright, R. J., Brennand-Roper, D. A., Cucni, T. A., Dowton, E., Hilson, A. J. W. and Maisey, M. N. (1979). Cold pressor test in detection of coronary heart disease and cardiomyopathy using technetium 99m gated blood pool imaging. *Lancet,* **2,** 320

57. Elliott, A. T., Dargie, H. J. and Gillen, G. J. *et al.* (1985). Production and clinical use of Gold-195m. In *Radiopharmaceuticals and Labelled Compounds 1984,* p. 117. (Vienna: IAEA)

58. Burow, R. D., Strauss, H. W., Singleton, R. *et al.* (1977). Analysis of left ventricular function from multiple gated acquisition cardiac blood pool imaging. Comparison to contrast angiography. *Circulation,* **56,** 1024

59. Dodge, H. T. and Sandler, A. (1968). The use of single plane angiocardiograms for the calculation of left ventricular volume in man. *Am. Heart J.,* **75,** 325

60. Greenberg, H., McMaster, P., Dwyer, E. M. and the Multicentre Post Infarction Research Group (1984). Left ventricular dysfunction after acute myocardial infarction: results of a prospective multicentre study. *J. Am. Coll. Cardiol.,* **4 No. 5,** 867

61. Dewhurst, N. G. and Muir, A. L. (1983). Comparative prognostic value of radionuclide ventriculography at rest and during exercise in 100 patients after first myocardial infarction. *Br. Heart J.,* **49,** 111

62. Berger, H. J. and Zaret, B. L. (1981). Nuclear cardiology (second of two parts). *N. Engl. J. Med.,* **305 No. 15,** 855

63. Massie, B. M., Kramer, B. L., Gertz, E. W. and Henderson, S. G. (1982). Radionuclide measurement of left ventricular volume: comparison of geometric and count based methods. *Circulation,* **65,** 725

64. Bonow, R. D., Leon, M. B., Rosing, D. R. *et al.* (1981). Effects of verapamil and propranolol on left ventricular systolic function and diastolic filling in patients with coronary artery disease. Radionuclide studies at rest and during exercise. *Circulation,* **65,** 1337

65. Passamani, E., Davis, K. B., Gillespie, M. J. and Killip, T. (1985). A randomized trial of coronary artery bypass surgery. Survival of patients with a low ejection fraction. *N. Engl. J. Med.,* **312,** 1665

66. Eleven-year survival in the Veterans Administration randomized trial of coronary bypass surgery for stable angina. (1984). The Veterans Administration Coronary Artery Bypass Surgery Cooperative Study Group. *N. Engl. J. Med.,* **311,** 1333

67. Mock, M. B., Ringovist, I. and Fisher, L. D. (1982). Survival of medically treated patients in the Coronary Artery Surgery Study (CASS) Registry. *Circulation,* **66 No. 3,** 562

68. Carr, E. A., Beierwaltes, W. H., Wengst, A. V. and Barlett, J. D. (1972). *J. Nucl. Med.,* **13,** 76

69. Carr, E. A., Shaw, J. and Krontz, B. (1964). *Am. Heart J.,* **68,** 627

70. Hurley, P. J., Cooper, M., Reba, R. C., Poggenburg, K. J. and Wagner, H. N. (1971). ^{43}KCl. A new radiopharmaceutical for imaging the heart. *J. Nucl. Med.,* **12,** 516

71. Lebowitz, E., Greene, M. W., Bradley-Moore, P., Atkins, H., Ansari, A., Richards, P. and Belgrave, E. (1973). ^{201}Tl – For medical use. *J. Nucl. Med.,* **14,** 421

72. Mullins, L. J. and Moore, R. D. (1960). *J. Gen. Physiol.,* **43,** 759

73. Strauer, B. E., Burger, S. and Bull, U. (1978). *Bas. Res. Cardiol.,* **73,** 298

74. Strauss, H. W., Harrison, K., Langan, J. K. *et al.* (1975). Thallium-201 – for myocardial imaging – relation of thallium-201 to regional myocardial perfusion. *Circulation,* **51,** 641

75. McKillop, J. H. (1982). Myocardial perfusion: thallium and beyond. In Short M. D., Pay, D. A., Leeman, S., Harrison R. M. (eds.) *Physical Techniques in Cardiological Imaging,* p. 77. (Bristol: Adam Hilger)

76. McKillop, J. H., Murray, R. G., Turner, J. G. *et al.* (1979). Can the extent of coronary artery disease be predicted from thallium-201 myocardial images. *J. Nucl. Med.,* **20,** 715

77. Otto, C. A., Brown, L. E., Wieland, D. M. *et al.* (1981). Radio-iodinated fatty acids for myocardial imaging. Effects of chain length. *J. Nucl. Med.*, **22**, 613
78. Westera, G., Vand der Wall, E. E., Heidendal, G. A. K. *et al.* (1980). *Eur. J. Nucl. Med.* **5**, 339
79. Schang, S. J. and Peppine, C. H. (1977). Transient asymptomatic ST segment depression during daily activity. *Am. J. Cardiol.*, **39**, 396
80. Selwyn, A., Fox, K., Eves, M., Oakley, D. and Dargie, H. J. (1979). Myocardial ischaemia in patients with angina pectoris. *Br. Med. J.*, **2**, 1594
81. Deanfield, J. E., Ribiero, P., Oakley, K., Krikler, S. and Selwym, A. P. (1984). Analysis of ST-segment changes in normal subjects: implications for ambulatory monitoring in angina pectoris. *Am. J. Cardiol.*, **54**, 1321
82. Quyyumi, A. A., Wright, G. and Fox, K. (1983). Ambulatory electrocardiographic ST segment changes in healthy volunteers. *Br. Heart J.*, **50**, 46
83. Lynch, P., Dargie, H. J., Krikler, S. and Krikler, D. M. (1980). Objective assessment of antianginal therapy: a double blind comparison of nifedipine, propranolol and their combination. *Br. Med. J.*, **280**, 184
84. Quyyumi, A. A., Mockus, L., Wright, C. and Fox, K. M. (1985). Morphology of ambulatory ST segment changes in patients with varying severity of coronary artery disease. *Br. Heart J.*, **53**, 186
85. Deanfield, J. E., Shea, M., Ribiero, P. *et al.* (1984). Transient ST-segment depression as a marker of myocardial ischaemia during daily life. *Am. J. Cardiol.*, **54**, 1195
86. Chierchia, S., Smith, G., Morgan, M., Gallino, A., Deanfield, J. and Croom, M. (1984). Role of heart rate in pathophysiology of chronic stable angina. *Lancet*, **2**, 1353
87. Chierchia, S., Brunelli, C., Simonetti, I., Lazzari, M. and Maseri, A. (1980). Sequence of events in angina at rest: primary reduction in coronary flow. *Circulation*, **61**, 759
88. Chierchia, S., Landucci, M. and Lazzari, A. (1978). A computerised beat by beat analysis and rational plots of ECG, ventricular and arterial pressure during transmural ischaemic episodes. In *IEEE Proc. Comput. Cardiol. Stanford*, p. 155
89. Maseri, A., L'Abbate Am Pesola, A. *et al.* (1977). Coronary vasospasm in angina pectoris. *Lancet*, **1**, 713
90. Quyyumi, A. A., Wright, C. A., Mockus, L. J. and Fox, K. M. (1984). Mechanisms of nocturnal angina pectoris: importance of increased myocardial oxygen demand in patients with severe coronary artery disease. *Lancet*, **1**, 1207
91. Fulton, W. F. M. (1982). Morphology and pathogenesis of coronary artery stenosis, relevant to intraluminal dilatation. In Kaltenbach *et al.* (eds.) *Transluminal Coronary Angioplasty and Intracoronary Thrombolysis.* (Berlin, Heidelberg: Springer-Verlag)
92. Nudermanee, K., Intarachot, V., Pinotek, M. *et al.* (1984). Silent myocardial ischaemia on Holter: has it clinical or prognostic significance? *Circulation*, **70**, 45
93. Long-term results of prospective randomised study of coronary artery bypass surgery in stable angina pectoris. *Lancet*, (1982). **2**, 1173
94. CASS Principal Investigators and their Associates. (1983). Coronary Artery Surgery Study (CASS): a randomized trial of coronary artery bypass surgery. Survival data. *Circulation*, **68**, 939
95. Takaro, T., Hultgren, H. N., Lipton, M. J., Detrek, M. and participants in the study group. (1976). The VA co-operative randomised study of surgery for coronary arterial occlusive disease II sub group with significant left main lesions. *Circulation*, **54** (Suppl. 3), 111–107
96. Salonen, J. K., Puska, P., Kottke, K. E., Thomilheto, J. and Nissinen, A. (1983). Decline in mortality from coronary heart disease in Finland from 1969 to 1979. *Br. Med. J.*, **1226**, 1857
97. Hjermann, I., Velve Byre, K., Holme, I. *et al.* (1981). The effect of diet and smoking intervention on the indices of coronary heart disease: report from the Oslo study group of a randomised trial in healthy men. *Lancet*, **2**, 1303

98. Deanfield, J., Wright, C., Krikler, S., Ribeiro, B. and Fox, K. (1984). Cigarette smoking and the treatment of angina pectoris with propranolol, atenolol and nifedipine. *N. Engl. J. Med.*, **310**, 951

99. The lipid research clinic coronary primary prevention trial results 1) Reduction in incidence of coronary heart disease. (1984). *J. Am. Med. Assoc.*, **251**, 351

100. Scheuer, J. and Tipton, C. M. (1979). Cardiovascular adaptations to physical training. *Annu. Rev. Physiol.*, **39**, 221

101. Northcote, R. J., Evans, A. D. B. and Ballantyne, D. (1984). Sudden death in squash players. *Lancet*, **1**, 148

102. Osler, W. (1910). The Lumleian lectures on angina pectoris II. *Lancet*, **1**, 839

103. Maseri, A., Parodi, O., Severi, S. *et al.* (1976). Transient transmural reduction of myocardial blood flow, demonstrated by thallium 201 scintigraphy, a cause of variant angina. *Circulation*, **54**, 280

104. Breckenridge, A. (ed.) (1985). *Drugs in the Management of Heart Disease*. (Lancaster: MTP Press)

105. Brunton, T. L. (1857). On the use of nitrite of amyl in angina pectoris. *Lancet*, **2**, 97

106. Murrell, W. (1879). Nitrylglycerine as a remedy for angina pectoris. *Lancet*, **1**, 80

107. Smith, E. R., Smiseth, O. A., King, M. A. I., Manyari, D., Balenkie, I. and Tyberg, J. V. (1984). Mechanism of action of nitrates. *Am. J. Med.* 2nd North American Conference on nitroglycerine therapy, pp. 14–22

108. Lewis, T. (1937). *Diseases of the Heart*. p. 54. (London: McMillan)

109. Ganz, W. and Marcus, H. L. (1972). Failure of intracoronary nitroglycerine to alleviate pacing induced angina. Circulation, **46**, 880

110. Needleman, P., Lang, S. and Johnston, E. M. Jr. (1972). Organic nitrates: relationship between biotransformation and rational angina pectoris therapy. *J. Pharmacol. Exp. Therap.*, **181**, 489

111. Findlay, I. N. and Dargie, H. J. (1985). Medical therapy for angina pectoris. *Pharm. J.*, (April) 445–447

112. Livesey, B., Catley, P. F., Campbell, R. C. and Oran, S. (1973). Double blind evaluation of verapamil, propanolol and isosorbide dinitrate against a placebo in the treatment of angina pectoris. *Br. Med. J.*, **1**, 375

113. Glancy, D. L., Ritcher, M. A., Ellis, E. V. and Johnson, W. (1977). Effect of swallowed isosorbide dinitrate on blood pressure, heart rate and exercise capacity in patients with coronary artery disease. *Am. J. Med.*, **62**, 39

114. Dahany, D. T., Burrell, D. T., Aranoli, W. S. and Prakash, R. (1977). Sustained haemodynamic and antianginal effects of high oral dose isosorbide dinitrate. *Circulation*, **55**, 381

115. Markis, J. E., Gorlin, R., Mills, R. M. *et al.* (1979). Sustained effect of orally administered isosorbide dinitrate on exercise performance of patients with angina pectoris. *Am. J. Cardiol.*, **43**, 265

116. O'Neill, D., Dargie, H. J. and MacLeod, K. (1983). Are long acting nitrates effective in chronic stable angina? *Br. Heart J.*, **49**, 619

117. Lee, G., Mason, P. T. and De Maria, A. N. (1978). Effects of long term oral administration of isosorbide dinitrate on the anti-anginal response to nitroglycerine. *Am. J. Cardiol.*, **41**, 82

118. Thadani, U., Fung, H., Darke, A. C. and Parker, J. O. (1982). Oral isosorbide dinitrate in angina pectoris: Comparison of duration of action and dose response relation during acute and sustained therapy. *Am. J. Cardiol.* **49**, 411

119. Reichek, N., Boldstein, R. E., Redwood, D. R. and Epstein, S. E. (1974). Sustained effects of nitroglycerin ointment in patients with angina pectoris. *Circulation*, **50**, 348

120. Parker, J. O. and Ho-Leung Fung. (1984). Transdermal nitroglycerin in angina pectoris. *Am. J. Cardiol.*, **54**, 471

121. Sullivan, M., Sawides, M., Abouantoum, S., Madsen, E. B. and Froelicher, V. (1985). Failure of transdermal nitroglycerin to improve exercise capacity in patients with angina pectoris. *J. Am. Coll. Cardiol.*, **5**, 1220

122. Dickstein, K. and Knutsen, H. (1985). A double blind multiple crossover trial evaluating a transdermal nitroglycerin system vs placebo. *Eur. Heart J.*, **6**, 50

123. Parker, J. O., Vankoughnett, K. A. and Farrell, B. (1985). Comparison of buccal nitroglycerin and oral isosorbide dinitrate for nitrate tolerance in stable angina pectoris. *Am. J. Cardiol.*, **56**, 724

124. Chasseaud, L. F. (1983). Pharmacokinetics and bioavailability of different nitrate preparation. *Br. J. Clin. Pharmacol.*, Symposium supplement 26; 7–14

125. Black, J. W. (1876). Alquist and the development of beta adrenoceptor antagonists. *Postgrad. Med. J.*, **52** (Suppl. 4), 11

126. Cruickshank, J. M. (1980). The clinical importance of cardioselectivity and lipophilicity in beta blockers. *Am. Heart J.*, **100**, 2160

127. Feely, J., Wilkinson, G. R., Wood, A. R. (1980). Cimetidine administration results in increased effects of propranolol and higher propranolol levels. *Circulation*, **62** (Abstract) 982

128. Warrington, S. J., Holt, D., Johnston, A. and Fitzsimmons, T. J. (1984). Pharmacokinetics and pharmacodynamics of verapamil in combination with atenolol, metoprolol and propranolol. *Br. J. Clin. Pharmac.*, **17**, 37(s)

129. Medical Research Council Working Party. (1985). MRC trial of treatment of mild hypertension; principal results. *Br. Med. J.*, **291**, 97

130. Kendall, M. J. (1981) Are selective beta adrenoceptor blocking drugs an advantage? *J. R. Coll. Physicians*, **15**, 33

131. Harry, J. D. (1977). The demonstration of atenolol as a beta adrenoceptor blocking drug in man. *Postgrad. Med. J.* **53** (Suppl. 3) 65

132. Quyyumi, A. A., Wright, C., Mockus, L. and Fox, K. (1984). Effect of partial agonist activity in beta blockers in severe angina pectoris: a double blind comparison of pindolol and atenolol. *Br. Med. J.*, **289**, 951

133. Findlay, I. N., McLeod, K., Dargie, H. J., Ford, M., Gillen, G. and Elliott, A. T. (1986). The treatment of angina pectoris with nifedipine and atenolol; efficacy and effects on cardiac function. *Br. Heart J.*, **55**, 240

134. Norwegian Multicentre Study Group. (1981). Timolol-induced reduction in mortality and reinfarction in patients surviving acute myocardial infarction. *N. Engl. J. Med.*, **304**, 801–7

135. BHAT Study Group. (1982). A randomized trial of propranolol in patients with acute myocardial infarction. II. Mortality results. *J. Am. Med. Assoc.* **247**, 1707

136. ISIS Collaborative Group. (1985). Vascular mortality after early iv beta blockade in myocardial infarction. *Circulation*, **72** (Suppl. 3) III224, No. 893

137. Fleckenstein, A. (1964). *Verh. Dtsch. Ges. Inn. Med.*, **70**, 81

138. Fleckenstein, A. (1970/71). Specific inhibitors and promoters of calcium action in the excitation contraction coupling of heart muscle and their role in the prevention of production of myocardial lesions. In Harris, P. and Opie, L. (eds.) *Calcium and the Heart.* pp. 135–188 (London and New York: Academic Press)

139. Fleckenstein, A. (1977). Specific pharmacology of calcium in myocardium cardiac pacemakers and vascular smooth muscle. *Am. Rev. Pharmacol. Toxicol.* **17**, 149

140. Engel, H. J. and Lichtlen, P. R. (1981). Beneficial enhancement of coronary bloodflow by nifedipine. Comparison with nitroglycerine and beta blocking agents. *Am. J. Med.*, **71**, 658

141. Masseri, A. and Chierchia, S. (1981). A new rationale for the clinical approach to the patient with angina pectoris. *Am. J. Med.*, **71**, 639

142. Braunwald, E. (1982). Mechanism of action of calcium-channel-blocking-agents. *N. Engl. J. Med.*, **307**, 1618

143. Dargie, H. J., Rowland, E. and Krikler, D. M. (1981). Calcium antagonists in cardiovascular therapy. *Br. Heart J.*, **46**, 8

144. Parodi, O., Maseri, A., Simometti, I. (1979). Management of unstable angina at rest by verapamil. A double-blind cross-over study in the coronary care unit. *Br. Heart J.*, **41**, 146

145. Antman, E., Muller, J., Goldberg, S. *et al.* (1980). Nifedipine therapy for coronary-artery spasm. Experience in 127 patients. *N. Engl. J. Med.*, **302**, 1269

146. Feldman, R., Pepine, C., Whittal, J. and Conti, C. (1982). Short and long term responses to diltiazem in patients with a variant angina. *Am. J. Cardiol.* **49**(3), 554

147. Mehta, J., Pepine, C. J., Day, M., Guerrero, J. R. and Conti, C. R. (1981). Short-term efficacy of oral verapamil in rest angina. *Am. J. Med.* **71**, 977

148. Gertensblith, G., Ouyang, P., Achuff, S. C. *et al.* (1978). Nifedipine in unstable angina. A double-blind randomized trial. *N. Engl. J. Med.* **306**, 885

149. Zelis, R. (1982). Calcium-blocker therapy for unstable angina pectoris. *N. Engl. J. Med.,* **306**, 926

150. Kaltenback, M., Schutz, W. and Kober, G. (1979). Effects of nifedipine after intravenous and intra coronary administration. *Am. J. Cardiol.,* **44**, 832

151. Kurnik, P. B., Tierfenbrunn, A. J. and Ludbrook, P. A. (1984). The dependence of the cardiac effects of nifedipine on the responses of the peripheral vascular system. *Circulation,* **69**, 963

152. Robinson, D. F., Dobbs, R. J. and Kelsey, C. R. (1980). Effects of nifedipine on resistance vessels, arteries and veins in man. *Br. J. Clin. Pharmacol.,* **10**, 433

153. Emanuelsson, H. and Holmberg, S. (1983). Mechanisms of angina relief after nifedipine: a hemodynamic and myocardial metabolic study. *Circulation,* **68**, 124

154. Harris, L., Dargie, H. J., Lynch, P., Bulpitt, C. and Krikler, D. (1982). Blood pressure and heart rate in patients with ischaemic heart disease receiving nifedipine and propranolol. *Br. Med. J.,* **284**, 1148

155. Ebner, F. (1975). *Survey and summary of the results obtained during the world wide clinical investigations of Adalat (nifedipine). 2nd International Nifedipine Symposium,* pp. 348–360 (Berlin: Springer Verlag)

156. Sherman, L. G. and Liang, C. S. (1983). Nifedipine in chronic stable angina: A double blind placebo controlled crossover trial. *Am. J. Cardiol.,* **51**, 706

157. Jariwalla, A. G. and Anderson, E. G. (1978). Production of ischaemic cardiac pain by nifedipine. *Br. Med. J.,* **1**, 1181

158. Balasubramanian, V., Bowles, M. J., Davies A. B. and Raftert, E. B. (1982). Calcium channel blockade as primary therapy for stable angina pectoris. A double blind placebo controlled comparison of verapamil and propranolol. *Am. J. Cardiol.,* **50**, 1158

159. Findlay, I. N., Dargie, H. J., Gillen, G. and Elliott, A. T. (1984). The treatment of angina pectoris with calcium channel blockers; efficacy and effect on cardiac function. *J. Am. Coll. Cardiol.,* **3**, 482

160. Leon, M. B., Rosing, D. R., Bonow, R. O. and Epstein, S. E. (1985). Combination therapy with calcium-channel blockers and beta blockers for chronic stable angina pectoris. *Am. J. Cardiol.,* **55**, 69B–80B, 146

161. Chaffman, M. and Brogden, R. N. (1985). Diltiazem – A review of its pharmacological properties and therapeutic efficacy. *Drugs,* **29**, 387

162. Kenny, J., Kiff, P., Holmes, J. and Jewitt, D. E. (1985). Beneficial effects of diltiazem and propranolol, alone and in combination, in patients with stable angina pectoris. *Br. Heart. J.,* **53**, 43

163. Kenmure, A. C. F., Scrutton, J. H. (1980). A double blind controlled trial of the anti anginal efficacy of nifedipine compared with propranolol. *Br. J. Clin. Pract.,* **8**, 49

164. Ekelund, L. G. and Oro, L. (1979). Antianginal efficiency of nifedipine with and without a beta blocker studies with exercise test. A double blind randomised sub acute study. *Clin. Cardiol.* **2**, 203

165. Dargie, H. J., Lynch, P. G., Krikler, D., Harris, L. and Krikler, S. (1981). Nifedipine and propranolol; a beneficial drug interaction. *Am. J. Med.,* **71**, 676

166. Winniford, M. D., Huxley, R. L., Hillis, D. *et al.* (1983). Randomised double blind comparison of propranolol alone and a propranolol verapamil combination in patients with severe angina of effort. *J. Am. Coll. Cardiol.,* **1**(2), 492

167. Leon, M. B., Rosing, D. R., Bonow, R. O. and Epstein, S. E. (1981). Clinical efficacy of verapamil alone and combined with propranolol in treated patients with chronic stable angina pectoris. *Am. J. Cardiol.,* **48**, 131

168. Balasubramanian, V., Bowles, M. J., Davis, A. B. and Rafftery, E. B. (1982). Combined therapy with verapamil and propranolol in angina pectoris. *Am. J. Cardiol.*, **49**, 125

169. Johnston, D. L., Lesoway, R., Humen, D. P. and Kostuk, W. J. (1985). Clinical and haemodynamic evaluation of propranolol in combination with verapamil, nifedipine and diltiazem in exertional angina pectoris: a placebo controlled, double-blind, randomised, crossover study. *Am. J. Cardiol.*, **55**, 680

170. Hendry, P. D. (1980). Comparative pharmacology of calcium antagonists: nifedipine, verapamil and diltiazem. *Am. J. Cardiol.*, **46**, 1047

171. Singh, B. B. and Roche, A. H. G. (1977). Effects of intravenous verapamil on haemodynamics in patients with heart disease. *Am. Heart J.*, **94**, 593

172. Joshi, P. I., Dalal, J. J., Ruttley, M. S. J., Sheridan, D. J. and Henderson, A. H. (1981). Nifedipine and left ventricular function in beta-blocked patients. *Br. Heart J.*, **45**, 457

173. Rowland, E., Razis, P., Sugrue, D. and Krikler, D. M. (1983). Acute and chronic haemodynamic and electrophysiological effects of nifedipine in patients receiving atenolol. *Br. Heart J.*, **50**, 383

174. McInnes, G. T., Findlay, I. N., Murray, G., Cleland, J. G. F. and Dargie, H. J. (1985). Cardiovascular responses to verapamil and propranolol in hypertensive patients. *J. Hypertension*, **3** (Suppl. 3), S219

175. Johnstone, D. L., Gebhardt, V. A., Donald, A. and Kostuk, W. J. (1983). Comparative effects of propranolol and verapamil alone and in combination on left ventricular function and volumes in patients with chronic exertional angina: a double blind, placebo controlled, randomized cross over study with radionuclide ventriculography. *Circulation*, **68**, 1280

176. Anastassiades, C. J. (1980). Nifedipine and beta blocker drugs. *Br. Med. J.*, **281**, 1251

177. Opie, L. H. and White, D. A. (1980). Adverse interaction between nifedipine and beta blockade. *Br. Med. J.*, **281**, 1462

178. Robson, R. H. and Vishwanath, M. C. (1982). Nifedipine and beta blockade as a cause of cardiac failure. *Br. Med. J.*, **284**, 104

179. Wayne, V. S., Harper, R. W., Laufer, E., Federman, J., Anderson, S. T., Pitt, A. (1982). Adverse interaction between beta adrenergic blocking drugs and verapamil – report of three cases. *Aust. N.Z. J. Med.*, **12**, 285

180. Hutchison, S. J., Lorimer, A. R., Lakhdar, A. and McAlpine, S. G. (1984). Beta blockers and verapamil a cautionary tale. *Br. Med. J.*, **289**, 659

181. Winniford, M. D., Markham, R. V., Firth, B. G., Nicole, P. and Hillis, L. D. (1982). Haemodynamic and electrophysiologic effects of verapamil and nifedipine in patients on propranolol. *Am. J. Cardiol.*, **50**, 704

182. Dargie, H. J. (1986). Combination therapy with B-adrenoceptor blockers and calcium antagonists. *Br. J. Clin. Pharmacol.*, **21** (In Press)

183. Sirnes, P. A., Overskeid, K., Pedersen, T. R. et al. (1984). Evolution of infarct size during the early use of nifedipine in patients with acute myocardial infarction: The Norwegian Nifedipine Multicenter Trial. *Circulation*, **70 No. 4**, 638

184. Muller, J. E., Morrison, J., Stone, P. H. et al. (1984). Nifedipine therapy for patients with threatened and acute myocardial infarction: a randomized, double-blind, placebo-controlled comparison. *Circulation*, **69 No. 4**, 740

185. The Danish Study Group (1984). Verapamil in acute myocardial infarction. *Eur. Heart J.*, **5**, 516

186. Favorolo, R. G. (1968). Saphenous vein autograft replacement of severe segmental coronary artery occlusion. *Ann. Thorac. Surg.*, **5**, 334

187. Killip, T. and Ryan, T. J. (1985). Randomized trials in coronary bypass surgery. *Circulation*, **71 No. 3**, 418

188. Rahimtoola, S. H. (1982). Coronary bypass surgery for chronic angina – 1981: a perspective. *Circulation*, **65**, 225

189. Hampton, J. R. (1984). Coronary artery bypass grafting for the reduction of mortality: an analysis of the trials. *Br. Med. J.*, **289**, 1166

190. Detre, K., Hultgren, H., Takaro, T. (1977). Veterans Administration cooperative study of surgery for coronary arterial occlusive disease III methods and baseline characteristics, including experience with medical treatment. *Am. J. Cardiol.,* **40,** 212

191. Coronary Artery Surgery Study (CASS): a randomised trial of coronary bypass surgery. (1983). Quality of life in patients randomly assigned to treatment groups. *Circulation,* **63,** 951

192. European Coronary Surgery Study Group. (1985). Prospective randomised study of coronary artery bypass surgery in stable angina pectoris: a progress report on survival. *Circulation,* **65 (Suppl. 2),** 67

193. Gersh, B. J., Kronnmal, R. A., Hartzell, V. *et al.* (1985). Comparison of coronary artery bypass surgery and medical therapy in patients 65 years of age or older. *N. Engl. J. Med.,* **313,** 217

194. Kennedy, J. W., Kaiser, G. C., Fisher, L. D. *et al.* (1981). Clinical and angiographic predictors of operative mortality from the collaborative study in coronary artery surgery (CASS). *Circulation,* **63,** 793

195. Murphy, M. L. and the VA co-op study group: myocardial infarction in the VA co-operative study of bypass surgery. (1984). *Circulation,* **70 (Suppl. 2),** 453

196. Myocardial infarction and mortality in the coronary artery surgery study (CASS) randomised trial. (1984). *N. Engl. J. Med.,* **310,** 750–8

197. Shaw, P. J., Bates, D., Hartledge, N. E. S., Heaviside, D., Julian, D. G. and Shaw, D. A. (1985) Early neurological complications of coronary artery bypass surgery. *Br. Med. J.,* **291,** 1384

198. Smith, P. L. C., Newman, S. P., Ell, P. J. *et al.* (1986). Cerebral consequence of cardiopulmonary bypass. *Lancet,* **i,** 823

199. Chesebro, J. H., Fuster, V. and Elveback, L. R. (1984). Effect of dipyridamole on late vein graft patency after coronary bypass operations. *N. Engl. J. Med.* **310,** 209

200. Pumphrey, C. W., Dhesebro, J. H., Dewanjee, M. K. *et al.* (1983). *In vivo* quantitation of platelet deposition on human peripheral arterial bypass grafts using indium 111 labelled platelets: effect of dipyridamole and aspirin. *Am. J. Cardiol.,* **51,** 796

201. Campeau, L., Enjalbert, M., Lesperance, J. *et al.* (1984). The relation of risk factors to the development of atherosclerosis in saphenous vein bypass grafts and the progression of disease on the native circulation. A study 10 years after aorto-coronary bypass surgery. *N. Engl. J. Med.* **311,** 1329

202. Vineberg, A. M. (1946). Development of an anastamosis between the coronary vessels and a transplanted internal mammary artery. *Can. Med. Assoc. J.,* **55,** 117

203. Vineberg, A. M. and Walker, J. (1964). The surgical treatment of coronary artery heart disease by internal mammary artery implantation: report of 140 cases followed up to 13 years. *Dis. Chest* **45,** 190

204. Green, G. E. (1972). Internal mammary to coronary artery anastomosis. Three year experience with 165 patients. *Ann. Thorac. Surg.,* **14,** 260

205. Grondin, C. M., Campeau, L., Lesperance, J., Enjalbert, M. and Bourassa, M. G. (1984). Comparison of late changes in internal mammary and saphenous vein grafts in two consecutive series of patients 10 years after operation. *Circulation,* **70 (Suppl. 1),** 1

206. Loop, F. T., Lytle, B. W. and Cosgrove, D. M. (1986). Influence of the internal mammary artery graft on 10 year survival and other cardiac events. *N. Engl. J. Med.,* **314,** 1

207. Dotter, C. T. and Judkins, M. P. (1964). Transluminal treatment of atherosclerotic obstruction: Description of a new technique and a preliminary report of the application. *Circulation,* **30,** 654

208. Gruentzig, A. R., Senning, A. and Siegenthaler, W. E. (1979). Nonoperative dilatation of coronary artery stenosis. *N. Engl. J. Med.,* **301,** 61

209. Sanborn, T. A., Faxon, D. P., Haudenschild, C., Gottinsman, S. B. and Ryan, T. J.

(1983). The mechanism of transluminal angioplasty: evidence for formation of aneurysms in experimental atherosclerosis. *Circulation,* **68,** 1136

210. Block, P. C., Myler, R. K., Stertzer, S. and Fallon, J. T. (1981). Morphology after transluminal angioplasty in human beings. *N. Engl. J. Med.,* **305,** 382

211. Bonow, R. O., Kent, K. M., Rosing, D. R., Lipson, L. C., Bacharach, S. L., Green, M. V., Epstein, S. E. (1982). Improved left ventricular diastolic filling in patients with coronary artery disease of the percutaneous transluminal coronary angioplasty. *Circulation,* **66,** 1159

212. Kent, K. M., Bonow, R. O., Rosing, D. R., *et al.* (1982). Improved myocardial function during exercise after successful percutaneous transluminal coronary angioplasty. *N. Engl. J. Med.,* **306,** 442

213. Vliestra, R. E., Holmes, D. R. Jr., Reeder, G. S. *et al.* (1983). Balloon angioplasty in multivessel coronary artery disease. *Mayo Clin. Proc.,* **58,** 563

214. Detre, K. M., Mylery, R. K., Kelsey, S. F., Van Raden, A. A., To, T. and Mitchell, H. (1984). Baseline characteristics of patients in the National Heart, Lung and Blood Institute Percutaneous Transluminal Coronary Angioplasty Registry. *Am. J. Cardiol.,* **53,** 7C

215. Cowley, M. J., Danos, G., Kelsey, S. F., Van Radan, M. and Detre, K. M. (1984). Acute coronary events associated with percutaneous transluminal coronary angioplasty. *Am. J. Cardiol.,* **53,** 12C

216. Danos, G., Cowley, M. J., Janke, L., Kelsey, S. F., Mullen, S. M. and Van Radan, M. (1984). In hospital mortality rate in the National Heart, Lung and Blood Institute Percutaneous Transluminal Coronary Angioplasty Registry. *Am. J. Cardiol.,* **53,** 17C

217. Murphy, D. A., Craver, J. M., Jones, E. L. *et al.* (1984). Surgical management of acute myocardial ischaemia following transluminal coronary angioplasty. *J. Thorac. Cardiovasc. Surg.,* **87,** 332

218. Willman, V. L. (1985). Percutaneous transluminal coronary angioplasty, a 1985 perspective. *Circulation,* **71,** 189

219. Consensitive Development Conference: coronary artery bypass grafting. (1984). *Br. Med. J.,* **289,** 1527

7
Investigation and management of unstable angina

P. A. CREAN

INTRODUCTION

Unstable angina is a clinical term used to describe a number of syndromes of varying aetiology. The need to identify patients with unstable angina is obvious as it frequently leads to myocardial infarction and death[1,2]. The definition of unstable angina is angina pectoris that is increasing in either frequency, duration or intensity in the absence of myocardial necrosis. This definition includes rest angina, variant angina, and angina of recent onset in addition to increasing symptoms in patients whose angina was previously stable. Although by definition a patient who has stable angina and then gets one extra episode of angina per week may be said to have unstable angina, this is not what is meant in clinical practice. Similarly, by definition, every patient must go through an 'unstable' phase when their angina starts but if it only occurs on walking five miles it can hardly be said to be unstable. Thus the practical definition should include a modification, which requires a change in angina symptoms of significant severity to require hospital admission.

The pathophysiology of unstable angina has been addressed in detail in an accompanying chapter. From a practical point of investigating and managing, it is necessary to highlight just a few points. Firstly, nearly all patients have significant fixed coronary artery disease. Secondly, the mechanism which leads to the instability of angina may be due to a worsening of the fixed coronary disease or to the superimposition of an element of coronary spasm. In a patient with a 90% coronary artery stenosis a minor further reduction in the coronary diameter due to alteration in coronary tone will lead to a critical reduction in myocardial blood supply and angina; whereas, in a patient with only a minimal coronary stenosis it requires a major degree of change in coronary tone to affect myocardial perfusion. Although arguments in the literature would suggest that fixed coronary disease and coronary spasm are mutually exclusive conditions it appears likely that in unstable angina

219

the spectrums overlap considerably. Some patients have a major component of fixed disease, while others have a major variable element, and between these two extremes lie patients with a combination of both. From a practical point of view it is important to direct the investigations to determine where in each patient the balance between fixed and variable stenosis lies. The investigation of unstable angina must include tests to determine why the condition has become unstable and to establish the presence and severity of the underlying coronary artery disease. When these factors have been established, a rationalized treatment plan can be devised for each individual patient.

MANAGEMENT OF UNSTABLE ANGINA

The overall management of unstable angina should include: initial stabilization of the condition with medical therapy; search for the reversible or initiating factors; assessment of the functional coronary reserve; documentation of the state of the underlying coronary disease and left ventricular function by arteriography; and finally a decision regarding long term therapy, be it medical therapy, angioplasty or coronary artery bypass surgery.

INVESTIGATIONS IN UNSTABLE ANGINA

Tests on admission

On admission the patient must have at least a resting ECG, chest X-ray and blood tests. Whether the resting ECG is abnormal, confirming the clinical impression of coronary artery disease, or normal, as it frequently is once the pain has resolved, the initial recording must be obtained for comparison against subsequent recordings. The chest X-ray must be obtained to look for cardiac enlargement and signs of left ventricular failure, which indicate extensive damage to the left ventricle and hence a poor prognosis. To exclude a myocardial infarction a series of normal cardiac enzymes is mandatory. These investigations should be repeated if symptoms recur after treatment.

Search for reversible non-cardiac causes of unstable angina

In all cases, simple causes for a deterioration in the patient's symptoms should be sought. Thyrotoxicosis, arrhythmia and anaemia should be easily detected and treated as illustrated in Figure 7.1. A 73-year-old man with previously stable angina complained of progressively increasing chest pain over three months. His exercise test was stopped during the warm up stage with chest pain and 3 mm ST segment depression at a peak heart rate of 110 beats per minute. At this time the patient had a microcytic anaemia with a haemaglobin level of 8.5 g and when this returned to his previously normal level of 15.3 g. his angina settled and

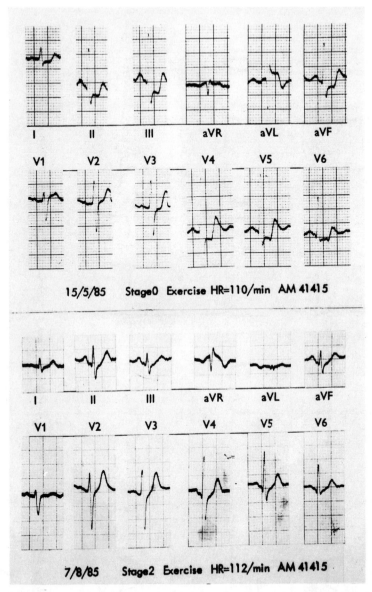

Figure 7.1 Twelve lead ECG at peak exercise, in a patient with significant left anterior descending coronary stenoses and anaemia. The exercise test in the top panel shows significant ST depression that accompanied chest pain at Stage 0 and at a heart rate of 110 beats/min. Three months later, when the Hb increased from 8 to 15 g/dl, the patient reached Stage 3 of a modified Bruce protocol without chest pain and minimal ST change (bottom panel)

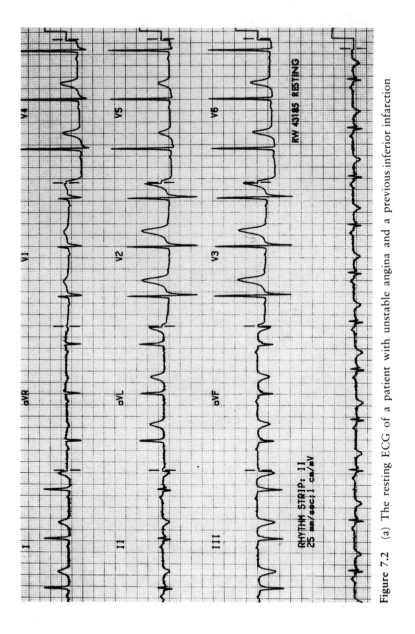

Figure 7.2 (a) The resting ECG of a patient with unstable angina and a previous inferior infarction

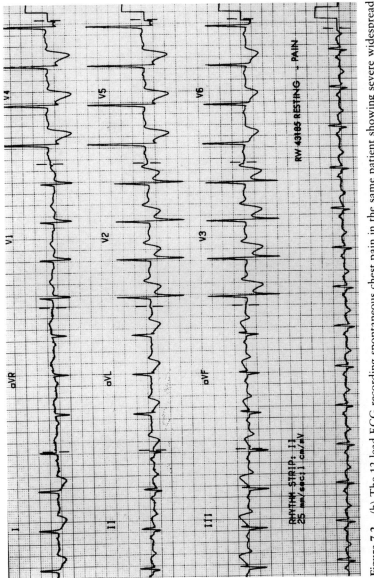

Figure 7.2 (b) The 12 lead ECG recording spontaneous chest pain in the same patient showing severe widespread ST segment depression. Coronary angiography demonstrated left main stem disease and a blocked right coronary artery

223

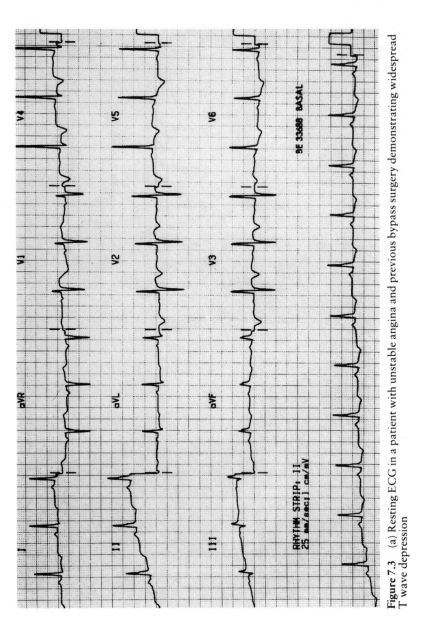

Figure 7.3 (a) Resting ECG in a patient with unstable angina and previous bypass surgery demonstrating widespread T wave depression

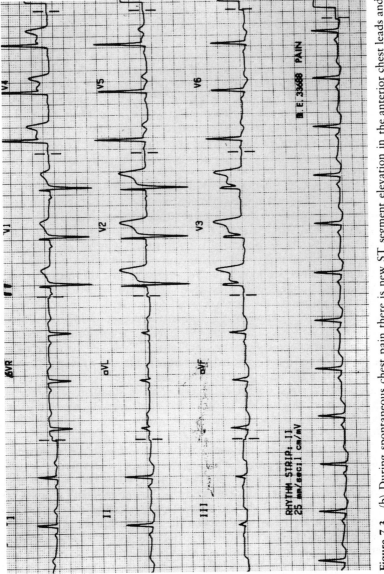

Figure 7.3 (b) During spontaneous chest pain there is new ST segment elevation in the anterior chest leads and pseudonormalization of previous inverted T waves

the corresponding exercise test to Stage 3 and a peak heart rate of 112 beats per minute shows minimal ST depression (lower panel).

Investigations during initial hospitalization

Electrocardiogram during pain

Patients with unstable angina should be monitored in a ward where a 12 lead ECG can be obtained once the pain occurs preferably before and after sublingual nitrates are given. The ECG recordings during chest pain provide valuable information as to the pathogenesis of the condition. Transient electrocardiographic changes may indicate the site and indeed the extent of underlying coronary disease. In addition the direction and magnitude of ECG changes during pain provide a guide to treatment.

If the basal ECG is normal and fails to show any changes during the patient's typical chest pain it is unlikely that the pain is cardiac in origin and further investigations including provocative tests should be pursued. Having stated this, particular care must be paid to look for transient T wave changes (such as peaking, pseudonormalization or inversion), which in unstable angina are as significant as ST segment changes.

ST segment depression or T wave inversion are the most frequent accompanying changes with chest pain. The site where ECG changes are observed point to the coronary artery in which disease may be expected. Widespread anterior ST segment depression during pain suggests significant stenosis in the proximal part of the left anterior descending or left main coronary artery. In Figure 7.2 the electrocardiogram during spontaneous pain demonstrates new transient widespread severe ST segment changes in a patient who had a severe left main stenosis and an occluded right coronary artery. The mechanism causing pain with ST segment depression is more likely to be due to severe fixed coronary narrowings especially if the ischaemia is not preceded by an increase in the heart rate[3].

In those patients with unstable angina due to a major degree of coronary spasm during pain the ST segment may be elevated, depressed or associated with only minor T wave changes[4]. However, ST elevation, T wave peaking or pseudonormalization during pain all suggest coronary spasm[4]. Figure 7.3 shows transient ST segment elevation in the anterior leads in a patient with spasm in the proximal part of the left anterior descending coronary artery. Ventricular arrhythmias are a frequent accompaniment with spontaneous pain and ST segment change[5]. These arrhythmias usually resolve with the relief of the pain, however. Figure 7.4 shows a 24 hour tape recording of a patient with angina ST segment depression and sudden death. The atrial fibrillation had been present for some time but new ST segment depression can be seen to precede the onset of chest pain, the rhythm then degenerated into ventricular tachycardia and later fibrillation.

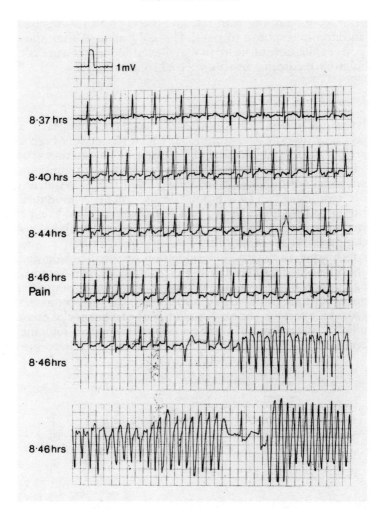

Figure 7.4 Continuous strip from a 24 hour recording in a patient with longstanding atrial fibrillation and unstable angina. ST segment depression and chest pain precede a number of ventricular ectopics, which initiated the onset of ventricular tachycardia

The heart rate during chest pain has been used by some groups as a guide to treatment[6]. If ST segment depression is associated with an increase in heart rate or blood pressure (rate pressure product) it indicates that ischaemia is secondary to increased myocardial oxygen demand, which is therefore best treated with beta-blocking agents. Should the pain and ECG changes not be associated with an increase in rate pressure product, then a primary reduction in coronary flow may be suspected and treated with calcium antagonist[7]. To implement this approach, continuous recordings of the heart rate must be obtained prior to and at the onset of pain; because if a single recording is made after the onset of pain, the heart rate and blood pressure will be elevated as an autonomic response to pain. The only method that allows this continuous evaluation of heart rate and even blood pressure is the use of ambulatory recording devices referred to later[8].

Ambulatory ST segment monitoring

Ambulatory 24 hours monitoring of ST segment changes is a comparatively new investigative technique, which has mainly been used as a research device to understand the pathogenic mechanisms of chest pain[26]. The American Heart Association has laid down minimum standard guidelines for the equipment used so that the ST segment can be faithfully reproduced[27]. Two bipolar leads, usually a modified CM5, and an inferior lead are recorded and a patient activated event marker and timer are also recorded. The tape is replayed and analysed visually[28] or by computer[8].

This technique allows the determination of the direction and magnitude of ST segment shifts and the estimation of their frequency. By studying patients in this way it has shown that most episodes (80%) of ST segment shift are not associated with pain, thus symptom recording alone provides a serious underestimation of the frequency of myocardial ischaemia[26,29]. When used in a patient population with a high incidence of coronary artery disease, the ST segment shifts have been proven to

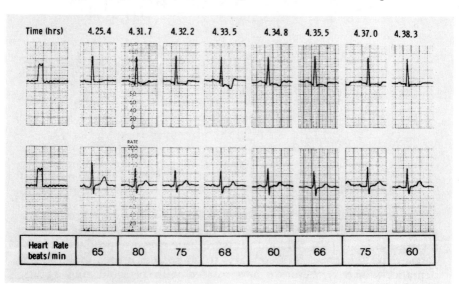

Time (hrs)	4.25.4	4.31.7	4.32.2	4.33.5	4.34.8	4.35.5	4.37.0	4.38.3
Heart Rate beats/min	65	80	75	68	60	66	75	60

Figure 7.5 Simultaneous ECG complexes from an anterior and inferior lead using FM 24 hour monitoring during an episode of painful ST segment depression. The top row shows the time of each complex and the lower row shows the heart rate at that time. This system provides useful information regarding the pathological mechanisms and treatment of the condition

be due to myocardial ischaemia[29]; although in each patient, the records must be examined carefully to exclude posture induced changes which characteristically start and terminate rapidly. The episodes of silent and painful myocardial ischaemia are similar in nearly all respects except that painful episodes have a tendency to be of longer duration and more extensive ST shifts[26,30].

Analysis of the behaviour of the heart rate response in association to the ST segment changes provides useful information as to the pathogenesis of angina (Figure 7.5). The characteristic feature of angina due to fixed coronary disease is that heart rate increases before the onset of ST shift, caused by an increased demand for oxygen[3]. In variant angina, the heart rate does not increase before the onset of ST shift (usually ST elevation) although it does increase when ischaemia has been established for some minutes. This later type of ischaemia is presumably due to decreased coronary flow and implies a degree of coronary spasm in the pathogenesis of the condition provided the blood pressure remains constant[7].

Exercise testing

Stress testing electrocardiography in stable angina is a useful non-invasive test, which provides an important guide to the presence and severity of coronary artery stenosis[9] and also a guide to subsequent prognosis[10]. Exercise testing following myocardial infarction is also a safe test, which provides useful prognostic information[11]. Until recently, exercise tests were avoided in unstable angina as it was feared that infarction may be provoked by the stress. It has now been shown that patients may exercise safely some days following stabilization using a gentle protocol[12,13] with the exercise terminated by the onset of 1 mm ST change, a drop in blood pressure, angina, frequent ectopic beats or a heart rate of 70% of the age predicted maximal[14,15] (Figure 7.6).

Early exercise tests performed 4 days after the last episode of chest pain in 72 patients provided a good long term guide to symptomatic status. Twenty nine of 32 patients (90%) with a positive test had severe angina (Grade 3–4 NYHA), while only 7 of 32 (21%) with a negative exercise test had severe angina at follow up one year later[14]. Similar findings with regard to the prediction of symptomatic status six months after discharge were also reported by Nixon *et al.* in a study of 55 patients[15]. Submaximal exercise testing also provided a guide to the severity of coronary disease present with 27/29 positive tests being in patients with multivessel disease[14]. The high incidence of false negative tests in that report further emphasizes the need for angiography in patients with unstable angina[14]. When combined with clinical findings and angiographic results, exercise tests may be used to define a rationale plan for those who may need early intervention by either coronary angioplasty or bypass surgery.

In patients with rest angina due to coronary artery spasm, stress

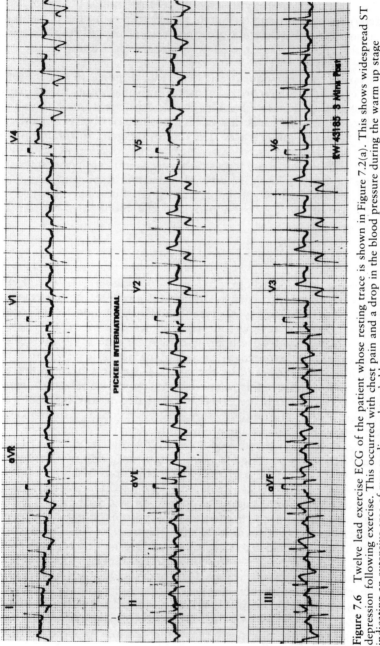

Figure 7.6 Twelve lead exercise ECG of the patient whose resting trace is shown in Figure 7.2(a). This shows widespread ST depression following exercise. This occurred with chest pain and a drop in the blood pressure during the warm up stage indicating an extensive area of myocardium subtended by a severe coronary stenosis

testing may be used to induce myocardial ischaemia. The changes induced by exercise are also due to induced coronary spasm but do not give a reliable guide to the severity of the underlying coronary disease or prognosis. In a study of patients reported by Waters *et al.* one third of patients had ST segment elevation, one third ST segment depression, and the remainder no ST change. The results had very poor correlation with the extent of underlying coronary artery disease but related closely with the disease activity[16,17]. In a recent paper, however, when patients with variant angina were tested while on treatment with calcium antagonists to block any exercise induced spasm the results obtained were indicative of the severity of fixed underlying coronary stenoses. In 57 patients who exercised on treatment reported by Araki *et al.* 48 were negative and 9 positive. All 9 patients with a positive exercise test had significant stenoses, while only 2 of 48 patients with a negative test had significant disease (sensitivity 100%, specificity 96%)[18].

CORONARY ARTERIOGRAPHY

Coronary arteriography should be performed on all patients with unstable angina prior to hospital discharge. Ideally the angiographic examination should be performed some days after the patient has been rendered free of chest pain or earlier in those patients in whom spontaneous pain persists despite oral and parenteral therapy. Arteriography is only contraindicated when an intervention such as angioplasty or surgery is not a viable mode of treatment because of advanced age, systemic disease or known inoperable coronary disease. The examination may be performed via the femoral or brachial routes with adequate heparinization. In severe cases, a low ionic concentration contrast medium is preferable. Patients frequently experience pain during the procedure, which is best avoided by the continuous infusion of nitrates throughout the test.

The cause of unstable angina is multifactorial with a common element of fixed coronary arterial stenoses in over 90% of cases. Coronary arteriography in patients presenting with unstable angina reveals a high incidence of occluded or severely narrowed coronary arteries[19]. This high incidence of coronary disease has been confirmed by widespread intervention studies in patients with refractory chest pain and in the early stages of myocardial infarction[20]. The presence of multiple severe strictures alone does not explain the instability of unstable angina as a similar pattern of coronary arterial disease is observed in those patients undergoing elective investigation for the presence of chronic stable angina[21]. There are, however, a number of interesting angiographic observations to be noted. The incidence of normal coronary arteries in patients with unstable angina is approximately 10% and appears to be higher in those with recent onset angina. Disease of a single vessel (usually the left anterior descending) was found in 31 of 75 patients with recent onset angina[22], while triple vessel disease was present in only

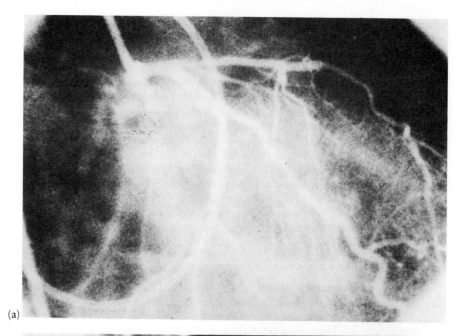

(a)

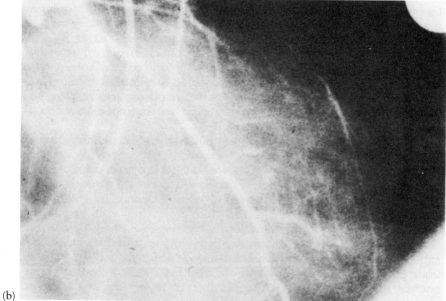

(b)

Figure 7.7 (a) selective left coronary angiogram in the right anterior oblique projection with a significant proximal stenosis in the left anterior descending artery

(b) Repeat angiography in the same projection following hyperventilation which induced chest pain and ST elevation shows near total occlusion of the left anterior descending artery. The changes resolved completely following nitrate administration

10% of cases. In contrast to this a much higher incidence of multiple and/or multisegment vessel disease was found in those patients who had previous anginal symptoms[23]. Further interesting data comes from a careful retrospective study from the Montreal Heart Institute. They demonstrated that progression of coronary artery disease was significantly more common in patients with unstable angina compared to those with stable angina, both groups being comparable for other variables[24].

In patients with normal coronary arteries and myocardial infarction, spasm of a large epicardial artery is a frequent finding. This has been elegantly demonstrated by continuous electrocardiographic and haemo-dynamic monitoring during spontaneous chest pain in patients who have subsequently been shown to have coronary spasm at arteriography, either spontaneous or induced by various physical or pharmacological stimuli[4]. The prevalance of spasm in patients with fixed coronary stenoses and unstable angina has been estimated at between 5 and 90% depending largely on the referral pattern to the reporting centres. Even in the presence of a large atherosclerotic plaque there is nearly always a non-diseased portion of the arterial wall, which can contract normally. This finding has been shown by Brown *et al.* in cases of both stable angina with fixed coronary artery disease and unstable angina where there may be a critical reduction in the diameter in addition to an already tight stenosis[4,25]. An example of the latter is shown in Figure 7.7, which shows the angiograms of a patient with recent onset unstable angina. The basal angiogram demonstrates a tight proximal left anterior descending artery stenosis. The patient's typical chest pain and anterior ST segment elevation were reproduced by hyperventilation and the stenosed artery was seen to occlude. All of these changes resolved with intra-coronary nitrates leaving a tight residual stenosis. In patients like this, minor changes in coronary diameter superimposed on a fixed stenosis are often sufficient to cause myocardial ischaemia.

PROVOCATIVE TESTS IN UNSTABLE ANGINA

The provocative tests outlined below should only be performed with knowledge of the patient's anatomy, and patients in whom continuous observation has failed to yield a changing electrocardiogram during chest pain. Hence, the indications for such tests are (a) atypical chest pain with normal electrocardiogram, (b) a history suggestive of variant angina but no spontaneous episodes observed, and (c) as a research test to assess the effect of treatment in variant angina. No patient with left main, triple vessel disease or poor left ventricular function should undergo these tests.

Hyperventilation test

The patient is asked to breathe deeply and fast for at least two minutes and preferably five. Arterial samples may be taken before and after to ensure adequate shift of the pH to >7.5. During the test, the patient frequently experiences tingling in the fingers and light-headedness. As the test progresses, the heart rate increases slightly but the induction of coronary spasm usually occurs in the first two minutes after hyperventilation. The standard criteria for ST segment shift are used to determine a positive result. The test should be terminated with intravenous nitrates[31].

Cold pressor test

The aim of this test is to provoke a potent increase in alpha sympathetic output and hence reduce coronary artery diameter. One hand should be immersed in ice cold water to the level of the wrist for two minutes[32]. The alteration in heart rate and blood pressure may be accompanied by ST segment depression in patients with fixed coronary disease or ST elevation in those with coronary spasm.

Ergonovine test

This test is a sensitive test for the diagnosis of coronary artery spasm, which reproduces the chest pain and ST changes of a spontaneous episode in nearly all cases[33]. The test has been associated with fatalities but may be done safely in either the coronary care unit or at arteriography, provided an incremental dosage technique is used and nitrates are given as soon as diagnostic electrocardiographic changes are seen[33-35]. Whilst the test is performed, the patient should have his blood pressure and a 12 lead ECG recorded every minute during and for 10 minutes after the test. Nitrates, atropine and lignocaine should be drawn up ready to inject and full resuscitation equipment should be available.

Ergonovine causes a 20% reduction in normal coronary arteries, while an abnormal response is interpreted as a focal narrowing with >50% reduction in coronary diameter. The electrocardiographic changes most often observed are ST segment elevation in patients with variant angina, which starts abruptly, while in patients with fixed severe lesions, the ST segment depression is more likely due to the increase in left ventricular volume and minor reduction in coronary diameter rather than focal coronary spasm.

TREATMENT OF UNSTABLE ANGINA

Patients should be initially confined to bed and monitored in a coronary care unit. A simple step-wise approach to treatment in each case rather than the routine use of a large number of drugs in all cases is the best approach.

NITRATES

The first line of treatment in unstable angina must include a short acting nitrate preparation. Nitroglycerin will relieve the acute ischaemic episode irrespective of whether it occurs at rest or is exercise induced and whether it is associated with fixed or dynamic coronary obstruction. Nitrates when given by different routes exert the same haemodynamic effects but over a different time span and to a different magnitude.

The beneficial effects of nitrates are shown in Figure 7.8. The peripheral vasodilating effect results in a fall in systemic vascular resistance (afterload). The venous pooling effect decreases the ventricular end-diastolic volume (preload). Both effects are additive in reducing myocardial oxygen demand[36]. In unstable angina the direct coronary arterial dilating effect is probably the most important effect as most episodes occur at rest and are often not preceded by an increase in myocardial oxygen consumption. Nitrates dilate all the coronary arterial tree including the stenotic areas and indeed probably the stenoses to a greater degree than the normal artery[25].

Intravenous nitrates should be started at a low dose and increased as necessary. The dose should be titrated against the systolic blood pressure and symptoms. The maximal dose that can be administered is limited by the side effects of excessive vasodilators, i.e. headache and hypotension. In those patients in whom there is severe multiple coronary stenoses and little coronary reserve and in whom minimal exertion produces myocardial ischaemia, intravenous nitrates should be used with beta-adrenergic blockers because the tachycardia and hypotensive effects of large doses of nitrates may be detrimental.

In variant angina, intravenous nitrates and placebo have been compared in a randomized double blind cross-over study of 12 patients. The number of episodes of ST segment shift fell from a mean of 97 during placebo to 16 during a similar time interval with intravenous nitrates. Active treatment was as effective in reducing episodes of ischaemia, both silent and with pain, and equally in episodes that were associated with either ST elevation or depression[37]. In all 12 cases the authors reported an improvement in symptoms. Intravenous nitrates either on their own or as combined therapy can be expected to render over 60% of patients asymptomatic.

CALCIUM ANTAGONISTS

The introduction of calcium antagonists has added a potent new regime for the treatment of angina. The three major calcium channel agents presently available in this country have similar basic properties but many differing effects that make one or other more suitable in certain conditions. Nifedipine is a potent vasodilator with little depressant effect on contractility and conduction, whereas verapamil potently depresses these two functions and diltiazem lies somewhere in between in its

235

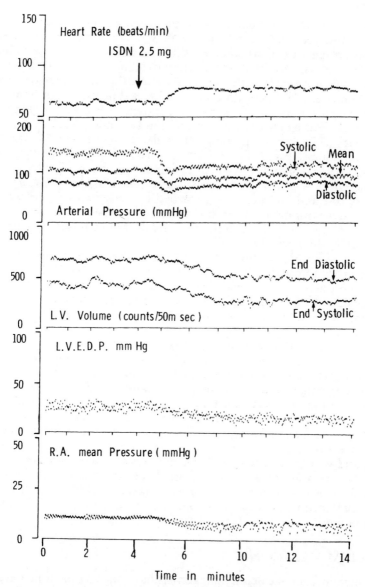

Figure 7.8 Continuous computer analysed recordings of heart rate, arterial pressure, left ventricular end diastolic pressure, LV volume using red cell labelling and right atrial pressure before, during and after the administration of nitrates. Following nitrate injection there is a decrease in left ventricular volume and filling pressure (preload) in association with a fall in blood pressure (afterload). There is a minimal rise in heart rate and fall in aortic diastolic pressure

spectrum of effects. All three agents are given orally thrice daily and are effective in improving exercise tolerance in patients with chronic stable angina[38].

In addition, calcium channel blocking drugs have been shown to block coronary artery spasm, either spontaneous or induced by ergonovine, with similar degrees of success both in the short term and during long term follow up[39]. Verapamil was reported as effective in controlling rest pain and has subsequently been demonstrated to be an effective treatment of angina in a randomized prospective trial by Parodi[40] in a double blind cross-over trial of alternating placebo and verapamil 480 mg daily in 12 patients. The number of episodes of ST segment shift per 48 hour treatment period fell from a mean of 127 with placebo to 27 with verapamil, a highly significant effect. Metha reported a similar beneficial effect of verapamil in 15 patients with unstable angina studied in a further placebo controlled randomized trial[41]. Nifedipine has also been shown as effective in controlling symptoms in a randomized trial of 128 patients reported by Gerstenblith[42]. In this study, the addition of nifedipine to conventional medical therapy significantly reduced the incidence of death, surgery and infarction compared to placebo treatment. The three previous studies included patients with rest angina and both ST segment elevation and depression; whereas the overall effect of nifedipine and verapamil appears similar, it is important to note that verapamil was equally effective irrespective of the direction of the ST segment shift while nifedipine was only effective in those patients with elevation. Diltiazem in common with the other calcium antagonists is excellent in controlling spontaneous or ergonovine induced coronary artery spasm[39]. When patients with variant angina were excluded from a randomized trial in unstable angina Diltiazem showed a significant reduction in the number of daily episodes of chest pain from 0.75 with placebo to 0.25 with therapy[43]. With long term follow up (4 to 5 months) diltiazem alone controlled symptoms in 42% of patients, while nifedipine in addition to propranolol, controlled 39% of patients satisfactorily[42,43].

Nifedipine should be started in a dosage of 10 mg tds and increased to 20 mg tds if necessary. Further increase in therapy is likely to result in side effects such as headache, hypotension and ankle swelling and other therapeutic regimes should be sought. Nifedipine has no effect on intra-cardiac conduction and thus may be safely combined with a beta-adrenergic blocking effect. This combination is often effective as the beta-blocker will prevent the reflex tachycardia induced by the potent vasodilator effect. Verapamil is an agent with many properties similar to beta-blockers in its depressant effect on the atrioventricular node and on myocardial contractility. Thus, verapamil and beta blockers should not be combined except in carefully monitored situations. Verapamil should be avoided in patients with atrioventricular block or heart failure. The initial dosage of 40 mg tds may be augmented to 120 mg tds as required to gain symptomatic relief. Diltiazem, the latest of these agents to be used in this country, has a spectrum of effects that lie somewhere between nifedipine and verapamil. It should be used in a dosage of 90 mg tds at least for effective control of angina but this may be increased to 120 mg tds. Unfortunately, only 60 mg tablets are available in this country, thus tablets have to be split, a practice the manufacturers should soon rectify.

BETA-ADRENERGIC BLOCKING AGENTS

Beta-adrenergic blocking drugs reduce the oxygen demands of the contracting myocardium by reducing the rate and force of myocardial contraction. At rest the heart rate and blood pressure are lowered, while on exercise the rate of increase of both of these indices is delayed. Hence they are effective in reducing exercise induced myocardial ischaemia, although it appears to be achieved by a more complicated mechanism than that which is simply outlined above[44]. Whatever their exact mode of action, they improve total exercise duration by approximately 30% in chronic stable angina and are equally effective in reducing episodes of ST segment depression and angina which are not preceded by an increase in heart rate as those episodes which occur following a rise in heart rate[44].

Since their introduction, beta-blocking agents have been used either on their own or with nitrate preparations in order to treat unstable angina with good results. Indeed beta-blockers have been accepted as effective therapy to such a degree that this type of treatment is the yardstick against which any new intervention (such as new drugs, surgery or coronary dilatation) must be evaluated[43,45]. With the realization that beta-blockers may worsen symptoms in certain cases that have a vasospastic component, a number of studies have suggested that calcium antagonists are more effective than beta-blockers in unstable angina. In the report by Gerstenblith, the addition of a calcium blocker to the already prescribed beta-blocker resulted in improved success rate of medical therapy, however, this improvement was confined to those with ST elevation at rest[42]. In Parodi's study, the failure of propranolol to improve symptoms in unstable angina, as compared to the significant effect of verapamil, was due to the high percentage of patients with coronary spasm included in the study.

Given that clinicians now avoid beta-blockers in variant angina, it is unfair to compare the results of treatment with calcium antagonists and beta-blockers in unstable angina when a large proportion of the patients have variant angina. In the report by Theroux, in which treatment with propranolol was compared to diltiazem in patients with unstable angina specifically excluding patients with variant angina, the results of the two drug treatments were comparable. During hospital admission, the number of anginal attacks per day fell from 0.75 with placebo to 0.25 with diltiazem and 0.29 with propranolol. In the long term follow up of 5.1 months the control of symptoms, rates of myocardial infarction or death were similar in both groups[43]. Thus beta-blocking agents are effective in controlling unstable angina when variant angina is excluded.

In unstable angina beta-blockers should be started in a small dose. We prefer to use propranolol, which is a short acting agent that offers easy changes in dosage. A change to a cardiospecific agent or one which can be administered once daily may be carried out once the condition has been stabilized. Beta-blocking agents are contraindicated in heart failure and heart block and should be used with caution in those patients with diabetes, obstructive airways disease and obviously variant angina. In variant angina, beta-blockade may potentiate the role of alpha receptors in which case their unopposed action may lead to enhanced coronary vasoconstriction. Worsening of angina after starting beta-blockers should raise the possibility of coronary spasm.

Anticoagulants and antiplatelet agents in unstable angina

Antiplatelets

Evidence supporting a role of platelets in unstable angina is derived from the observation of an increase in the breakdown products of thromboxane A2 (a potent vasoconstrictor) in the coronary sinus compared to the aortic levels. This gradient across the coronary bed increases during chest pain and pacing. In addition, platelet activation could be the unifying event that leads to coronary vasospasm or thrombosis in the region of a ruptured atherosclerotic lesion.

In variant angina due to spasm there is convincing evidence to suggest that platelet activation is not the cause of coronary spasm. Firstly, in a series of observations increase in thromboxane B2 levels occurred at least 30 seconds after ST segment elevation suggesting platelet aggregation in a secondary rather than a primary event[46]. In two clinical trials, antiplatelet agents failed to reduce the incidence of spontaneous attacks as monitored by 24 hours ST segment analysis. Indomethacin, 50 mg eight hourly, prevents platelet aggregation but did not affect the frequency of angina – neither did low dose aspirin therapy or dipyridamole[47]. Prostacyclin given by intravenous infusion prevents platelet aggregation and reduces blood pressure by a direct vasodilating effect but again produced no improvement in spontaneous angina[48].

Antiplatelet agents given following myocardial infarction produce no reduction in mortality. This could be viewed as similar to patients with a completed stroke receiving antiplatelet drugs; whereas unstable angina, with its evidence of distal platelet infarcts, is more analogous to a transient ischaemic attack in which aspirin has been successful in preventing further events[49]. This theory has been borne out in clinical practice. Lewis et al. reported a study randomizing 1266 men with unstable angina given 324 mg aspirin or placebo daily[50]. As early as three months following unstable angina mortality was reduced by 50% in the aspirin compared to the placebo group and this difference was highly significant at one year being 5.5 and 9.6% in the respective groups

($p = 0.008$). The incidence of death and myocardial infarction was also significantly decreased by aspirin. In a subsequent trial in Canada 555 patients were randomized to aspirin, sulphinpyrazone, both or neither. No significant effect was observed with sulphinpyrazone, aspirin reduced the incidence of death by 71% ($p < 0.004$) and the incidence of deaths and myocardial infarctions by 51% ($p < 0.0008$)[51].

Anticoagulants

The role of formal anticoagulants with either heparin alone or with warfarin in unstable angina is difficult to evaluate because of the lack of controlled clinical studies. The vogue for treating all myocardial infarcts or impending infarcts with anticoagulants is based on the logic that intracoronary thrombosis leads to infarction and followed early impressive results in unfortunately uncontrolled trials. Nichol et al. reported impressive data in 318 patients suggesting a role for anticoagulants in unstable angina[52]. After this, most coronary care units in Europe used anticoagulants routinely and further controlled clinical trials were judged unethical and not performed. The few trials of anticoagulation in unstable angina, although suggesting a beneficial effect, are fraught with design flaws.

CORONARY ARTERY BYPASS SURGERY

In chronic stable angina coronary artery bypass surgery relieves angina and improves survival in certain subgroups of patients with specific coronary stenoses, while having a low mortality and morbidity[53,54]. Emergency bypass surgery in unstable angina was initially performed with a high mortality rate but this has now been reduced to less than 2%, thus rendering it a possible option for the treatment of unstable angina[54].

There have been a number of randomized prospective studies comparing surgical and medical therapy in unstable angina, the largest of which, the National Cooperative Unstable Angina Study, randomized 288 patients[45]. This trial excluded patients with left main stenosis, severe triple vessel disease and poor left ventricular function. The results of the study demonstrated an in hospital mortality of 3% in the medical group and 5% in the surgical group and a late mortality (68 months) of 16% and 15% for the respective groups ($p = $ ns). The incidence of infarction was higher in the surgical group compared to the medical group for both early 17% vs 8% and late results 33% vs 18% ($p < 0.05$). These results of no significant improvement in mortality with surgery in unstable angina are supported by similar findings from Seldon et al. and Pugh et al.[55,56]. One study from Bertolasi suggested that what they classified as an intermediate syndrome showed better results when managed surgically but this may have been due to the inclusion of left main stem and other subgroups known to require surgery[57].

Although these studies showed no overall mortality benefit of surgery in unstable angina, they demonstrated that if necessary surgery may be performed with low mortality. They also showed a clear long term improvement in symptoms for those undergoing early surgery and also a high cross over from the medical to surgical group during follow up. In addition, other studies have identified simple clinical markers, which point towards a high risk group that may benefit from surgery. These include the presence of previous infarction or hypertension, ST segment abnormalities on the resting electrocardiogram or >3mm ST depression on exercise, and severe symptoms.

The overall policy in unstable angina should include urgent surgery in the early stages for angina, which fails to settle on maximal medical therapy (approximately 3%). In the remaining patients who settle, a high risk group may be identified using the above mentioned clinical criteria combined with angiographic findings of left main stem, triple vessel or proximal left anterior descending and right coronary stenoses. These high risk patients should be operated upon, preferably during that hospital admission. In those patients in whom the symptoms settle and do not appear to be a high risk, surgery may be performed at any time in the future for symptomatic benefit.

CORONARY ANGIOPLASTY

The initial limited clinical indications and narrow spectrum of suitable coronary anatomy for percutaneous balloon dilatation has been expanded because of the impressive initial and long term success[58]. Double or triple vessel stenoses may be dilated and total occlusions reopened. Unstable angina was considered a contraindication to angioplasty but except in a limited number of cases with variant angina, it now appears an attractive and effective form of treatment. This is particularly so in the case of recent onset angina or worsening angina without a long preceding history – in these cases, angiography is likely to show severe single vessel stenoses. Angioplasty is indicated in patients with unstable angina and proximal stenoses in one or two of the major coronary arteries.

Because of the existence of plaque fissuring and the potential for coronary spasm, certain precautions should be followed. All patients should be treated with calcium antagonists before the procedure and beta-blockers should be withdrawn. The patient should be stabilized and symptom free for a few days, if at all possible. Intravenous nitrates should be given by infusion throughout the procedure and full heparinization during and following the dilatation. The control angiogram should be repeated after intracoronary nitrates to ensure the stenosis is not due to reversible coronary spasm before dilatation is contemplated.

The results of coronary angioplasty in unstable angina show a high primary success rate in excess of 75% and a low incidence of emergency surgery for complications[59]. In the large series reported by Bentivoglio

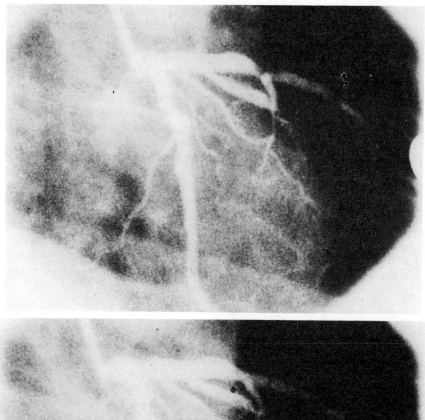

(a)

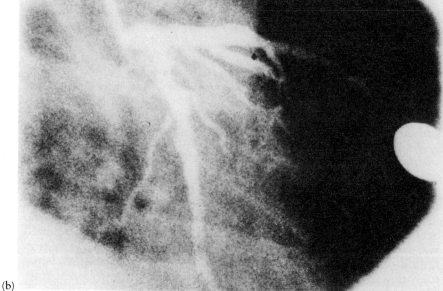

(b)

Figure 7.9 (a) Selective left coronary angiograms in the right anterior oblique view of a patient with unstable angina. A severe stenosis in the proximal portion of the left anterior descending artery is clearly visualized

(b) Control angiogram in the same projection immediately following uncomplicated angioplasty with relief of the coronary stenosis the results are similar in unstable and stable angina with regards to early and long term success and complications including infarction, emergency surgery and mortality[60,61]. The improved results have resulted from the development of low profile balloon dilatation catheters and steerable guide wires. In Figure 7.9(a) the coronary arteriogram from a 60-year-old man with a two week history of unstable angina shows a severe proximal left anterior descending coronary artery stenosis. Following dilatation the artery looks normal (Figure 7.9(b)). The patient became asymptomatic and angiography six months later demonstrated no recurrence of the stenosis.

A particularly cautionary note must be made with respect to patients with variant angina. The experience of the Montreal Heart Institute suggests that although a good angiographic result may be obtained at the time of dilatation, there is a 70% recurrence rate. Indeed their results of dilatation in this setting do not improve either the morbidity or mortality of the condition compared to its medical treated outcome with calcium antagonists[62].

ROLE OF THROMBOLYSIS IN UNSTABLE ANGINA

In recent years there has been considerable interest in the administration of thrombolytic agents in acute myocardial infarction. Studies in experimental animals and in man have shown that there is a limited 'time window' after the total occlusion of a coronary vessel before the onset of irreversible damage to the myocardium[63]. Thus any intervention to restore blood flow in an occluded artery must be performed early to ensure myocardial salvage. Following myocardial infarction, the incidence of total coronary vessel occlusion to the infarcted area decreases with time following infarction[64]. In the setting of myocardial infarction restoration of blood flow in an occluded vessel may be observed directly by coronary arteriography or indirectly by the observation of an early peak of the release of the enzyme creatinine phosphokinase or its MB isoenzyme fraction.

As unstable angina has been frequently observed to be a precursor of myocardial infarction, the pathological events leading to infarction are more than likely the same as those outlined before as the genesis in unstable angina. In a patient with unstable angina who has prolonged pain and ischaemic electrocardiographic changes, which are unrelieved by either intravenous nitrates and/or calcium antagonists, one must assume that there has been total occlusion of a coronary vessel and steps should be taken to restore blood flow. Ideally this should be performed in the cardiac catheterization laboratory. Selective intra-coronary injection of the coronary arteries allows for the visualization of the occluded vessel. If the vessel remains closed after intra-coronary nitrates, the occlusion may be assumed to be thrombotic in nature. Intra-coronary streptokinase should then be infused through an angiographic catheter or through a smaller bore catheter advanced down the main coronary vessels to the site of the occlusive lesion. Streptokinase is given until the vessel is re-opened or until some other intervention is decided upon. It should be remembered that vascular spasm and thrombosis often co-exist and in addition to the thrombolytic agent, nitrates should be administered by the intra-coronary route to improve the chances of restoration of blood flow[65].

The combination of thrombolytic agents with percutaneous dilatation at the same time has been advocated by many centres to ensure a higher rate of patency[66]. These interventions may be safely combined in patients with recent total vessel occlusion but the obvious sequelae should be anticipated and can either be avoided or quickly corrected. Thrombolytic agents may induce a shock like state and thus steroids should be administered systematically to avoid this reaction. Reperfusion causes frequent ventricular ectopics leading to ventricular tachycardia and fibrillation, which normally responds to DC cardioversion or anti-arrhythmic agents. The major late complication of thrombolytic agents is bleeding caused by the systemic thrombolytic state. Careful attention to possible bleeding sites and avoidance of arterial puncture, except for the cardiac catheter insertion, is mandatory.

In acute myocardial infarction there have been numerous randomized trials of intravenous and intracoronary administration comparing mortality and the indices of infarct size in the treated and control group. A large multicentre study was recently completed in Italy where 1200 patients with myocardial infarction were randomized to receive either placebo or a single intravenous injection of 1.5 million units of streptokinase within 12 hours of infarction. They reported a significant reduction (18%, $p = 0.0002$) in mortality in the treated group compared to the placebo group, with the most striking effect observed in those treated early[67]. Thrombolytic agents given at the time of cardiac catheterization also reported a short term improvement in mortality, although the one year mortality in the treated and untreated groups were similar. One logical conclusion from these studies must be that thrombolytic therapy will restore patency in a high percentage of occluded vessels but in those in whom a high degree of residual stenoses remains, some other intervention – either coronary dilatation or bypass surgery – should be performed in the days following to avoid the high incidence of reocclusion. A further promising development is the availability of tissue plasminogen activator (TPA). This agent induced lysis of the thrombus within the coronary vessel without inducing a systemic thrombolytic state, thus offering the prospect of thrombolysis without the serious complications of bleeding. The initial results appear promising but the final results of the large studies in both Europe and America are awaited[68].

INTRA-AORTIC BALLOON PUMPING

Intra-aortic balloon counterpulsation is a mechanical assist device introduced in the early 1960s for the support of patients with severe heart failure. The 30 ml balloon is introduced either at an open surgical procedure or percutaneously into the femoral artery and advanced to the thoracic aorta. The balloon is triggered by the patient's R wave on the electrocardiagram to inflate in diastole and deflate at the onset of systole. By deflating at the onset of systole the heart can contract against reduced systemic vascular resistance (afterload), which reduces the work the heart must perform. The peak aortic systolic pressure is reduced but the mean arterial pressure is usually elevated, thus improving organ perfusion. When the balloon inflates in diastole it raises the aortic diastolic pressure and as 80% of coronary perfusion occurs in diastole, the coronary blood flow is augmented.

In patients with unstable angina who are refractory to medical therapy, the use of the intra-aortic pump frequently allows stabilization of the condition and the safer performance of cardiac catheterization and coronary artery bypass surgery. In a prospective randomized trial in patients with unstable angina comparing balloon pumping to intravenous nitrate therapy there was no difference in symptom control or mortality by using intra-aortic counterpulsation[71]. When balloon pumping is used in those patients resistant to medical therapy it appears to offer a clear benefit. Weintaub et al. reported 60 cases of refractory angina pectoris treated with balloon counterpulsation and emergency surgery with only five peri-operative infarcts and two deaths[69]. In a non-randomized study of 130 patients in whom 75 received balloon pumping, the results were compared to 55 patients in whom the balloon could not be inserted (control group). Langou et al. reported a 5.6% mortality and 5.1% infarction rate in those patients treated by balloon counterpulsation prior to surgery compared to a 14.5% mortality and 29% infarction rate for those with surgery and no prior counterpulsation[70]. The selection of patients as controls by failure to insert a balloon pump means that these patients had more extensive atherosclerosis and thus were more likely to be older and with a worse prognosis; however, this selection bias is unlikely to explain the large difference between the treated and untreated groups. The major haemodynamic effect of balloon counterpulsation in unstable angina is a reduction of the left ventricular end-diastolic pressure with a decrease in aortic systolic pressure and increased aortic diastolic pressure[67].

Before an intra-aortic balloon pump is inserted the high rate of complications must be considered. These complications are mostly local vascular problems with thrombus, embolic formation or ischaemia of the lower limb. The serious complications of aortic dissection and rupture are rare events. In all cases systemic heparinization with its attendant coagulation problems must be performed. In balance, intra-aortic balloon counterpulsation in medially refractory angina pectoris often allows stabilization of the condition prior to coronary arteriography and coronary artery bypass surgery.

References

1. Conti, C. R., Brawley, R. K., Griffith, L. S. C., Pitt, B., Humphries, J., Gott, V. L. and Ross, J. R. (1973). Unstable angina pectoris. Morbidity and mortality in 57 consecutive patients evaluated angiographically. *Am. J. Cardiol.* **32**, 745–50

2. Mulcahy, R., Daly, L., Graham, I., Hickey, N., O'Donoghue, S., Owens, A.,Ruane, P.,and Tobin,G.(1981).Unstable angina natural history and determinants of prognosis. *Am. J. Cardiol.*, **48**, 525–82

3. Quyyumi, A. A., Wright, C. A., Mockus, L. T., and Fox, K. M. (1984). Mechanisms of nocturnal angina: Importance of increased myocardial oxygen demand in patients with severe coronary artery disease. *Lancet*, **1**, 1207–9

4. Maseri, A., Severi, S., De Nes, M., L'Abbate, A., Chierchia, S., Marzilli, M., *et al.* (1978). Variant angina: one aspect of a continuous spectrum of vasospastic myocardial ischaemia. Pathogenic mechanisms, estimated incidence and clinical and coronary arteriographic findings in 138 patients. *Am. J. Cardiol.*, **42**, 1019–35

5. Araki, H., Koiwaya, Y., Nakagaki, O. and Nakamura, N. (1983). Diurnal distribution of ST-segment elevation and related arrhythmias in patients with variant angina. A study by ambulatory ECG monitoring. *Circulation*, **67**, 995–1000

6. Conti, R., Hall, J.A., Feldman, F.L., Metha, J. L. and Pepine, C. J. (1983). Nitrates for treatment of unstable angina pectoris and coronary vasospasm. *Am. J. Med.*, **74**, 40–4

7. Chierchia, S., Brunelli, C., Simonetti, I., Lazzari, M. and Maseri, A. (1980). Sequence of events in angina at rest. Primary reduction in flow. *Circulation*, **61**, 759–68

8. Gallino, A., Chierchia, S., Smith, G., Croom, M., Morgan, M., Marchesi, C. and Maseri, A. (1984). Computer system for the analysis of ST segment changes on 24-hour holter monitor tapes: Comparison with other available systems. *J. Am. Coll. Cardiol.*, **4**, 245–52

9. Goldschlaher, N., Selzer, A., and Cohn, K. (1976). Treadmill stress tests as indicators of presence and severity of coronary artery disease. *Ann. Int. Med.*, **85**, 277–86

10. Dagenais, G. R. (1982). Survival of patients with a strongly positive exercise electrocardiogram. *Circulation*, **65**(3), 452–6

11. Theroux, P., Waters, D. D., Halpen, C., Debaisieux, J. C. and Mizgala, H. F. (1979). Prognostic value of exercise testing soon after myocardial infarction. *N. Engl. J. Med.*, **301**, 341–5

12. National Exercise and Heart Disease Project: (1975). Common protocol. (Washington DC: George Washington Medical Center)

13. Fox, S. M., Naughton, J. P. and Haskell, W. L. (1971). Physical activity and the prevention of coronary heart disease. *Ann. Clin. Res.*, **3**, 304–10

14. Butman, S., Piters, K. M., Olson, H. G., Schiff, S. M. and Gardin, J. M. (1983). Early exercise testing in unstable angina: angiographic correlation and prognostic value. *J. Am. Coll. Cardiol.*, **1**, 638

15. Nixon, J. V., Hillert, M. C., Shapiro, W. and Smitherman, T. C. (1980). Submaximal exercise testing after unstable angina. *Am. Heart J.*, **99**, 772–8

16. Waters, D. D., Szlachicic, J., Bourassa, M. G., Scholl, J. M. and Theroux, P. (1982). Exercise testing in patients with variant angina: results, correlation and angiographic features and prognostic significance. *Circulation*, **65**, 265–74

17. Crean, P. A. and Waters, D. D. (1984). Interpreting the exercise ECG in the patient with variant angina. *Pract. Cardiol.*, **10**, 107–13

18. Araki, H., Hayata, N., Matsuguchi, T., Takeshita, A. and Nakamura, M. (1986). Value of exercise tests with calcium antagonist to diagnose significant fixed coronary stenosis in patients with variant angina. *Br. Heart J.* (in press)

19. Alison, H. W., Russell, R. O. Jr., Mantle, J. A., Kouchoukos, N. T., Moraski, R. E. and Rackley, C. E. (1978). Coronary anatomy and arteriography in patients with unstable angina pectoris. *Am. J. Cardiol.*, **41**, 204–9

20. Holmes, D. R. Jr., Hartzler, G. O., Smith, H. C. and Foster, V. (1981). Coronary artery thrombosis in patients with unstable angina. *Br. Heart J.*, **49**, 1146–51

21. Balcon, R., Brooks, N., Warnes, C. and Cattell, M. (1980). Clinical spectrum of unstable angina. In Raffenbeul, W., Lichteln, P. R., and Balcon, R. (eds.) *Unstable*

angina pectoris. International Symposium. Hanover pp. 42–44 (New York: Thieme-Stratton)

22. Victor, M. F., Likoff, M. J., Mintz, G. S. and Likoff, W. (1981). Unstable angina pectoris of new onset: A prospective clinical and arteriographic study of 75 patients. *Am. J. Cardiol.* **47**, 228–32

23. Rotnick, G. D. (1981). Unstable angina: what the symptoms tell you. *Cardiovasc. Med.*, **6**, 499

24. Moise, A., Theroux, P. Taeymans, Y., Descoins, B., Lesperance, J., Waters, D. D., Pelletier, G. B. and Bourassa, M. G. (1983). Unstable angina and progression of coronary atherosclerosis. *N. Engl. J. Med.*, **309**, 685–9

25. Brown, G. B., Lee, A. B., Bolson, E. L. and Dodge, H. T. (1984). Reflex constriction of significant coronary stenosis as a mechanism contributing to ischemic left ventricular dysfunction during isometric exercise. *Circulation*, **70**, 18–25

26. Chierchia, S., Davies, G., Berkenboom, G., Crea, F., Crean, P. and Maseri, A. (1984). Alpha adrenergic receptors and coronary spasm: an elusive link. *Circulation*, **69**, 8–14

27. Bragg-Remschel, D. A., Anderson, C. H. and Winkle, R. A. (1982). Frequency response characteristics of ambulatory ECG monitoring systems and their implication for ST segment analysis. *Am. Heart J.*, **103**, 20–31

28. Crean, P. A., Ribeiro, P., Crea, F., Davies, G. J., Ratcliffe, D. and Maseri, A. (1984). Failure of transdermal nitroglycerin to improve chronic stable angina: A randomized placebo-controlled, double-blind, double cross trial. *Am. Heart J.*, **108**, 1494–1500

29. Deanfield, J. E., Selwyn, A. P., Chierchia, S., Maseri, A., Ribeiro, P., Krikler, S. and Morgan, M. (1983). Myocardial ischaemia during daily life in patients with stable angina: its relation to symptoms and heart rate changes. *Lancet*, **1**, 753–8

30. Deanfield, J. E., Shea, M., Ribeiro, P., Landsheere, C. M., Wilson, R. A., Horlock and Selwyn, A. P. (1984). Transient ST segment depression as a marker of myocardial ischaemia during daily life. *Am. J. Cardiol.*, **54**, 1195–1200

31. Yasue, H., Nagao, M., Omote, S., Takizawa, A., Miwa, K. and Tanaka, S. (1978). Coronary arterial spasm and Prinzmetals variant form of angina induced by hyperventilation and tris-buffer infusion. *Circulation*, **58**, 56–62

32. Raizner, A. E., Chahine, R. A., Ishimore, T., Verani, M. S., Zacca, N., Jamal, N., Mil, R. and Luchi, R. J. (1980). Provocation of coronary artery spasm by the cold pressor test. Hemodynamic, arteriographic and quantitative angiographic observation. *Circulation*, **62**, 925–32

33. Waters, D. D., Theroux, P., Szlachcic, J., Dauwe, F., Crittin, J., Bonan, R. and Mizgala, H. F. (1980). Ergonovine testing in a coronary care unit. *Am. J. Cardiol.*, **46**, 922–30

34. Bertrand, M. E., La Blanche, J. M., Tilmant, P. Y., Thieuleux, F. A., Deforge, M. R. A. G., Asseman, P., Berzin, B., Libersa, C. and Laurent, J. M. (1982). Frequency of provoked coronary spasm in 1089 consecutive patients undergoing coronary arteriography. *Circulation*, **65**, 1299–1306

35. Crean, P. A., Waters, D. D., Roy, D., Pelletier, G. B., Bonan, R. and Theroux, P. (1985). Sensitivity and safety of ergonovine testing inside and outside the catheterisation laboratory. *J. Am. Coll. Cardiol.*, **5**(2), 431

36. Crean, P. A., Crow, J. and Davies, G. J. (1984). Sequential changes in ventricular function following intravenous isosorbide dinitrate. *Vasc. Med.*, **2**, 205–9

37. Distante, A., Maseri, A., Severi, S., Biagini, A., Chierchia, S. (1979). Management of vasospastic angina at rest with continuous infusion of isosorbide dinitrate. *Am. J. Cardiol.*, **44**, 533–9

38. Theroux, P. and Waters, D. D. (1983). Calcium anatagonists. Clinical use in the treatment of angina. *Drugs*, **25**(2), 178–95

39. Waters, D. D., Theroux, P., Szlachcic, J. and Dauwe, F. (1981). Provocative testing to assess the efficacy of treatment with nifedipine, diltiazem and verapamil in variant angina. *Am. J. Cardiol.*, **48**, 123–30

40. Parodi, O., Maseri, A. and Simonetti, I. (1979). Management of unstable angina by verapamil: a double blind cross over study in the CCU. *Br. Heart J.*, **41**, 167–74

41. Mehta, J., Pepine, C. J., Day, M., Guerrero, J. R. and Conti, C. R. (1981). Short term efficacy of oral verapamil in rest angina. A double blind placebo controlled trial in CCU patients. *Am. J. Med.*, 71, 977–82
42. Gerstenblith, G., Ouyang, P., Achuff, S. C., Buckley, B. H., Becker, L. C., Mellits, D. *et al.* (1982). Nifedipine in unstable angina. *N. Engl. J. Med.*, 306, 885–9
43. Theroux, P., Taeymans, Y., Morissette, D., Bosch, Z., Pelletier, G. and Waters, D. (1985). A randomised study comparing propranolol and diltiazem in the treatment of unstable angina. *J. Am. Coll. Cardiol.*, 5, 717–22
44. Glazier, J. J., Chierchia, S., Smith, G. C., Berkenboom, G., Crean, P. A., Gerosa, S. and Maseri, A. (1986). Beta blockers for angina pectoris: how do they really work? (abstract) *Clin. Sci.*, 70, 1p
45. Co-operative Unstable Angina Study Group (1978). Unstable angina pectoris: National co-operative study group to compare medical and surgical therapy. In hospital experience and initial follow up results in patients with one, two and three vessel disease. *Am. J. Cardiol.*, 42, 839–48
46. Robertson, R. M., Robertson, D., Friesinger, G. C., Timmons, S. and Hawiger, J. (1980). Platelets aggregates in peripheral and coronary sinus blood in patients with spontaneous coronary artery spasm. *Lancet*, 2, 829–31
47. Robertson, D., Mass, R. L. and Roberts, L. J. (1980). Antiplatelet agents in vasospastic angina: a double blind cross-over study. *Clin. Res.*, 28, 242A
48. Chierchia, S., Patrono, C., Crea, F., Giabattoni, G., de Caterina, R., Cinotti, G. A. *et al.* (1982). Effects of intravenous prostacyclin in variant angina. *Circulation*, 65, 470–7
49. Canadian Cooperative Study Group (1978). A randomized trial of aspirin and sulpinpurazone in threatened stroke. *N. Engl. J. Med.*, 299, 53–9
50. Lewis, H. D., Davis, J. W., Archibald, D. A., Steinke, W. E., Smitherman, T. C., Dohert, J. E. *et al.* (1983). Protective effect of aspirin against acute myocardial infarction and death in men with unstable angina. *N. Engl. J. Med.*, 309, 396–405
51. Cairns, J. A., Gent, M., Singer, J. *et al.* (1984). A study of aspirin and sulphinpyrazone in unstable angina pectoris. *Circulation*, 70, 415
52. Nichol E. S., Phillips, W. C. and Casten, C. G. (1959). Virtue of prompt anticoagulation therapy in impending myocardial infarction: experience with 318 patients during a 10 year period. *Ann. Intern. Med.*, 50, 1158
53. European Coronary Surgery Study Group (1982). Long term results of prospective randomized study of coronary artery bypass surgery in stable angina pectoris. *Lancet*, 11, 1173–80
54. Conti, R., Becker, L., Biddle, T., Hutter, A. and Resnekov, L. Unstable angina. NHLBI co-operative study group to compare medical and surgical therapy: long term morbidity and mortality. *Am. J. Cardiol.*, (abstract) 49, 1007
55. Selden, R., Neill, W. A. and Ritzman, L. W. (1975). Medical versus surgical therapy for acute coronary insufficiency. A randomised study. *N. Engl. J. Med.*, 293, 1329–33
56. Pugh, B., Platt, M. R. and Mills, L. J. (1978). Unstable angina pectoris: a randomized study of patients treated medically and surgically. *Am. J. Cardiol*, 41, 1291–99
57. Bertolasi, C. A., Tronge, J. E. and Riccitelli, M. A. (1976). Natural history of unstable angina with medical or surgical therapy. *Chest*, 70, 596–605
58. Bourassa, M. G., David, P. R. and Guiteras, V. P. Percutaneous transluminal coronary angioplasty. In Rowalds, D. J. (ed.) *Recent Advances in Cardiology* Vol. 9, pp. 193–213 (Edinburgh: Churchill Livingstone)
59. Williams, D. O. Riley, R. S., Singh, A. K., Genirtz, H. and Most, A. S. (1981). Evaluation of the role of coronary angioplasty in patients with unstable angina. *Am. Heart J.*, 102, 1–9
60. De Feyter, P. J., Serruys, P. W., Van der Brand, M., Balakumaran, K., Mocht Soward, A. L., Arnold, A. E. R. and Hugenholtz, P. G. (1985). Emergency coronary angioplasty in unstable angina. *N. Engl. J. Med.*, 313, 342–6
61. Bentivoglio, L. G. (1983). Personal communication: Data from the NHLBI registry presented at the 1983 Bethesda workshop on PTCA. Bethesda, Maryland.

62. Corcos, T., David, P. R,., Bourassa, M. G., Guiteras, P. V., Robert, J., Mata, L. A. and Waters, D. D. (1985). Percutanous transluminal angioplasty for the treatment of variant angina. *J. Am. Coll. Cardiol.*, **5**, 1046–54
63. Reduto, L. A., Freund, G. C., Gaeta, J. M., Smalling, R. W., Lewis, B. and Gould, K. L. (1981). Coronary artery reperfusion in acute myocardial infarction: Beneficial effect on left ventricular salvage and performance. *Am. Heart J.*, **102**, 1168–78 .
64. De Wood, M. A., Spores, J., Notske, R., Mouser, L. T., Burroughs, R., Golden, M. S. and Lang, H. T. (1980). Prevalence of total coronary occlusion during the early hours of transmural myocardial infarction. *N. Engl. J. Med.*, **303**, 897–902
65. Kennedy, J. W., Ritchie, J. L. Davies, K. B. and Fritz, J. K. (1983). Western Washington randomized trial of intracoronary streptokinase in acute myocardial infarction. *N. Engl. J. Med.*, **309**, 1477–82
66. Melzer, R. S., Van der Brand, M., Serruys, P. W., Fioretti, P. and Hugenholtz, P. G. (1982). Sequential intracoronary streptokinase and transluminal angioplasty in unstable angina with evolving myocardial infarction. *Am. Heart J.*, **104**, 1109–11
67. GISSI (1986). Effectiveness of intravenous thrombotic treatment in acute myocardial infarction. *Lancet*, **1**, 397–401
68. Van de Werf, F., Ludbrook, P. A., Bergmann, S. R., Tiefenbrunn, A. J., Fox, K. A. A., Geest, H. *et al.* (1984). Coronary thombolysis with tissue type plasminogen activator in patients with evolving myocardial infarction. *N. Engl. J. Med.*, **310**, 609–14
69. Weintaub, R. M., Voukydis, P. C., Aroesty, J. M., Cohen, S. I., Ford, P., Kurland, G. S., Raia, P. J., Morkin, E. and Paulin, S. (1974). Treatment of preinfarction angina with intraaortic balloon counterpulsation and surgery. *Am. J. Cardiol.*, **34**, 809–14
70. Langou, R. A., Geha, A. S., Hammond, G. L. and Cohen, L. S. (1978). Surgical approach for patients with unstable angina pectoris: Role of the response to initial medical therapy and intraaortic balloon pumping in perioperative complications after aortocoronary bypass graft. *Am. J. Cardiol.*, **42**, 629–33
71. Flaherty, J. T., Becker, L. C., Weiss, J. L., Brinker, J. A., Buckley, B. H., Gerstenbli, G., Kallman, C. H. and Weisfeld, M. L. (1985). Results of a randomised trial of intraaortic balloon counterpulsation and intravenous nitroglycerin in patients with acute myocardial infarction. *J. Am. Coll. Cardiol.* **6**, 434–46

8
Investigation and management of acute myocardial infarction

C. D. J. ILSLEY AND M. B. ABLETT

INTRODUCTION

In the initial hours following a 'heart attack', as many as 50% of subjects die from ventricular fibrillation or acute left ventricular failure. For the survivors who reach hospital, or who are treated at home, left ventricular function, reflecting the amount of viable myocardium that remains, is the single most important determinant of both short and long term morbidity and mortality. Patients with large infarctions will tend to demonstrate poor left ventricular function and a high percentage will develop cardiogenic shock, late ventricular tachyarrhythmias, or subsequent (often unheralded) ventricular fibrillation. Though coronary care units, introduced in the early 1960s, have decreased the in-hospital mortality from arrhythmias, in the 1970s there was only a slight reduction in mortality from the other principal causes of death, such as cardiogenic shock, heart failure or further myocardial infarction. The recent introduction of an aggressive early interventional approach to the management of acute myocardial infarction offers some hope for future patients.

Considerable effort in current research relating to myocardial infarction is aimed towards the recognition of high risk groups, particularly those at the high risk of early sudden death. The coronary care unit does not merely fulfil the function of an arrhythmia detection centre, but is necessarily a starting point for ongoing research and the development of a more rational approach to the management of patients with acute myocardial infarction and indeed other cardiac diseases. Patients who have unequivocal evidence of acute myocardial infarction, or those in whom a strong suspicion that a myocardial infarction is an evolution, should be admitted to a coronary care unit for the first 48 hours of their illness.

It is nearly 20 years since it was suggested that the quantity of myocardium that becomes necrotic following coronary artery occlusion might be limited by specific interventions[1]. Since then, evidence has become available from studies in experimental animals indicating that an infarct was not a sudden catastrophic event but rather one that evolved and was therefore subject to modification. Experimental studies suggest that substantial quantities of myocardium can be salvaged by treatment with beta-adrenergic blockers, nitrates, hyaluronidase and other agents[2]. More recently, direct revascularization with thrombolysis, percutaneous transluminal coronary angioplasty and aorto-coronary bypass surgery has been advocated. Despite apparently unequivocal laboratory findings in experimental animals, there have been no clear guidelines for the use of any modality designed to protect ischaemic myocardium in patients with acute myocardial infarction. Perhaps the single most important factor hampering such research is the inability to predict the infarct size in patients with evolving myocardial infarction and perhaps more importantly the inability to assess the amount of ischaemic myocardium salvaged by intervention. Such predictions may be difficult, or indeed impossible, at the present time; but it is likely that there are several interventions, which are clinically useful.

CLINICAL FEATURES OF ACUTE MYOCARDIAL INFARCTION[3]

Chest pain, evolving electrocardiographic changes and elevated serum enzymes remain the necessary building blocks to establish a diagnosis of acute myocardial infarction. The chest pain is variable in intensity but in most patients, is severe, typically lasting for more than 30 minutes and resembles classic angina pectoris. A prodromal history can be elicited in up to 60% of patients with myocardial infarction and though the onset is often at rest (in over 50%) severe exertion, emotional stress, trauma or surgical procedures are well known precipating factors. Up to one quarter of non-fatal myocardial infarctions may be unrecognized by the patient and discovered only on routine electrocardiography. Unrecognized or silent infarction occurs but rarely in patients with angina pectoris and is more common in patients with diabetes and hypertension.

Patients with myocardial infarction are usually classified into two groups on the basis of well known electrocardiographic criteria: 'transmural', Q wave infarction; and 'non-transmural', non Q wave infarction occurring without the development of Q waves with associated isolated ST or T wave changes. Both types of myocardial infarction may occur in the absence of significant electrocardiographic changes.

Irreversibly injured myocardial cells release enzymes causing the serum creatinine phosphokinase (CPK) activity to exceed the normal range within about 6 hours of infarction, elevating the aspartate transaminase (AST) levels within 12 to 14 hours and elevating the serum hydroxybutyric dehydrogenase (HBD) activity beyond the normal within 24–28 hours. Peak activity in these enzymes occurs at approximately 24 hours, 48 hours and 4-5 days respectively (Figure 8.1).

Patients with acute myocardial infarction are usually anxious and in considerable pain. The heart rate may vary from a marked bradycardia – either naturally occurring or induced by therapy, such as beta-adrenergic blockade or morphine – or may be rapid and regular or irregular depending on the underlying rhythm and the degree of left ventricular failure. The blood pressure is usually normal or low, but a minority of patients may show a hypertensive response with the arterial pressure exceeding 160/90 mmHg. Patients with a tachycardia and elevated blood pressure are at greater risk, presumably as a consequence of adrenergic

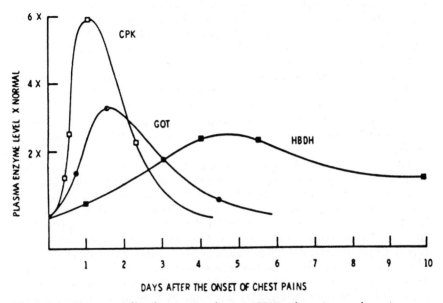

Figure 8.1 Plasma profiles for creatine kinase (CPK), glutamine–oxaloacetic transaminase (GOT) and hydroxybutyrate dehydrogenase (HBDH, LDH) activities following the onset of acute myocardial infarction

discharge secondary to pain and agitation. Arrhythmias are common and some abnormality of cardiac rhythm is noted in 75% patients. Moreover, many arrhythmias occur prior to hospitalization and thus the overall incidence of rhythm disturbance in acute myocardial infarction may be as high as 100%. Sinus bradycardia is the commonest arrhythmia; but 1 in 3 patients will have a sinus tachycardia at some stage in the early period following infarction and atrial premature extrasystoles, supraventricular tachycardia, atrial flutter, ventricular extrasystoles and ventricular tachyarrhythmias are all common.

Ventricular extrasystoles are so frequent as to be almost universal. 'Warning arrhythmias' have been defined as frequent ventricular extrasystoles (more than $5\,min^{-1}$), multiform configuration, early coupling (the R on T phenomenon) and repetitive extrasystoles in the form of couplets or salvos. However, primary ventricular fibrillation (ventricular fibrillation in the absence of congestive failure, pulmonary oedema and cardiogenic shock) occurs without warning arrhythmias in as many as 80% of cases and frequent and complex extrasystoles are commonly observed in patients with acute myocardial infarction, who never develop ventricular fibrillation. Although the suppression of ventricular premature beats is traditional, most physicians treat simple unifocal extrasystoles (whatever the frequency), conservatively. Conduction disturbances, particularly atrioventricular block, carry varying prognostic importance depending on site and haemodynamic consequences of the myocardial infarction. It is well known that complete atrio–ventricular block in association with an anterior myocardial infarction carries a grave prognosis; whereas mild degrees of heart block in inferior infarction carry little additional risk.

The major haemodynamic derangement in acute myocardial infarction is consequent on left ventricular dysfunction. However, catastrophic events such as the development of acute ventricular septal defect, papillary muscle rupture, and left ventricular free wall rupture in a small proportion of patients and are associated with a very high mortality.

The investigation of a patient presenting with chest pain consistent with acute myocardial infarction is designed to confirm the diagnosis and provide an indirect estimate of infarct size. The management is directed at limiting infarct size as much as possible and in treating the haemodynamic disturbance, whatever the mechanism, with appropriate therapy. Myocardial infarction is the result of acute coronary thrombosis. Experimental evidence suggests that early and full reperfusion offers a logical and most likely the best method of reducing infarct size. However, it appears that mortality related to large infarcts can be reduced by a host of different agents and since these agents act through independent mechanisms, combinations of all or some of them are likely to be more beneficial than any single treatment modality. As such, modern treatment may make a considerable impact upon the risk of death due to left ventricular failure associated with acute myocardial infarction.

Estimation of infarct size[2]

Myocardial infarct size can be estimated indirectly by the use of electrocardiographic changes, enzyme release, myocardial scintigraphy and 2 dimensional echocardiography. Although these techniques have been validated experimentally, each method has its limitations.

ST segment elevation obtained from multiple precordial ECG leads are a useful indicator of the extent of myocardial ischaemia in patients with anterior infarction who have no conduction defect. A normal or near normal ECG on admission with suspected myocardial infarction carries a good prognosis[4]. Although ST segment mapping may be criticized for its lack of reproducibility or lack of correlation with other markers of necrosis, if very early peak ST segment elevation is compared with enzyme release or the development of subsequent Q waves, good correlations can be demonstrated. Loss of R wave amplitude and the development of Q waves have been shown to correlate well with pathological measurements in experimental infarction and total enzyme release.

Persistent ST segment depression or elevation (especially if the latter occurs without objective evidence of pericarditis), persistent T wave inversion and abnormal Q waves in multiple leads correlates with a poor prognosis following infarction. In addition, patients demonstrating persistent repetitive ventricular extrasystolic activity, atrioventricular and interventricular conduction defects, atrial fibrillation and left ventricular hypertrophy have an increased mortality.

A relationship exists between prognosis and high serum enzyme levels and several studies have demonstrated that infarct size estimated from serial CPK measurements correlates with pathological infarct size. In this regard, the measurement of the MB isoenzyme of CPK appears to be the most useful test for myocardial necrosis. However, highly elevated cardiac enzymes may be found in patients undergoing spontaneous or therapeutic thrombolysis and such patients may go on to have a good clinical result. Patients with cardiogenic shock, who may have poor blood flow through the infarct, demonstrate geater enzyme release than those without cardiogenic shock and thus it is possible that the size of the infarct has actually little effect on the kinetics of enzyme release.

Myocardial scintigraphy can be performed with a variety of techniques and it appears that infarct estimates using technetium-99 correlate well with infarct size in dogs and a good correlation has also been reported between thallium scanning and post mortem estimation of infarct size in man. Good correlations have been obtained between quantitative QRS scoring systems and ventricular function assessed by radionuclide studies.

With the advent of 2 dimensional echocardiography, repeated noninvasive measurements of left ventricular wall motion may be performed at the bedside. Though actual infarct size is overestimated by this technique, its very ready application to the coronary care setting makes it a more attractive clinical option than radionuclear methods.

Survival following myocardial infarction depends on a number of factors, the most important of these being the state of left ventricular function. Overall, there appears to be an in-hospital mortality of 15% in patients admitted with acute myocardial infarction, though in the absence of clinically apparent cardiac failure on admission mortality is 8% or less. In the smaller number of patients admitted with established left ventricular failure or shock, mortality is 45% and 75–100% respectively.

The Norris coronary prognostic index (CPI) is a useful and clinically relevant index derived from the patient's age, the admission ECG, blood pressure, heart size and pulmonary vasculature. The major value of the Norris index, however, lies in the stratification of groups of patients rather than the ability to define any individual course. Such factors as male sex, increasing age, history of diabetes mellitus, hypertension, prior angina pectoris or previous myocardial infarction have been considered related to a worse prognosis, but are not predictive (apart from increasing age) of in-hospital mortality according to Norris' data.

MANAGEMENT OF ACUTE MYOCARDIAL INFARCTION[6]

Bed rest, the establishment of electrocardiographic monitoring, analgesia for the relief of chest pain and the provision of oxygen (when necessary) may be regarded as routine measures in all patients admitted with chest pain in whom myocardial infarction is suspected. In addition, all patients should be anticoagulated with systemic administration of full dose heparin therapy, most frequently at a dose of 5000 units 4 hourly. The initial management of chest pain is to administer morphine, supplemented by intravenous nitroglycerine infusion and beta-adrenergic blockade. Therapy with calcium antagonists in our unit is related to the presence of ongoing angina in patients in whom beta-adrenergic blockade is contraindicated, or where antianginal therapy is required in addition to established beta-blockade. Oxygen is only administered when clear arterial hypoxaemia has been demonstrated. An ECG is taken on admission and subsequently every 12 hours, or more frequently if the patient's progress is complicated. Blood is taken for haemoglobin, white count, renal function, glucose and serially for cardiac enzymes estimation.

Anticoagulation in the early stages of acute myocardial infarction has three main benefits. Since acute coronary thrombosis is usually responsible for infarction, herapin may enhance natural thrombolytic mechanisms. Anticoagulants also diminish the formation of intracardiac thrombi and therefore the risk of systemic embolization – especially in acute anterior myocardial infarction. Anticoagulant therapy certainly exerts a favourable effect on survival in patients with a high risk of embolism – i.e. those with ventricular aneurysm and/or demonstrable intraventricular thrombus, patients with marked obesity, low output state, or a past history of deep vein thrombosis or pulmonary embolism. However, the long term benefit of anticoagulants remains controversial.

It is pertinent that this 'routine' management has been available for two decades with little demonstrable improvement in patient survival. For example, an analysis of results of all the coronary care units in Boston, Massachussetts, has failed to show any demonstrable improvement in hospital mortality calculated for the years 1973/74 and compared to 1978/79 – a period in which the United States mortality for ischaemic heart disease was consistently falling. Overall admission rates with approximately 8500 patients admitted in both years, were accompanied by similar mortalities of 22% and 23% respectively[7]. Most attention during this period related to the consequences of myocardial infarction rather than its cause.

Interventions that may be expected to limit infarct size revolve around the basic principles of supply and demand. It is obviously attractive to remove the initiating thrombus and re-establish coronary arterial perfusion in the infarct related vessel; but an equally favourable result might be obtained by improving collateral flow from non-obstructed arterial beds. Alternatively, the provision of metabolites – such as glucose, insulin and potassium – may limit the effects of hypoxaemia, if sufficient perfusion exists to deliver them to the site of infarction. Indirectly, oxygen demand may be reduced by beta-adrenergic blockade or decreasing the 'load' on the heart by systemic arteriolar or venous vasodilation. All of these approaches have been evaluated and demonstrated as effective in the experimental laboratory but perhaps only a few have been properly evaluated in man[2].

Acute myocardial infarction usually occurs as thrombosis on an established coronary atherosclerotic plaque. Thrombosis leading to infarction may also occur in apparently normal epicardial vessels. Equally, although spontaneous thrombolysis is recognized, it may not occur until irreversible damage has been sustained. Activation and augmentation of the thrombolytic system offers the prospect of effective reperfusion within a sufficiently short time frame to allow for some or complete myocardial salvage. If instituted very early in the evolution of a myocardial infarction, complete recovery is possible. After several small scale studies supported this hypothesis, the recent publication of the GISSI study may be seen as a major stimulus to change what has previously been regarded as 'routine' therapy for myocardial infarction[8]. The further implication is that the greatest benefit will come from the earliest form of intervention. It is unlikely that streptokinase will be freely given in the community but in the not too distant future thrombolysis with tissue plasminogen activator may be readily available. The specificity of these agents might also be improved by the use of specific antifibrin antibody. However far we progress in the in-hospital treatment of myocardial infarction, a major effect on mortality will not occur until active thrombolytic therapy is delivered to patients in the community. The parallel between thrombolytic therapy and the experience with out-of-hospital cardio-pulmonary resuscitation for ventricular fibrillation is obvious.

EARLY IN-HOSPITAL INTERVENTION IN ACUTE MYOCARDIAL INFARCTION

Although patients receive what might be termed 'routine' care, the specific management in any individual depends upon the clinical presentation. Figure 8.2 outlines the basic scheme of management under-

Figure 8.2 Outline of the typical management provided at Dunedin Hospital

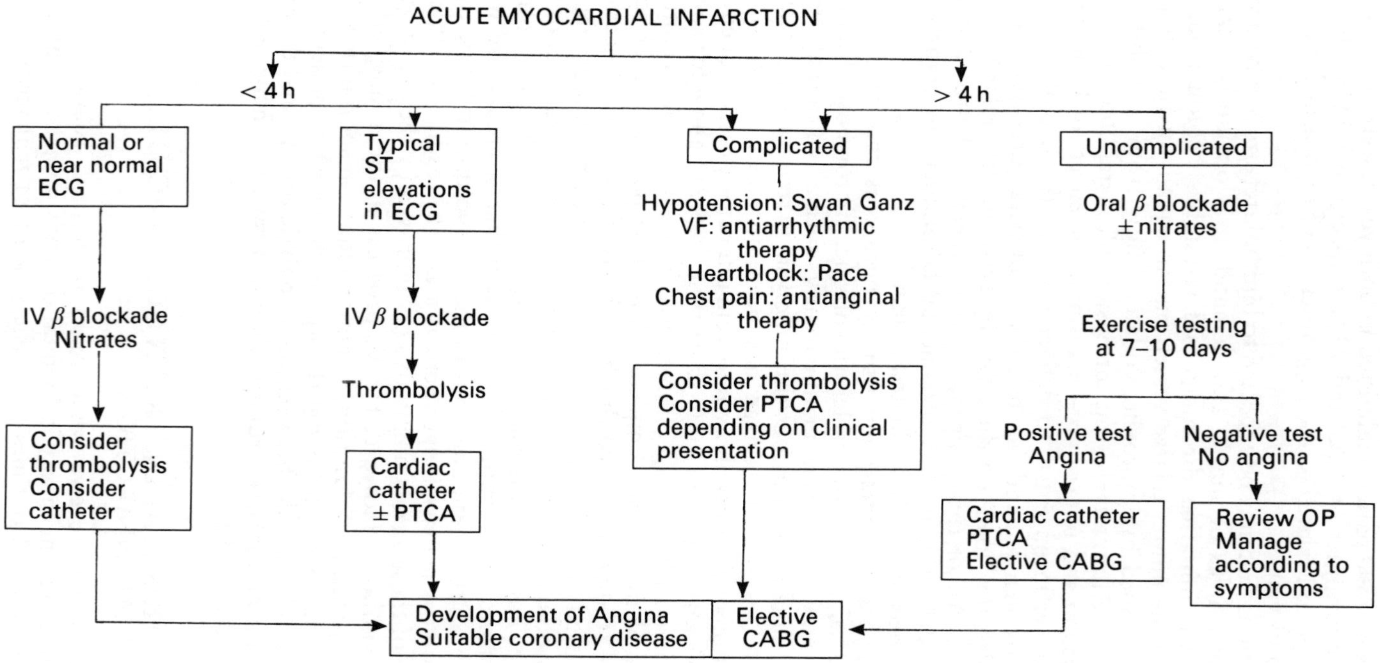

ACUTE MYOCARDIAL INFARCTION

CABG = coronary artery bypass grafting, OP = outpatient, VF = ventricular fibrillation, PTCA = percutaneous transluminal coronary angioplasty

taken for patients admitted to the coronary care unit (CCU) at Dunedin Hospital. Our coronary care unit is supported by an intermediate care unit and telemetry for post-infarction monitoring is available in the general cardiology ward. In addition to routine tests we place an emphasis on the non-invasive assessment of infarct size by use of 2 dimensional echocardiography (2D-echo). We also have a cardiac catheter laboratory situated on the same floor as the CCU. The procedures outlined below depend on open access to both these non-invasive and invasive facilities.

Traditionally, the diagnosis of acute myocardial infarction relies on history, serial ECG changes and a characteristic enzyme pattern. Once all these criteria are satisfied that infarction has occurred, the time for active intervention has long passed. Therefore the history and ECG changes on admission are best supported by the use of 2D-echo demonstrating regional wall motion abnormalities. Once a diagnosis of acute myocardial infarction has been made, it is possible to consider the various therapeutic options.

The role of thrombolytic therapy in acute myocardial infarction

At Dunedin we currently use streptokinase in all patients presenting within four hours of the onset of pain (1) in which the electrocardiogram demonstrates typical ST segment elevation (2) in some individuals with relatively normal ECGs (those with a convincing history within one to two hours of the onset of pain), and (3) occasional patients with myocardial infarction complicated by hypotension or ongoing chest pain (Figure 8.2). In patients selected for streptokinase therapy, a dose of corticosteroids (either 200 mg of hydrocortisone or 2 g of methylprednisolone, depending on physician preference) is given followed by 1.5 million units of streptokinase administered by intravenous infusion over 20 minutes. Streptokinase may also be administered either directly, or during cardiac catheterization into the infarct related vessel where a much lower dose may be given – an initial 40 000 units and then 10 000 units each minute (up to a maximum of 250 000 units) until restoration of blood flow in the infarct vessel has been demonstrated. However, many studies are available to suggest that the rate of coronary thrombolysis (either recanalization or reperfusion, depending on coronary dye flow) is similar. As peripheral administration is logistically easier, this is likely to have more widespread appeal.

Despite the vast literature produced in the first half of this decade, many questions remained[9,10]. In their review of intravenous and intracoronary fibrolytic therapy in myocardial infarction, Yusuf and his colleagues have summarized all the available information on the mortality, the infarction rate and side effects from 33 randomized controlled trials from 1959–85[11]. Whilst the wisdom of pooling results from several trials is questionable, Yusuf and his colleagues did draw some interesting conclusions. Whilst 10–15% of patients suffered minor bleeding, only a very small percentage had a significant haemorrhage. A moderate reduction in mortality appeared to be gained from thrombolytic therapy (streptokinase or urokinase) and the rate of reinfarction was also lower. However, there were many questions left unanswered, some of which have been addressed in four recent major studies involving thrombolytic therapy: The Western Washington Study[12]; the TIMI (thrombolysis in myocardial infarction) study[13]; the Dutch Multicentre study[14]; and the most recent GISSI (Gruppo Italiano per lo Studio della Streptochinasi nell'infarcto Miocardio) study[8].

Several elements of the Western Washington randomized trial of intracoronary streptokinase in acute myocardial infarction have been published. The main results, however, were published in 1983 and demonstrated a three fold improvement in the 30 day mortality in those patients receiving streptokinase as compared to the control population[12]. One hundred and thirty-four of 250 patients were assigned to the treatment group with a 30 day mortality of 3.7% compared to 11.2% in the 116 control patients ($p = 0.02$). The greatest benefit was observed in patients with anterior infarction. Unfortunately, however, there was an apparent inequality in the distribution of patients with baseline hypotension and shock in the control patients, perhaps favouring the streptokinase treatment group. Also, there appeared to be no significant improvement in left ventricular ejection fraction (as measured by gated blood pool scanning and technetium-99m labelled red cells) in all patients after catheterization and at two weeks in the streptokinase treated patients.

The TIMI study randomized intravenous recombitant tissue type plasminogen activator (r-tPA) vs intravenous streptokinase carried out under the auspices of the National Heart, Lung and Blood Institute in the United States of America[13]. There was an observed reperfusion rate of only 35% in the streptokinase group, compared to 60% following r-tPA at 90 minutes. Of 290 patients, 76 were excluded because of the incomplete coronary occlusion before drug infusion, demonstrating the natural thrombolytic tendency in many patients with acute myocardial infarction. Mortality, analysed by intention to treat, was 5% (7/143) and 8% (12/147) of those originally assigned to r-tPA and streptokinase therapy respectively. Despite the theoretical advantages of r-tPA over streptokinase, it was important to note that haemorrhagic problems were not demonstrably eliminated with r-tPA. Once again, methodological criticisms are easy to assemble and it should be noted that the mean time from onset of pain to the initiation of treatment was nearly five hours in the TIMI trial. In contrast to the Western Washington trial, there was no control group and despite the apparent better reperfusion rates there was no difference in mortality between the two treatments. An additional study from the European Cooperative study group for r-tPA published in the *Lancet*, also in 1985, showed essentially similar results[15].

In the GISSI trial, 11 806 patients in 177 units were enrolled over 17 months[8]. Patients admitted within 12 hours after the onset of pain were randomized with respect to streptokinase but otherwise had additional 'usual treatment'. At 21 days there was an 18% reduction in overall mortality ($p = 0.0002$) with reported mortality of 10.7% (628/5860) in the streptokinase treated patients compared with 13% (758/5852) in the control group.

In contrast to our own practice, and that advocated by others, it should be remembered that the GISSI study enrolled patients within 12 hours of the onset of symptoms and the authors conclude that:

> In view of the high consistency of our findings with those obtained in small, more rigidly controlled studies, intravenous infusion of 1.5 million units of streptokinase can be recommended as a safe treatment for all patients with no positive contraindication, who can be treated within six hours from the onset of pain.

But within the trial, subgroup analysis clearly demonstrated greatest mortality reduction in patients treated within one hour and no reduction in those treated after six hours.

In terms of our practice in Dunedin, the most interesting of the recent studies was the Dutch Multicentre study from Simoons and colleagues published in the *Lancet* in 1985[16]. Although the paper is entitled *Improved survival after thrombolysis in acute myocardial infarction*, many of the streptokinase treated patients actually underwent associated percutaneous transluminal coronary angioplasty (PCTA) and thus was a comparison of two 'strategies' for treatment of myocardial infarction. Two hundred and sixty four patients were allocated to conventional treatment and 269 patients to a strategy aimed at rapid reperfusion. Initially, therapy was intracoronary streptokinase only, though in the later part of the study with supplementation by early intravenous streptokinase and subsequent PTCA in patients with residual coronary stenosis demonstrated following thrombolysis. As so often in trials of myocardial infarction in man, all the other therapies associated with infarction differ in the two groups – with patients receiving thrombolytic therapy also receiving such drugs as nitroglycerine, heparin, aspirin and prednisolone and patients treated with PCTA also receiving calcium antagonists. Cumulative one year survival was 91% after thrombolysis and 84% in the 'control group' ($p = 0.01$). Those in the thrombolytic group followed a better clinical course than control patients with a lower incident of ventricular fibrillation (38 vs 61, $p < 0.01$), 14 day mortality (14 vs 26, $p < 0.05$) and heart failure during convalescence (37 vs 53, $p < 0.05$).

The role of percutaneous transluminal coronary angioplasty (PTCA) in acute myocardial infarction

Interest in streptokinase therapy and other forms of therapeutic thrombolysis began three decades ago. Whilst the failure to demonstrate clinical improvement with therapeutic thrombolysis may be ascribed to many causes, the fundamental problem with early studies can be summed up by the aphorism 'too little, too late' – small doses of streptokinase, delivered peripherally, and often many hours following the onset of infarction. Whilst the efficacy of thrombolysis in evolving acute trans-mural infarction has been established to some extent, 'reperfusion' is achieved in only 75% of patients (ranging from 35–90% in different studies). The relative safety has also been established. However, improvement does not occur in all patients and is dependent on a number of factors including the quality of reperfusion – ranging from simple recanalization, implying the restoration of a degree of flow past a severe lesion; to full reperfusion, implying restoration of adequate coronary flow – the duration and completeness of occlusion, the pres-ence of collateral flow, infarct location, prior left ventricular function, the occurrence of later reocclusion with or without reinfarction and the extent of reperfusion injury. Usually coronary flow may be re-established in the infarct related vessel revealing the atherosclerotic plaque upon which the acute thrombosis occurred. The residual stenosis and on going thrombotic tendency related to that stenosis represents an important problem after reperfusion, occurring in 15–35% of patients in many studies. These limitations of thrombolysis have stimulated interest in use of early or primary PTCA in an attempt to improve the immediate and long term results of acute intervention to the infarction process.

Percutaneous transluminal coronary angioplasty is now totally estab-lished as a valid method of treatment for coronary artery disease, since its introduction by Andreas Grunzig who performed the first case in September 1977. The first report of immediate PTCA after successful intracoronary thrombolysis was reported by Meyer and colleagues in 1982[16]. In their study 17 of 21 patients (81%) underwent successful PTCA within 24 hours of successful thrombolysis and the results compared favourably to a retrospective control group of 18 patients with similar clinical characteristics that had been treated with intracoronary strep-tokinase alone. Similar results have been described from other centres, though usually with relatively small numbers of patients and accepting the fact that it is exceedingly difficult to provide a scientifically sat-isfactory control group in such studies. In this regard it may be seen that the recent open study from Simoons and colleagues, who reported the Dutch experience, provides a reasonable clinical framework for the use of PTCA in acute infarction[16]. They performed an open study comparing a highly invasive approach with both thrombolysis and PTCA in some patients and compared the results to patients treated with more conventional management without acute catheterization or the use of thrombolytic drugs. Of 44 patients who underwent PTCA immediately after thrombolysis, three had non-fatal reinfarctions and one died. Overall, the long term survival was much improved, with their invasive approach compared to 'conservative management'.

In 1983, Hartzler and colleagues provided the first study in which PTCA was used without associated thrombolytic therapy for myocardial infarction[17]. PTCA alone was performed in 37 patients and was successful in 78%. Streptokinase was applied as the primary intervention in 39 patients (50%) and in the 80% for whom streptokinase produced coronary recanalization, PTCA was performed with a high grade residual stenosis with an 81% success. The instance of early ischaemic events was only 6% after acute PTCA and the late reocclusion rate of 17% at a mean follow up of 6 months.

In our experience, we have performed PTCA on 36 patients in the acute stages of myocardial infarction, 33 of which were performed without associated streptokinase therapy. In the 19 patients undergoing PTCA within four hours of the onset of chest pain (11 anterior and 8 inferior infarctions) successful dilatation was achieved in 91%; although there were three deaths, each in a patient with a proximal occlusion of the anterior descending artery in which ventricular function was severely compromised to the point of cardiogenic shock, despite successful dilatation and restoration of coronary flow. Two of these three deaths occurred in patients who were dilated within two hours of the onset of myocardial infarction. On the other hand, five of these 19 patients undergoing PTCA within three hours of the onset of pain had complete reversal of the infarction process with demonstrated late patency, normal left ventricular function and peak cardiac enzyme estimations

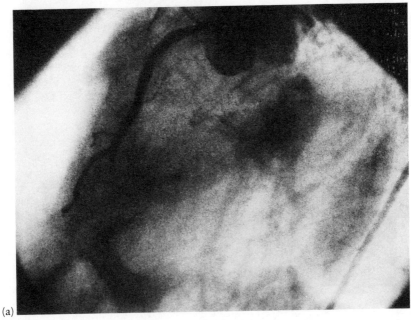

(a)

Figure 8.3
(a) Acute inferior infarction: Right coronary angiogram taken in a 48-year-old man. He presented with chest pain and the ECG demonstrated hyperacute ST segment elevation in leads II, III, aVF. The artery is completely occluded. Taken 1.5 hours after the onset of pain

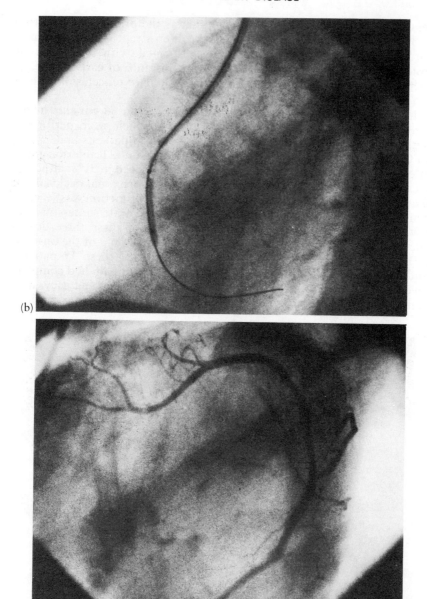

(b) The occlusion was probed and crossed with a guide wire, which allowed the balloon dilation catheter to be positioned and inflated

(c) After PTCA, showing complete restoration of right coronary flow. In this patient there were no other stenoses in the coronary arterial system, the ECG and left ventricular function returned to normal. Peak enzyme 'rises' were within the normal range

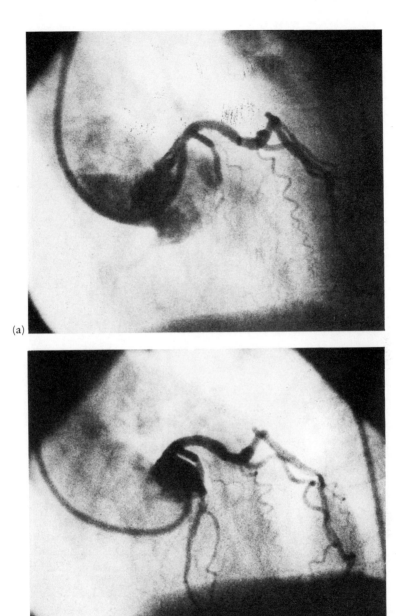

(a)

(b)

Figure 8.4
(a) Acute anterior infarction. Left coronary angiogram (left anterior oblique view) in a 63-year-old woman who presented with chest pain 2 hours prior to angiography. The anterior descending artery shows a moderate proximal stenosis with subsequent total occlusion
(b) After streptokinase (40 000 units intracoronary, followed by 10 000 units per minute for 10 minutes) the acute thrombus has disappeared to reveal a ragged, moderately severe stenosis just proximal to the diagonal artery. PTCA was then performed [see Figure 8.3(c)]

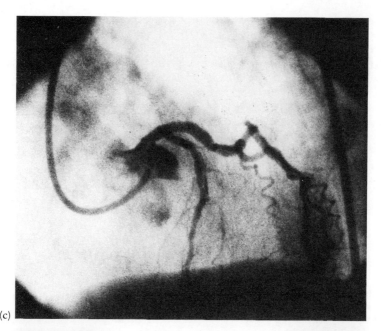

(c)

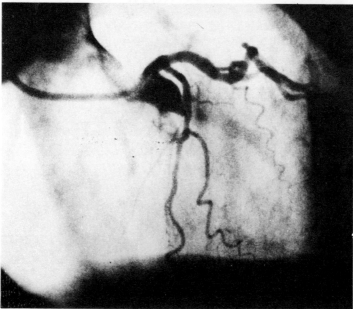

(d)

Figure 8.4 (cont.)
(c) After PTCA – dilatation of both anterior descending arteries with a 2.5 mm balloon catheter. Note good perfusion in anterior descending artery, but relatively poor flow in the diagonal. There is an easily visible intimal tear
(d) Same patient – elective restudy at six months following the acute intervention. The anterior descending artery remains widely patent, the intimal tear has healed and diagonal flow excellent. The ECG showed Q waves in VI-3 left ventricular function remained well preserved with an ejection fraction of 63%

remaining within the normal range (Figures 8.3, 8.4). We have seen no late deaths in our small series in a mean follow up period of 10 months.

The same logistic considerations limiting the value of intracoronary streptokinase also limit the use and value of PTCA as a primary method of myocardial infarction salvage. Many studies point to the major influence of survival being early intervention and yet there are few CCUs in which a majority of patients arrive within four hours from the onset of pain and there is a necessary further delay before cardiac catheterization is possible.

It is possible that 'more elective' PTCA, about 48 hours after the acute infarction, may allow for an improved prognosis in terms of both morbidity and mortality in a potentially much larger group of patients since patients in the 'higher risk' groups can be transferred to the units performing PTCA. Patients with ongoing angina pectoris, dilatation of the infarct related vessel, even in the presence of multivessel disease, may provide stabilization of the infarct zone.

The role of cardiac surgery in acute myocardial infarction

Despite the relatively high risk in patients with established myocardial infarction undergoing cardiac surgery, a small number of such patients will inevitably require cardiac surgery for the treatment of ongoing unstable angina, residual stable angina pectoris or mechanical complications of the infarction.

Revascularization of acute myocardial infarction

Whilst the benefits and risks for the aggressive application of coronary bypass surgery in an acute evolving myocardial infarction have not been clearly defined, some centres report an early surgical mortality of 2% if surgery is performed less than six hours after onset of chest pain[18]. This compares to a mortality of about 11.5% with conventional medical therapy at the same institutions. One surgical group also reported an extremely low first year mortality of only 1.4%. Although these results appear superficially to be very favourable, the absence of proper control groups makes it difficult to draw any conclusions other than if surgery is necessary, for example, for persistent angina, then it may be performed with an acceptable risk.

Threatened extension of myocardial infarction

The clinical presentation of this syndrome may be varied. Broadly, but perhaps oversimply, it could be represented as either a partial thickness infarction threatening to extend to a full thickness infarction or an established Q wave infarction that threatens to extend laterally. The essence of diagnosis is the presence of continued pain with additional ECG changes. Early cardiac catheterization is important and many such patients demonstrate left main coronary artery disease or extensive disease involving all three of the major epicardial coronary arteries, which may not be suitable for PTCA. If aggressive medical therapy, comprising continuous nitroglycerin infusion with or without intra-aortic balloon pumping, fails to control the pain, then surgery is indicated. The risks of surgery in this setting are relatively high, possibly as high as 20% depending on the age and state of left ventricular function[19]. This must be compared to studies that have demonstrated that the 'natural history' of post infarction angina is very gloomy with as much as a 70% mortality at six months in patients treated conservatively[20].

Mechanical complications of acute myocardial infarction[21]

Mitral regurgitation in association with myocardial infarction may be caused by dilatation of the left ventricle and papillary muscle dysfunction. Less frequently, infarction may produce rupture of some or all of the papillary muscle, resulting in torrential acute mitral regurgitation and severe pulmonary oedema. Rupture of the papillary muscle is usually fatal, with death in a few hours occurring in a third and within 24 hours in 50% of these patients without surgical intervention. Mitral valve replacement in this group itself carries a 20–25% risk but surgery is inevitable in the face of the otherwise gloomy prognosis – assuming that sufficient ventricular function is demonstrated to allow post-operative recovery.

Rupture of the ventricular septum is a complication occurring in about 1% of acute myocardial infarctions and most usually occurs between 7–10 days. This sudden appearance of a loud murmur with clinical deterioration may make it difficult to distinguish acute ventricular septal rupture from acute mitral regurgitation but in cases of doubt, the diagnosis of septal rupture can be confirmed by right heart catheterization with associated 2 dimensional echocardiography. Clinically, it is useful to note that patients with acute mitral regurgitation demonstrate extremely severe pulmonary oedema, whereas the majority of those with ventricular septal defects can lie at least semi-prone with less marked pulmonary oedema. Defects in the distal ventricular septum are usually amenable to surgical repair; defects which develop high in the ventricular septum, usually in the context of extensive infarction, tend to have a high mortality irrespective of surgical intervention. In those patients in whom the haemodynamic consequences of septal rupture can be controlled, surgery should be delayed for about four weeks.

Ventricular free wall rupture

This occurs in about 8% of acute Q wave infarction and is perhaps responsible for about 10% of post-infarction deaths in hospital. It usually occurs in older patients and appears to be more common in women. Death is the most common sequel but surgical successful repair has followed 'subacute heart rupture' and the prognosis for such patients appears to be surprisingly good if they survive the surgery.

Left ventricular aneurysm

This may develop after acute infarction, classically acute Q wave anterior infarction. It presents usually several weeks or possibly months later with either tachyarrhythmias, left ventricular thrombus and embolism or the signs and symptoms of left ventricular failure. Excision of left ventricular aneurysm will remove the thrombus, improve ventricular function where sufficient viable muscle exists to provide for an adequate left ventricular cavity post surgery, and many patients (but by no means all) may lose their recurrent ventricular tachyarrhythmia. In this latter situation, tachycardia control might be provided by alternative surgical techniques, such as endocardial resection or the encircling ventriculotomy approach.

Beta adrenergic blocking drugs in acute myocardial infarction

Following the initial observations from Snow in 1966, there is a wealth of literature pertaining to the use of nearly all of the currently available beta-blockers in the context of myocardial infarction[22]. Studies with various intravenous beta-blockers given within 4 to 12 hours of the onset of pain have reliably demonstrated an average reduction in enzyme release by about a third and there is also greater preservation of the R wave in treated compared to control groups. These apparently beneficial effects, linked and attributed to reduction in infarct size, have been accompanied by reduction in chest pain, ventricular tachyarrhythmias and in particular ventricular fibrillation and present a persuasive case that early intravenous beta-blockade is likely to be beneficial in the absence of any contraindications. However, randomized placebo controlled trials in acute myocardial infarction are notoriously difficult to set up and the results of the available data are open to the criticism that a majority of apparently 'high risk' patients (i.e. those with significant left ventricular failure or cardiogenic shock) are consistently excluded from such trials. Reduced infarct size by the early administration of intravenous metoprolol and timolol published recently show a 10% reduction in mortality.

The recent MIAMI (metoprolol in acute myocardial infarction) trial provides a representative example of such studies[23]. Between December 1982 and March 1984, 5778 patients with suspected acute infarction were randomized for treatment with intravenous followed by oral metoprolol (n = 2877) or placebo (n = 2901). The trial was double blind and conducted at 104 centres in 17 countries. Mortality rates for the 15 day study period were 4.9% (142 deaths) in the control group and 4.3%

(123 deaths) in those treated with metoprolol; representing a 13% mortality reduction in the treated group, which did not achieve statistical significance. Dunedin was one of those 104 centres and a local analysis of our own results underlined the fact that those people actually eligible for inclusion in the MIAMI trial (n = 56) had a low risk Norris coronary prognostic index (4.7 + / − 0.2) with no deaths in the 15 day follow up period. During the same period, 137 patients who fulfilled the basic entry criteria (age under 75 years, chest pain of at least 15 minutes duration) were excluded for one reason or another with a total of 16 deaths (12%, CPI 6.9 ± 0.3, $p < 0.01$). Subgroup analysis showed that only one of five patients (2%) who had pretreatment with beta-blockers prior to the onset of suspected infarction, died. We interpret these results as confirming beta blockade as a useful therapy in the context of acute myocardial infarction.

It must be acknowledged that definitive proof that substantial quantities of myocardium can be salvaged and prognosis thereby improved is not yet available. However, those that advocate that 'even a 10% mortality reduction' in patients with acute myocardial infarction treated world-wide, present an impressive (if somewhat emotive) message.

It appears certain that patients treated with the oral administration of a beta-blocker after an acute infarction carry a significantly lower mortality[22]. After initially impressive short term improvements in mortality with timolol (Norwegian study), metoprolol (Swedish studies) and propranolol (BHAT, beta-blocker heart attack trial) it would appear that long term benefits are maintained and continue with prolonged administration of therapy. Only the sotolol trial failed to show any statistical demonstrable improvement, though mortality was 18% less in the treated group.

Our recommendation is that all patients who are eligible for treatment with beta-blockers should receive them in the early stages of acute myocardial infarction.

Other therapeutic interventions

Although intravenous beta-blockers have been the most common therapeutic modality to be investigated, various agents have been shown to have an effect on different indices of infarct size. Many of these studies involve only small numbers of patients but are supported by good experimental evidence. Glucose-insulin-potassium therapy, the vasodilator drugs (nitroprusside and nitroglycerine), streptokinase and other thrombolytic agents and hyaluronidase have all been demonstrated to have efficacy. Several excellent detailed reviews of the results of all these trials are available but the question of reduced mortality in association with apparent reduction in infarct size is less clearly established[2,24]. On the other hand, the published early intervention studies with either verapamil[25] or nifedipine[26] have been disappointing.

THE ROLE OF TWO–DIMENSIONAL ECHOCARDIOGRAPHY IN ACUTE MYOCARDIAL INFARCTION

Two-dimensional echocardiography (2D-echo) has an important role to play in the management of patients presenting with acute chest pain[27]. The indications and expectations of 2D-echo in this context may be summarized as:

(1) The provision of diagnostic information as to the extent and site of regional areas of left ventricular dysfunction confirming the diagnosis of myocardial infarction. Whilst this will not necessarily distinguish between old and current infarction, increasing experience suggests that even subtle abnormalities of myocardial systolic performance can be appreciated and provide a clue that ischaemic heart disease underlies the symptoms rather than one of the many other causes of chest pain.

(2) Ejection fraction may be accurately assessed and in patients in whom multiple views are possible (about 85% in our experience) the estimated ejection fraction correlates closely with both angiography and radionuclide methods. An assessment of ejection fraction will necessarily provide an index of risk, especially when it is correlated to either clinical or haemodynamic information available from the same patient.

(3) Major complications, such as acute mitral regurgitation, right ventricular infarction and ventricular septal defects may be quickly and readily identified. In addition, the presence of interventricular thrombus may be appreciated and managed with extended anticoagulant therapy.

(4) The effect of interventions on left ventricular function may be established serially. In this regard, major regional hypokinetic segments recover to normal after successful PTCA and thrombolysis.

(5) In those patients requiring cardiac catheterization, knowledge of left ventricular function derived from 2D-echo data can simplify the procedure to involve only coronary angiography and thus remove the potential hazards involved in emergency left ventricular angiography.

The major limitation of 2D-echo is the fact that not all patients are suitable echocardiographic subjects and thus not all patients have entirely accurate evaluation of, for example, their ventricular function. On the other hand, the ease with which studies may be repeated as frequently as necessary, provides a major advantage over other methods of assessing the left ventricle.

In our experience, the patient at high risk can be identified from the admission 2D-echo. Multiple views allow for analysis of the left ventricular wall in 14 segments, each of which is ascribed a score (normal = 1, hypokinetic = 2, akinetic = 3). A wall motion score index (WMSI) is derived by dividing the sum of wall motion by the number of segments visualized. High risk patients are predicted as those with a WMSI > 2. In our first 50 consecutive patients undergoing echocardiographic assessment within 48 hours of acute infarction, 20% (4/20) of the high risk group died compared to none of the remaining 30 patients ($p < 0.02$). Thirteen of 18 anterior infarcts fell into the high risk group compared with only 7 of 31 with inferior infarction ($p < 0.01$).

Future developments with computer-assisted methods, such as edge detection and image processing, will increase objectivity and perhaps allow differentiation of ischaemic from infarcted myocardium. Doppler echocardiography will also help in detecting and quantifying intracardiac lesions (such as mitral regurgitation) and providing an estimation of cardiac output.

ROLE OF CARDIAC CATHETERIZATION IN HOSPITAL IN-PATIENTS AFTER MYOCARDIAL INFARCTION

The indications for cardiac catherization in patients with acute and recent myocardial infarction remain controversial. As the prognosis in these patients depends on left ventricular function and the extent of coronary artery disease, however, we currently advocate and practise an aggressive approach to early coronary angiography in acute infarction. The indications for coronary angiography in the setting of acute myocardial infarction include[28]:

(1) Chest pain with hyperacute ST segment elevation in patients presenting within four hours of the onset of pain
(2) Ongoing angina after either Q wave infarction or non-Q wave infarction
(3) 'High risk' patients (e.g. patients with occasional angina yet significantly reduced left ventricular function, those threatening to extend a previous infarction, those with recurrent ventricular tachyarrhythmias or survivors of the 'sudden death' syndrome)
(4) Patients requiring emergency surgery for other than ongoing angina
(5) Elective study at 7–10 days in those following a non-Q wave infarction in order to plan a future strategy.

Although patients can often be separated into high risk and low risk subsets by a non-invasive assessment during and after myocardial infarction, several other factors are also considered when making the decision to proceed – including the availability of accurate non-invasive tests at the particular institution (Figures 8.5 and 8.6).

Persistent angina pectoris following myocardial infarction is a bad prognostic sign. However, cardiac catheterization is not necessary for all patients if the left ventricular function is severely depressed, even though the prognosis is bad in this group, unless surgical therapy is contemplated. Patients with persistent ventricular arrhythmias, which are either symptomatic producing cardiac arrest or detected on post infarction monitoring, should be considered for further investigation

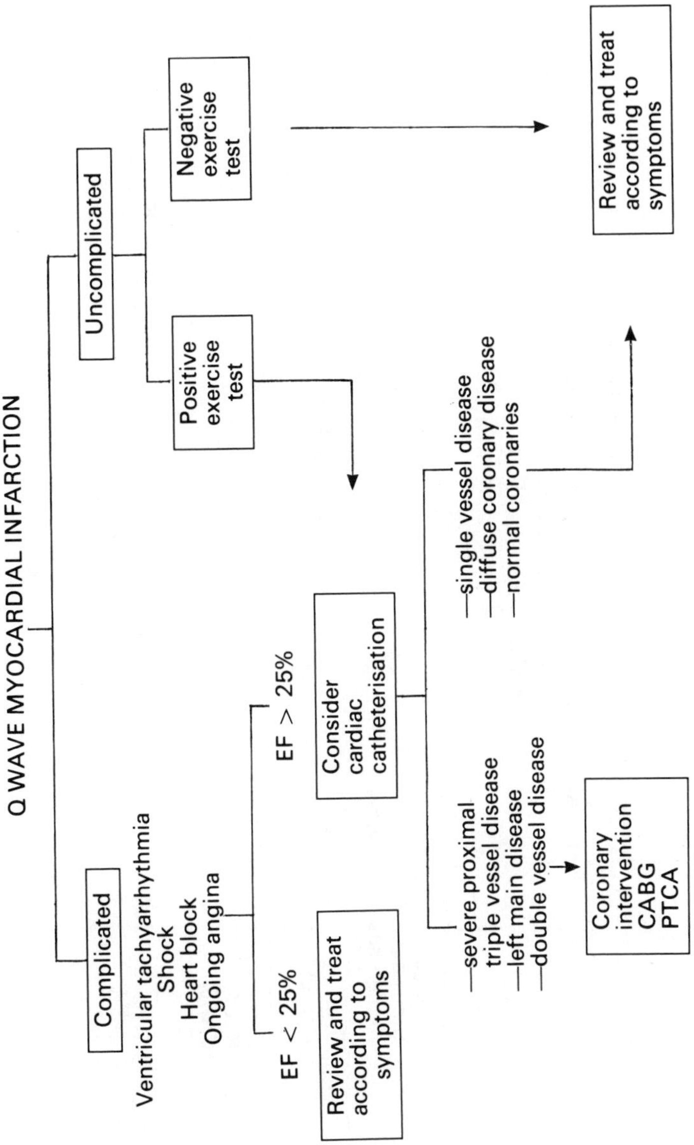

Figure 8.5 Strategy for the management of Q-wave infarction at Dunedin Hospital

Q WAVE MYOCARDIAL INFARCTION

Complicated

Ventricular tachyarrhythmia
Shock
Heart block
Ongoing angina

EF < 25%

Review and treat according to symptoms

EF > 25%

Consider cardiac catheterisation

—severe proximal triple vessel disease
—left main disease
—double vessel disease

Coronary intervention
CABG
PTCA

—single vessel disease
—diffuse coronary disease
—normal coronaries

Uncomplicated

Positive exercise test

Negative exercise test

Review and treat according to symptoms

273

Figure 8.6 Strategy for the management of non-Q wave infarction at Dunedin Hospital

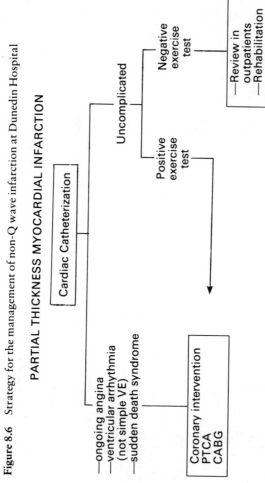

PARTIAL THICKNESS MYOCARDIAL INFARCTION

Cardiac Catheterization

Uncomplicated

—ongoing angina
—ventricular arrhythmia
 (not simple VE)
—sudden death syndrome

Positive exercise test

Negative exercise test

Coronary intervention
PTCA
CABG

—Review in outpatients
—Rehabilitation

since preliminary evidence suggests that even in the absence of angina pectoris, patients with severe coronary artery disease and associated ventricular tachyarrhythmias may have a better prognosis following surgery.

Though the acute hospital mortality for non-Q wave myocardial infarction is less than that of Q wave infarction, it has been shown repeatedly that patients with such 'minor infarctions' have a high instance of early complications[29]. This is particularly true in those with left ventricular main disease, proximal anterior descending artery lesions and patients with triple vessel involvement. With the advent of PTCA, it is now possible to treat a majority of patients with advanced coronary artery disease underlying the apparently minor infarction, but proof that this results in an objective improvement in prognosis remains to be demonstrated. As the apparent risk in such patients is within the first two months of the minor infarction, we see little merit in delaying cardiac catheterization beyond 7–10 days in such patients. We recently completed a study of early in-hospital angiography on a consecutive series of 103 patients following acute myocardial infarction: 39 had non-transmural infarctions and 14 were demonstrated to have triple vessel disease, 8 double and 17 single vessel disease. Of these 39 patients only 13 were asymptomatic and had negative exercise tests, ten underwent elective coronary bypass grafting, 8 PTCA and two declined the offer of intervention. Only one of these 39 patients died in over 12 months follow up and this patient had two vessel coronary artery disease with no residual angina and a negative exercise electrocardiogram.

MANAGEMENT OF COMPLICATED MYOCARDIAL INFARCTION

There are a number of potential complications that beset patients with established acute myocardial infarction[3,6]. In the main, however, the more common and clinically relevant ones are those that cause cardiac failure and rhythm disturbances.

Haemodynamic complications of acute myocardial infarction

Haemodynamic disturbance in association with acute infarction is usual; but in general terms, there are several ways in which abnormal haemodynamics present and it is possible to delineate several subsets with characteristic haemodynamic profiles. A convenient classification may be (1) hyperdynamic circulation, (2) hypovolaemic hypotension, (3) left ventricular failure due to left ventricular muscle damage and myocardial ischaemia, acute mitral regurgitation and rupture of the ventricular septum, and (4) cardiogenic shock.

Indications for invasive haemodynamic monitoring

Invasive monitoring is generally not necessary in the truly uncomplicated infarction or in patients with a hyperdynamic state, but it should be instituted early in patients in whom it is apparent that complications are developing or in patients in whom complications are very likely. Invasive monitoring consists of inserting an arterial line for continuous measurement of arterial pressure (most usually in a radial artery) and inserting a balloon flotation catheter (Swan Ganz) for measurement of pulmonary artery, pulmonary capillary wedge and right atrial pressures and cardiac output by thermodilution. In patients with severe haemo-dynamic impairment, a urinary catheter to provide accurate and continuous measurement of urinary output is also recommended.

We would suggest the following to be indications for invasive haemo-dynamic monitoring in patients with acute infarction:

(1) Hypotension where the cause is not obvious (such as excessive morphine administration or heart block)
(2) Evidence of left ventricular failure and hypoxaemia which does not respond immediately to simple diuretic and oxygen therapy
(3) Unexplained or frequent tachyarrhythmias requiring high dose anti-arrhythmic therapy or cardiac pacing in which Swan Ganz catheters can be inserted at the same time as a pacing catheter without additional risk
(4) Unexplained or severe cyanosis, hypoxia or acidosis
(5) Acute mitral incompetence
(6) Ventricular septal defect.

The importance of invasive haemodynamic monitoring is related to the difficulty of interpreting clinical and radiographic findings, especially in patients with left ventricular failure and hypotension in whom the usual cardiac therapies may be either beneficial or detrimental. Hypovolaemia and right ventricular infarction will be treated differently, as it is not usual to give a fluid load to patients following myocardial infarction. Haemodynamic monitoring of cardiac output and wedge pressure make therapeutic intervention with such agents as nitroprusside, dopamine and other vasoactive drugs a much more controlled intervention. It can be difficult to assess the severity and sometimes even the presence of acute mitral valve insufficiency and ventricular septal defect, especially when cardiac output and systemic pressure are reduced.

Hyperdynamic circulation

In patients with a high sinus rate, elevated arterial pressure and a high cardiac output occurring either singly or together, treatment with beta-adrenergic blockade is indicated. If hypertension is the prime problem, virtually irrespective of cardiac output, the treatment of choice is intra-venous nitroprusside therapy monitored by continuous haemodynamic measurement using a Swan Ganz catheter.

Hypovolaemic hypotension

Exclusion of hypovolaemia as the cause of hypotension requires documentation of reduced cardiac output despite an adequate left ventricular filling pressure (pulmonary capillary wedge pressure or pulmonary diastolic pressure in excess of 12–15 mmHg). In this situation, two-dimensional echocardiography is an extremely useful adjunct to therapy, since not only does it give a direct indication of the extent of left ventricular damage but it also provides data on right ventricular function. Significant right ventricular infarction[30] may be confused with hypovolaemia because both are characteristically associated with a low left ventricular filling pressure. The characteristic triad of hypotension in association with elevated right atrial or jugular venous pressure and a low left ventricular filling pressure often responds to the vigorous administration of fluid. Some patients may need additional support in this situation by means of dopamine (or dobutamine) infusion.

Left ventricular failure

All patients with established myocardial infarction have a degree of left ventricular failure as evidenced by mild sinus tachycardia, the presence of a gallop rhythm or clinical evidence of pulmonary congestion. Once failure has developed to the extent that the patient is hypoxaemic, invasive haemodynamic monitoring is particularly helpful. The intravenous administration of a diuretic reduces pulmonary vascular congestion and pulmonary venous pressure both by direct vasodilation and subsequent diuresis. Active vasodilator therapy, however, is very important and the judicious use of nitroprusside, with frequent monitoring of cardiac output and intracardiac pressures, is usually the treatment of choice. Depending on the haemodynamic profile and severity, intravenous nitroglycerin may be an equally acceptable and 'easier' alternative in CCUs not used to dealing with nitroprusside. In addition to vasodilator therapy, with either nitroprusside or nitroglycerin, inotropic support may be indicated to improve cardiac output. Dopamine is the drug most favoured in this situation and usually doses of 2–5 μg kg^{-1} min^{-1} are all that is necessary. Dopamine is particularly useful where the haemodynamics situation has been reasonably controlled and yet renal function, as evidenced by urinary output, is depressed. In such patients, the addition of dopamine usually provides immediate improvement in diuresis, especially if administered early in the course of left ventricular failure. Once the acute episode is under control the institution of oral vasodilator therapy is achieved early and we currently favour angiotensin converting enzyme inhibitors, such as captopril or enalapril, as drugs of choice in this situation. Digitalis is not administered routinely but in patients already taking digoxin is continued.

It is well known that beta-adrenergic blockade may cause or precipitate left ventricular failure in patients with extensive infarction, but in clinical practice this association is relatively uncommon. Occasional patients, especially those with inappropriate tachycardia in relation to reduced cardiac output, may actually improve with judicious use of small doses of beta-blocker.

Cardiogenic shock

Massive myocardial infarction, or a further myocardial infarction in patients with previous ventricular damage may produce global impairment of ventricular function, which is so profound that cardiogenic shock develops. Such shock is characterized by marked hypotension (systolic arterial pressure < 80 mmHg) and a marked reduction of cardiac output (cardiac index < 1.7 l min^{-1} m^{-2} in the face of elevated left ventricular filling pressure (pulmonary capillary wedge pressure in excess of 20 mmHg). Clinically, such patients in addition to pulmonary congestion will also demonstrate the signs of low output failure with cold, pale extremities, sweating and either poor or absent urinary output. In patients with hypotension, 2-dimensional echocardiography is particularly useful as this technique can either confirm the profound depression of left ventricular function or identify particularly reversible situations – such as hypovolaemia, right ventricular infarction (dilated right ventricle with reasonably good left ventricular function), acute mitral valve rupture (papillary muscle rupture) or evidence of ventricular septal defect. In patients presenting with profound hypotension, once left ventricular impairment has been demonstrated as the cause, invasive haemodynamic monitoring is set up with a radial arterial line, Swan Ganz catheterization and the insertion of a urinary catheter.

Inotropic agents are employed extensively in the treatment of cardiogenic shock, but provide only a short term improvement and have not been demonstrated to affect overall mortality. Similarly, vasodilatory therapy, particularly nitroprusside may provide a satisfactory improvement in haemodynamics early after administration, but such improvement is usually short lived in the absence of left ventricular recovery. In uncommon instances, the systemic vascular resistance may, instead of being elevated, actually be either normal or in some cases low. In these cases, noradrenaline or adrenaline are better inotropic agents compared to dopamine or dobutamine.

Intra-aortic balloon counter pulsation (IABCP) is rarely used but on occasions, can be lifesaving – particularly if used in the pre-operative resuscitation of surgically correctable, mechanical left ventricular failure. Although IABCP used to be advocated for the treatment of persistent and ongoing cardiac pain (augmenting coronary flow), since the introduction of nitroglycerin it is rarely needed. IABCP may be required for control of the patient undergoing emergency coronary angiography as a prelude to cardiac surgery.

Surgical intervention is most successful in patients where the circulatory collapse is due to such mechanical complications as ventricular septal defect, acute mitral regurgitation and (more rarely) left ventricular aneurysm. Emergency surgery in such acutely ill patients carries a high mortality.

Treatment or prophylaxis of arrhythmia

Any cardiac arrhythmia may be seen to complicate the early phase of acute myocardial infarction. Those of special significance comprise (1) sinus bradycardia, (2) atrioventricular block, (3) atrial fibrillation, (4) ventricular extrasystoles, (5) ventricular tachycardia, and (6) ventricular fibrillation.

Sinus bradycardia

Sinus bradycardia in the early few hours of the myocardial infarction occurs more commonly in patients with inferior and posterior infarctions, which are more likely to be associated with marked vagotonia. Atropine in small dosage, repeated as necessary, is indicated where the sinus bradycardia is associated with symptoms. Sinus bradycardia is also commonly caused by analgesic therapy with morphine and of course beta-blockade. Temporary cardiac pacing is not indicated for simple sinus bradycardia. Whereas atropine may be useful in the presence of sinus node dysfunction, temporary cardiac pacing (particularly atrioventricular sequential pacing) may be indicated if there is haemodynamic disturbance.

Atrioventricular block

First degree and Mobitz Type I, second degree AV block (Wenckebach) are seen but usually do not require specific therapy. Mobitz Type II, second degree AV block is relatively uncommon in acute myocardial infarction and it should be treated with a temporary cardiac pacemaker. Traditionally, these lower grades of heart block tended to be treated conservatively in patients with inferior myocardial infarction as they are often transient and related to relatively short lived ischaemia of the AV node, being consequent on its anatomic supply from the posterior descending artery. In patients with anterior myocardial infarction, however, even low grade atrioventricular block may indicate relatively extensive infarction and thus be associated with poorer prognosis. Although there is no evidence that temporary cardiac pacing affects mortality, in practice, temporary pacing is often used in second degree heart block in patients with anterior myocardial infarction. Ventricular or atrioventricular sequential pacing is indicated in patients with complete AV block in the early stages of an infarction. Atropine is of little use in such patients. The prognosis of patients with complete AV block associated with anterior infarction is very poor regardless of therapy.

Complete bundle branch block (either left or right) or the combination of right bundle branch block and axis deviation ('bifascicular' block) are more often associated with anterior than inferior or posterior infarction. Temporary cardiac pacing is not automatic in such patients, but one must review these with specific regard to progressive development of high grade AV block. The prognosis in these patients is worse, but again, temporary cardiac pacing has not been demonstrated to improve mortality.

The question of permanent cardiac pacing in survivors of myocardial infarction with associated conduction defects remains controversial. Clearly, patients with ongoing symptomatic sick sinus syndrome or high grade AV block will require permanent cardiac pacing. Although the survivors of infarction complicated by AV block or bundle branch block have a poorer prognosis, this is not necessarily due to subsequent recurrent complete heart block. These patients have a high instance of late in-hospital ventricular fibrillation and clearly, a cardiac pacemaker will have no effect on this situation. On the other hand, a retrospective multicentre study has demonstrated a reduced incidence of sudden death in patients treated by insertion of a permanent pacemaker having experienced transient high grade block during infarction. It is our practice not to insert a permanent cardiac pacemaker in the absence of symptomatic bradycardia.

Atrial fibrillation

Both atrial fibrillation and atrial flutter are relatively more common in the first 24 hours following myocardial infarction than subsequently and are associated with increased mortality, particularly in patients with anterior myocardial infarction. This association is probably not an independent risk factor, however, as atrial fibrillation is more common where there is clinical and haemodynamic evidence of extensive damage. Beta-adrenergic blockade is to be preferred to digitalis for heart rate control, but if there is acute haemodynamic deterioration related to the onset of atrial fibrillation, then DC cardioversion remains the treatment of choice. In view of the Danish multicentre study showing an increased mortality in patients given verapamil in the early stages of myocardial infarction, we currently do not favour this particular drug. On the other hand, flecainide, a new Class Ic anti-arrhythmic agent, is extremely potent and usually controls the heart rate often reverting the rhythm to sinus without electrical intervention. In patients with extensive infarction, however, flecainide may have major adverse haemodynamic consequences.

Ventricular extrasystoles

The suppression of ventricular extrasystoles in the early stages of myocardial infarction was based on the premise that ventricular extrasystoles trigger ventricular fibrillation. This is far from proven and indeed there are several studies to suggest that the ventricular fibrillation occurs as an unheralded event with no premonitory ventricular extrasystoles. The concept that ventricular extrasystoles are 'warning arrhythmias' for ventricular tachycardia, however, has much more merit and intravenous lignocaine (2 mg kg^{-1} as a bolus followed by continuous infusion of 1–4 mg min^{-1}) is the standard treatment for either frequent (in excess of 10 min^{-1}) unifocal extrasystoles or high grade extrasystoles. Hypokalaemia should be corrected. Large numbers of randomized trials have compared the routine administration of several Vaughan Williams Class I agents (lignocaine, quinidine, procainamide, disopyramide and mexilitine) against placebo. All of these agents reduced the frequency of ventricular extrasystoles and occasional studies show reduced incidence of ventricular fibrillation. However, none of these agents administered in this fashion demonstrate reduced in-hospital mortality. Arguably, the routine use of beta-blockade has reduced the frequency of ventricular extrasystoles seen in the coronary care unit and many studies have now been shown to demonstrate reduced mortality though the overall effect is small[31,32].

Lignocaine, or related drugs, are indicated if there are any extrasystoles following a previously documented ventricular arrhythmia – occasionally a clinically important negative inotropic effect occurs, especially with higher doses. In such circumstances, intravenous amiodarone with continued oral therapy may be used in selected cases.

Ventricular tachycardia

Accelerated idioventricular tachycardia (sequential ventricular complexes with a rate of between 60 and 100 beats per minute) do not require active drug therapy. However, since they are often seen in the presence of relative bradycardia and may degenerate to ventricular tachycardia or ventricular fibrillation, we use temporary pacing to 'overdrive' the rhythm if necessary. There is no evidence of increased mortality in association with an accelerated idioventricular arrhythmia.

Definite ventricular tachycardia (usually with a rate of between 120–160 beats per minute) requires immediate therapy. In instances of non-sustained ventricular tachycardia (less than 15 consecutive beats) lignocaine and associated beta-blockade are usually adequate to suppress the rhythm. Following intravenous suppression, a short term therapy with oral anti-arrhythmias, usually Class I agents is recommended. In cases of sustained ventricular tachycardia, DC cardioversion is the treatment of choice, with subsequent oral anti-arrhythmia therapy to suppress the rhythm. If ventricular tachycardia occurs in a coronary care unit, immediate treatment usually prevents severe hypoxia, hypotension, acidosis or electrolyte disturbance, but if these supervene they must be treated appropriately. Hypokalaemia (serum potassium < 4.2 mmol l^{-1}) is a frequent clinical association with ventricular tachycardia in acute myocardial infarction and simple potassium replacement may be all that is necessary to control the acute episodes. Digoxin at toxic levels, is an important iatrogenic cause of ventricular tachycardia in the early stages of myocardial infarction.

Ventricular fibrillation

Since the advent of well-appointed coronary care units, ventricular fibrillation as a primary cause of death is a rare phenomenon in ECG monitored patients. However, late in-hospital ventricular fibrillation (usually occurring after the third or fourth day) is much more common in patients with interventricular conduction defects, extensive anterior infarction, persistent sinus tachycardia, atrial flutter or fibrillation during the first 24 hours, or those who have demonstrated ventricular tachyarrhythmias in the period 12–36 hours following infarction[33].

The treatment of ventricular fibrillation is immediate DC cardioversion. The likelihood of success declines rapidly with time and with the development of acidosis and electrolyte imbalance consequent on severe hypoxia. Ventricular fibrillation often recurs rapidly and repeatedly when patients are metabolically instable or simply severely hypokalaemic. In patients with resistant ventricular fibrillation, assuming lignocaine has been tried, the administration of amiodarone intravenously (5 mg kg^{-1} to a maximum of 350 mg over 20 mins) or bretylium tosylate (5 mg kg^{-1} intravenously) may ultimately be successful but require prolonged cardio-pulmonary resuscitation to allow time for these drugs to work (at least 20 minutes). Amiodarone has a rather strange pharmacodynamic profile and may be better in the prevention rather than the treatment of ventricular fibrillation, but nevertheless is worthe trying especially in patients where echocardiography has demonstrated that cardiac function is preserved. In such individuals, even prolonged cardio-pulmonary resuscitation if administered adequately, can result in excellent patient salvage.

Bretylium tosylate is not available in oral form, therefore, there are three longer term therapeutic alternatives in patients who have suffered serious ventricular arrhythmias or ventricular fibrillation. Vaughan Williams Class I agents have not been demonstrated to be effective, but beta-blockers do reduce the incidence of late death following myocardial infarction. Patients who have ventricular fibrillation after the first 4–6 hours ('secondary' ventricular fibrillation) and have heart failure or cardiogenic shock have a poor prognosis irrespective of therapy. In those who have late in-hospital ventricular fibrillation with good left ventricular function, the prognosis may be excellent and this group of patients should have on-going cardiac therapy with either beta-blockade or amiodarone.

Role of electrophysiological testing after acute myocardial infarction

Although programmed ventricular stimulation of the heart has proved useful in the treatment of patients with recurrent sustained ventricular tachycardia in general, its role in the hospital phase immediately after an acute infarction is unclear. The Westmeade Group provide the only prospective analysis of routine detailed electrophysiological assessment in patients 7–28 days after an uncomplicated myocardial infarction[34]. All 228 clinically well survivors of acute myocardial infarction underwent both exercise electrocardiography and programmed stimulation. In the 62% of their patients in whom both tests were negative, only 1% died in the first year of follow up; but those patients in whom it was possible to induce ventricular arrhythmias during electrophysiological testing, had a poor prognosis. However, the specific role of electrophysiological testing remains in doubt. Despite the Westmeade experience, most physicians question the validity and logistic demands of routine electrophysiological testing.

THE ROLE OF EXERCISE TESTING IN THE EARLY PERIOD AFTER MYOCARDIAL INFARCTION

Exercise testing is a safe and non-invasive method that can provide information not only on residual ischaemia as evidenced by ST segment change, but also on prognostically important changes, such as an abnormal blood pressure response, exercise capacity and the presence of exercise induced ventricular arrhythmias. There are several excellent reviews of the status of exercise testing after myocardial infarction[35,36].

Exercise electrocardiography

Most reports on early exercise tests after myocardial infarction have analysed only data collected during exercise and have failed to take into account other prognostic variables such as patient age, history of previous infarction and left ventricular function. It would appear from several studies that the annual mortality of patients who develop ST segment depression during exercise testing approaches 20% compared to only about 2–3% in those who do not. A poor exercise tolerance, indicating poor residual left ventricular function, is a relatively non-specific variable, but in multivariate analysis it becomes a very significant prognostic indicator. For example in a study from Weld and colleagues in a series of 250 patients undergoing a nine minute treadmill test before hospital discharge, an exercise duration of less than six minutes was a powerful independent prognostic index – indeed, more so than the presence of ST segment depression[37]. Ventricular arrhythmias occurring during exercise have also been considered by many to indicate a poor prognosis but others have reported that they are not relevant.

Nuclear stress testing

Exercise thallium-201 scintigraphy may be regarded as more sensitive and specific than the exercise electrocardiogram per se, but few studies provide a comparison between the two. Radionuclide angiography at rest and particularly during exercise offer excellent information about left ventricular function.

Summary

A negative exercise test (normal electrocardiographic response or good left ventricular function on exercise determined by radionuclide angiography) is a better indicator of good prognosis than an abnormal exercise test is an individual prognostic index for a bad prognosis in a specific patient. We, therefore, limit the use of exercise tests after myocardial infarction to specific subgroups. In patients who have had an uncomplicated myocardial infarction, 12 lead bicycle or treadmill exercise testing is performed at 7–10 days; and if it is positive by ST segment criteria, or if exercise induced angina develops, then the patients may be considered for early cardiac catheterization possibly to proceed to PTCA or elective coronary bypass grafting depending on the coronary anatomy and the exercise test response. Patients in whom the early exercise test is negative are reviewed after discharge and managed according to the presence or absence of symptoms.

CONCLUSIONS

In the United Kingdom approximately 160 000 deaths occur each year as a direct result of coronary artery disease. A large variety of potential interventions, therapies and investigations are currently available for the investigation and management of patients presenting with acute myocardial infarction. There is no definite agreement, and probably never will be, on the exact treatment for all patients. However, physicians must continue to emphasize the importance of reducing primary risk factors, in particular – cessation of cigarette smoking, improved levels of exercise and modified diet. After a myocardial infarction, investigations should be aimed at identifying the high risk patient for coronary intervention and the low risk patient for life style modification and long term beta-adrenergic blockade therapy where possible. The incidence of ischaemic heart disease and myocardial infarction appears to be falling. However, we cannot be complacent – data from the Framingham study show that 1 in 5 men and 1 in 17 women under the age of 60 will suffer acute myocardial infarction and 1 in 3 of the population will die from ischaemic heart disease. Further investigation and research into the causes and treatment of myocardial infarction remain of paramount importance.

References

1. Braunwald, E. (1967). Pathogenesis and treatment of shock in myocardial infarction. *Johns Hopkins Med. J.*, **121**, 421–9

2. Rude, R. E., Muller, J. E. and Braunwald, E. (1981). Efforts to limit the size of myocardial infarcts. *Ann. Intern. Med.*, **95**, 736–61
3. Alpert, J. S. and Braunwald, E. (1984). Acute myocardial infarction: pathological, pathophysiological and clinical manifestations. In Braunwald, E. (ed.) *Heart Disease.* pp. 1262–1300 (Eastbourne: Saunders)
4. Brush, J. E., Brand, D. A., Acampora D., Chalmer B. and Wackers, F. J. (1985). Use of initial electrocardiogram to predict in-hospital complications of acute myocardial infarction. *N. Engl. J. Med.*, **312**, 1137–41
5. Norris, R. M., Brandt, P. W. T., Caughey, D. E., Lee, A. J. and Scott, P. J. (1969). A new coronary prognostic index. *Lancet*, **1**, 274–8
6. Sobel, B. E. and Braunwald, E. (1984). The management of acute myocardial infarction. In Braunwald, E. (ed.) *Heart Disease.* pp. 1301–1333 (Eastbourne: Saunders)
7. Goldman, L., Cook, F., Hashimoto, B., Stone, P., Muller, J. and Loscalzo, A. (1982). Evidence that hospital care for acute myocardial infarction has not contributed to the decline in coronary mortality between 1973–74 and 1978–79. *Circulation*, **65**, 936–42
8. Gruppo Italiano per lo studio della streptochinasi nell'infarcto miocardico (GISSI). (1986). Effectiveness of intravenous thrombolytic treatment in acute myocardial infarction. *Lancet*, **1**, 397–401
9. Rentrop, K. P. (1985). Thrombolytic therapy in patients with acute myocardial infarction. *Circulation*, **71**, 627–631
10. Laffel, G. L., Braunwald, E. (1984). Thrombolytic therapy. A new strategy for the treatment of acute myocardial infarction (2 parts). *N. Engl. J. Med.*, **311**, 710–17 and 770–6
11. Yusuf, S., Collins, R., Peto, R., Furberg, C., Stampfer, M. J., Goldhaber, S. Z. and Hennekens, C. H. (1985). Intravenous and intracoronary fibrinolytic therapy in acute myocardial infarction: Overview of the results on mortality, reinfarction and side effects from 33 randomised controlled trials. *Eur. Heart. J.*, **6**, 556–85
12. Kennedy, J. W., Richie, J. L., Davis, K. B. and Fritz, J. K. (1983). Western Washington randomised trial of intracoronary streptokinase in acyte myocardial infarction. *N. Engl. J. Med*, **309**, 1477–81
13. Thrombolysis in Myocardial Infarction Study Group. (1985). The thrombolysis in acute myocardial infarction (TIMI) trial. Phase 1 findings. *N. Engl. J. Med.*, **312**, 932–6
14. Simoons, M. L., Serruys, P. W., Brand, M. V., Bar, F., DeZwaan, C., *et al.* (1985). Improved survival after thrombolysis in acute myocardial infarction. *Lancet*, **2**, 578–81
15. Verstraete, M., Bory, M., Collen, D., Bernard, R., Brower, R. W. *et al.* (1985). Randomised trial of intravenous recombinant tissue-type plasminogen activator versus intravenous streptokinase in acute myocardial infarction. Report from the European study group for recombinant tissue-type plasminogen activator. *Lancet*, **1**, 842–7
16. Meyer, J., Merx, W., Schmitz, H., Erbel, R., Kiesslich, T., Dorr, R., Lanbertz, H. *et al.* (1982). Percutaneous transluminal coronary angioplasty immediately after intra-coronary streptolysis of transmural myocardial infarction. *Circulation*, **66**, 905–13
17. Hartzler, G. O., Rutherford, B. D., McConahay, D. R., Johnson, W. L. Jr, McCallister, B. D., Gura, G. M., Conn, R. C. and Crockett, J. E. (1983). Percutaneous transluminal coronary angioplasty with and without thrombolytic therapy for treatment of acute myocardial infarction. *Am. Heart. J.*, **106**, 965–73
18. DeWood, M. A. and Berg, R. Jr. (1984). The role of surgical reperfusion in myocardial infarction. In Roberts, R. (ed.). Prognosis after myocardial infarction. *Cardiology Clinics*, **2**: (1), pp. 113–22. (Philadelphia: W. B. Saunders Co)
19. Gray, R. J., Sethna, D. and Matloff, J. M. (1983). The role of cardiac surgery in acute myocardial infarction. II Without mechanical complications. *Am. Heart. J.*, **106**, 728–35

20. Schuster, E. H. and Bulkley, B. H. (1981). Early post infarction angina. *N. Engl. J. Med.*, **305**, 1101–5
21. Gray, R. J., Sethna, D. and Matloff, J. M. (1983). The role of cardiac surgery in acute myocardial infarction. I. With mechanical complications. *Am. Heart. J.*, **106**, 723–8
22. Yusuf, S., Peto, R., Lewis, J., Collins, R. and Sleight, P. (1985). Beta blockade during and after myocardial infarction: An overview of the randomised trials. *Prog. Cardiovasc. Dis.*, **27**, 335–71
23. The MIAMI trial research group. Metoprolol in acute myocardial infarction (MIAMI). A randomised placebo-controlled international trial. *Eur. Heart. J.* 1985; **6**, 199–226
24. Muller, J. E. and Braunwald, E. (1983). Can infarct size be limited in patients with acute myocardial infarction? *Cardiovasc. Clin.*, **13**(1), 147–61
25. The Danish Study Group on verapamil in acute myocardial infarction. Verapamil in Acute Myocardial Infarction. *Eur. Heart. J.*, 1984; **5**, 516–28
26. Muller, J. E., Morrison, J., Stone, P. H., Rude, R. E., Rosner, B. *et al.* (1984). Nifedepine therapy for patients with threatened and acute myocardial infarction: a randomised, double blind, placebo controlled comparison. *Circulation*, **69**, 740–7
27. Quinones, M. A. (1984). Echocardiography in acute myocardial infarction. *Cardiol. Clin.*, **2**(1), 123–34
28. Epstein, S. E., Palmeri, S. T. and Patterson, R. D. (1982). Evaluation of patients after acute myocardial infarction. Indications for cardial catheterisation and surgical intervention. *N. Engl. J. Med.*, **307**, 1487–92
29. Maisel, A. S., Ahvre, S., Gilpin, E., Henning, H., Goldberger, A. L., Collins, D., LeWinter, M. and Ross, J. Jr. (1985). Prognosis after extension of myocardial infarct: the role of Q wave or non-Q wave infarction. *Circulation*, **71**, 211–17
30. Roberts, R. and Marmor, A. T. (1983). Right ventricular infarction. *Ann. Rev. Med.*, **34**, 377–90
31. May, G. S., Furberg, C. D., Eberlain, K. A. and Geraci, B. J. (1983). Secondary prevention after acute myocardial infarction: a review of the short term acute phase trials. *Prog. Cardiovasc. Dis.*, **25**, 335–59
32. May, G. S., Eberlein, K. A., Furberg, C. D., Passamani, E. R. and DeMets, D. L. (1982). Secondary prevention after myocardial infarction. A review of long-term trials. *Prog. Cardiovasc. Dis.*, **24**, 331–52
33. Graboys, D. B. (1975). In hospital sudden death after coronary care unit discharge: A high risk profile. *Arch. Intern. Med.*, **135**, 512–4
34. Denniss, A. R., Baaijens, H., Cody, D. V., Richards, D. A., Russell, P. A., Young, A. A., Ross, D. L. and Uther, J. B. (1985). Value of programmed stimulation and exercise testing in predicting one year mortality after acute myocardial infarction. *Am. J. Cardiol.*, **56**, 213–20
35. Baron, D. B., Light, J. R. and Ellestad, M. H. (1984). Status of exercise stress testing after myocardial infarction. *Arch. Intern. Med.*, **144**, 595–601
36. Cohn, P. F. (1983). The role of non-invasive cardiac testing after an uncomplicated myocardial infarction. *N. Engl. J. Med.*, **308**, 90–3
37. Weld, F. M., Chu, K. L. and Bigger, J. T. (1981). Risk stratification with low level exercise testing two weeks after acute myocardial infarction. *Circulation*, **64**, 306–14

9
Electrical consequences of myocardial infarction

E. ROWLAND

INTRODUCTION

Ischaemic heart disease represents one of the major scourges of the present day, being not only the leading cause of sudden death; but also, because of its various forms of expression, being a major cause of morbidity. While the predominant expression may be angina, persistent or transient electrical abnormalities play an important role in all aspects of the disease. As the epidemic of coronary artery disease has been growing, our knowledge of the electrical consequences of the problem has been expanding at a dramatic rate. This has developed particularly from the ability to monitor the ECG during and following the development of chest pain as well as for prolonged periods in the chronic phase of ischemic heart disease.

Following directly from these observations has been the realization that many patients 'rescued' from the potentially fatal consequences of their ischaemic heart disease may have had electrical complications that may well be amenable to therapeutic interventions. While such capabilities have clearly been demonstrated in the context of acute myocardial infarction, there remain many other important areas in which the benefits of therapeutic intervention have not been proven.

The electrical consequences of coronary artery disease are dominated by the vast problem of sudden cardiac death. Approximately 60% of the annual deaths from coronary artery disease occur suddenly. Whether viewed from the community – sudden cardiac death accounts for approximately 20% of all natural fatalities – or from the hospital coronary unit – 60% of those dying suddenly following myocardial infarction do so in the first hour – the problem is of immense proportions.

SUDDEN DEATH

A precise definition of sudden death has not been universally agreed –

it encompasses death that occurs instantaneously and death that occurs up to 24 hours after the onset of symptoms. The 1979 Task Force of the International Society and Federation of Cardiology and WHO on Nomenclature and Criteria for diagnosis of IHD opted to define cardiac arrest, and thereby allow 'sudden death' to be applied where either resuscitation failed or was not attempted[1]. This definition had the justification of taking cardiac arrest, which is the real clinical manifestation of ischaemic heart disease, as its basis and implying that the interval between time of death and onset of symptoms should be recorded. Whether an interval as long as 24 hours remains tenable for the diagnosis of sudden death is debatable. However the diagnosis seems tenable when death as a natural process, occurs unexpectedly and develops rapidly. An equally compelling area for precise definition has become the definition of survivors of sudden cardiac death – given the rapidly expanding use of community cardio–pulmonary resuscitation and the increasing number of studies performed on survivors of sudden cardiac death. The majority of studies have included as a prerequisite only those who have required DC countershock for ventricular fibrillation (VF) or sustained hypotensive ventricular tachycardia (VT).

Observations from epidemiological and pathological studies indicate that sudden cardiac death is most frequently due to coronary artery disease, the majority of cases showing severe occlusive disease of major coronary arteries[2-4]. Recent occlusive vascular lesions are uncommon and indeed only 10–30% have histological evidence of associated acute myocardial infarction. Corroborative evidence for these pathological observations has been derived from the study of survivors of sudden cardiac deaths. These studies have not only demonstrated the common findings of significant coronary artery disease, despite the absence of prior suggestive history, but also confirmed the low incidence of associated acute myocardial infarction[5,6].

From the clinical standpoint the relationship between sudden cardiac death and coronary artery disease exhibits 2 distinct patterns, of differing prognostic and clinical implications, and based on the presence or absence of associated myocardial infarction. It is, however, not always possible to separate patients resuscitated from sudden death clearly into 2 groups – as a minority will not clearly demonstrate whether infarction preceded sudden death or arose as a consequence of arrhythmia.

Sudden death in association with acute myocardial infarction

The preceding symptoms are apparently identical to those who have acute coronary occlusion without fatal consequences. The prodromal symptoms result in many of these patients seeking medical attention and thus being admitted to hospital. There remain however a majority of those with warning symptoms, who either do not seek medical advice or who succumb before they are admitted to hospital. It has been demonstrated that 40% of cases of sudden death occur within 4 hours of the onset of chest pain[7]. Thereafter the incidence of sudden death falls abruptly, illustrating that a substantial delay in patients reaching hospital will result in the major proportion of lethal consequences occurring out of hospital rather than in the coronary care units, which are designed specifically to deal with them.

The modes of sudden cardiac death in the context of acute myocardial infarction may be ventricular fibrillation, bradycardia or electromechanical dissociation. Primary ventricular fibrillation (i.e. occurring in the absence of cardiac failure) tends to occur in younger patients, particularly when there is a relatively large area of anterior damage. Paradoxically these patients seem to retain good cardiac function and the prognosis after resuscitation, which is generally straightforward, is similar to those with uncomplicated infarction. Recurrences are unlikely and are limited to the ensuing 2 to 3 days.

Asystole or complete heart block are the primary mode of cardiac arrest in relatively few patients with acute myocardial infarction. A similar temporal pattern occurs with these arrhythmias, as is seen with primary VT – the majority of cases occur within a short time of the onset of symptoms. However, those with inferior infarction develop bradyarrhythmias more commonly than those with other sites of infarction.

The least common form of sudden death and the least amenable to treatment is electromechanical dissociation. It may occur as a primary event or may follow resuscitation from secondary VF complicating severe cardiac failure. Although satisfactory ventricular depolarizations are present at first, there is no associated cardiac output and eventually even cardiac electrical activity ceases.

Further subgroups of patients at risk of sudden death are those with severe cardiac failure or shock (secondary VF) and a minority of those in the convalescent phase of acute myocardial failure. The outlook for those with secondary VF is dismal – even if resuscitation is successful, advancing cardiac failure usually exerts its toll within weeks. Convalescent sudden death occurs in an appreciable number – up to 20% of those dying in hospital may succumb in this phase[8]. As the initial course of their hospital stay has usually been uncomplicated, these patients have often been transferred to general wards. Ventricular fibrillation is the almost universal mode of death in these patients, who do have certain features that are associated with this risk. Amongst these are anteroseptal infarction (especially when accompanied by right bundle branch block), development of new bundle branch block, complex ventricular arrhythmia (soon but not immediately after infarction) and persisting sinus tachycardia. Approaches to the appropriate treatment of these patients has floundered on the inability of antiarrhythmic drugs to prevent the arrhythmia. At the present time, close monitoring and observation of those considered to be at greatest risk offers the only useful approach.

While resuscitation is effective in the vast majority, a preferred approach would be primary prevention. But there is an immediate problem – should all patients receive prophylaxis or can we identify the minority at high risk? The concept of warning arrhythmias has been developed in the expectation that VF will be preceded by a period of increasing arrhythmogenicity. However, none of the arrhythmias postulated has been shown to have sufficient sensitivity or specificity. Complex ventricular extrasystoles do indeed occur with increasing frequency prior to the onset of VF but they occur in equal frequency in those not prone to this lethal consequence and are therefore of no value as warning signs[9]. Also a significant proportion of those who do go on to develop VF do not have preceding arrhythmias. The only possible exception is an increase in the frequency of R on T ventricular extrasystoles within the 12 hours preceding the onset of VF, although sophisticated electronic ECG monitoring is required to show a slowly developing trend that the eye can easily miss[10].

So if there is no satisfactory warning sign that VF is about to occur, can prophylactic antiarrhythmic therapy prevent it? Lignocaine has led the way and been shown to reduce the incidence of primary VF (although the mortality was the same as the control group), when used in the coronary care unit[11]. Other studies have failed to demonstrate a significant reduction, although in most studies the overall trend has been towards a reduction[12,13].

When used as mass prophylaxis (being administered to all admissions to the CCU in order to protect a small minority) there clearly has to be considerable concern about toxicity. Additionally, patients may be admitted to coronary care units with suspected infarction and prove not to have had an infarction but will have still received lignocaine. Both cardiac and neurotoxicity are significant problems with lignocaine. None of the newer anti-arrhythmic drugs has demonstrated a significant reduction in the incidence of ventricular fibrillation.

Prophylactic anti-arrhythmic drugs given in the coronary care unit suffer the same drawback as CCU monitoring itself – if there is significant delay between onset of pain and hospital admission, the majority of salvable cases have already been missed. Therefore interest has developed in the administration of these drugs by community paramedics, soon after the onset of chest pain[14]. Providing that increased recruitment of those at-risk is not accompanied by an increase in the number who subsequently prove not to have had an infarction, this approach seems highly desirable.

Sudden death remote from myocardial infarction

Although the risk of sudden death declines within increasing duration after infarction, the first year mortality is in the region of 5%. Two directions have been followed in an attempt to deal with the problem. Perhaps the most impressive has been the development of community-based resuscitation programmes aimed at getting experienced medical and paramedical staff to a sudden death victim within the vital seconds of an event[15]. Such an approach has the benefit of incorporating the community in general more closely into health care but has the major limitation of dealing with the problem after the event. Clearly the second approach of identifying those at risk of sudden death and using prophylactic measures to prevent the lethal outcome is preferable. Various markers have been evaluated for such a role.

Ambulatory monitoring has revealed that many patients who have had myocardial infarction have ventricular arrhythmia that occurs spontaneously during normal daily activities. The most frequently observed arrhythmia is the presence of ventricular extrasystoles, the incidence depending on the duration of ECG monitoring. In all the studies that have examined the relationship there is an increased prevalence of sudden death during follow-up in those with ventricular arrhythmia[16]. But there is also a relationship between the presence of arrhythmia and non-sudden cardiac death, arguing that ventricular arrhythmias relate to the severity of heart disease, the latter being the important determinant of survival. Indeed further studies have confirmed the association between the presence of advanced grades of ventricular extrasystoles and the degree of left ventricular impairment. The relationship can be extended further – similar findings have been noted with exercise testing – in that the severity of ventricular arrhythmia is related to the severity of coronary artery disease[17]. Interestingly in a study examining both the grade of arrhythmia and ejection fraction sudden death occurred in those with low ejection fraction and high grade arrhythmia, but not in those with low ejection fraction and low grade arrhythmia[18].

Angiographic studies on a population who had been resuscitated from ventricular fibrillation but who had prior myocardial infarction, demonstrated that the vast majority had extensive left ventricular impairment and stenosis of at least 2 major coronary arteries[19]. It might therefore not be regarded as surprising that no study has yet managed to demonstrate that controlling ventricular extrasystoles by drug therapy can prevent sudden death.

Even if the grade of ventricular arrhythmia (extra systoles, couplets etc) revealed by ambulatory ECG monitoring is important, the arrhythmic event immediately leading to sudden cardiac death is ventricular fibrillation with or without antecedent rapid ventricular tachycardia. Treatment of a marker present on ambulatory monitoring may well differ in pharmacological responsiveness to the major target[20].

There have therefore been alternative approaches, based on an attempt to define directly the degree of electrical instability of the ventricular myocardium. This approach has been generated by the development of programmed electrical stimulation for the study of supraventricular and ventricular tachycardia. Study of patients with ventricular tachycardia has defined stimulation protocols necessary for induction of clinical arrhythmias. These protocols have been applied prospectively to populations of patients recovering from myocardial infarction in an attempt to define the group at risk of sudden death.

Initial studies concentrated on the repetitive ventricular response (a non-stimulated ventricular extrasystole after a single ventricular extra-stimulus introduced during atrial pacing) as an index of ventricular electrical instability and demonstrated that it predicted both VT and sudden death after myocardial infarction[21]. Subsequent studies[22,23] questioned the validity of this relationship and more recent approaches have used more vigorous stimulation protocols in an attempt to discriminate high risk from low risk patients. However, the results obtained so far are conflicting. Denniss et al.[24] demonstrated that the combination of programmed stimulation and exercise testing predicted virtually all deaths occurring within the first year after myocardial infarction, as well as identifying, when both tests were negative, a population with an excellent prognosis in the first year. However, Roy et al.[25] failed to identify a high risk group using programmed stimulation, although both sudden death and the occurrence of spontaneous VT were predicted by low ejection fraction, ventricular aneurysm and exercise-induced ventricular extrasystoles. Interestingly the rates of inducibility of ventricular arrhythmias in the two studies were similar, suggesting that differences in stimulation protocols and in the numbers receiving beta-blockers were not relevant. Further evaluation will be necessary on these and similar methods of assessing electrical instability before their value as routine investigations is established.

VENTRICULAR TACHYCARDIA

The distinction between patients who die suddenly as a result of a lethal ventricular arrhythmia and those who present with sustained ventricular tachycardia is narrow. It seems likely that the electrical characteristics of a spontaneously occurring arrhythmia determine the haemodynamic response, although susceptibility to ischemia may also be relevant. In a comparison of patients with aborted sudden death and those with sustained VT Stevenson et al.[26] noted a faster rate of induced VT at electrophysiological study and multiple sites of infarction in those with the 'lethal' form of arrhythmia. These findings correlated with a higher incidence of syncope during induced VT in the aborted sudden death group and agree with another study[27], which noted the importance of tachycardia cycle length as a major determinant of syncope during VT. Although these data suggest that modification of the induced VT cycle length by antiarrhythmic drugs may prevent the tendency for rapid rates to degenerate into VT – such evidence remains lacking.

The absence of direct evidence that anti-arrhythmic therapy improves prognosis in patients with ventricular arrhythmia remains a tantalizing hurdle. Clinical observation indicates that VT is associated with sudden death, that anti-arrhythmic drugs can prevent VT, but there is no evidence from population studies that the prognosis is improved. This discrepancy may in part be explained by the tendency of anti-arrhythmic drugs to have pro-arrhythmic actions as well, with the end-result that those who benefit from the drugs are balanced by those who suffer the ill-consequences. It remains to be seen whether newer techniques of treatment, such as surgical resection or electrical techniques based on the implantable defibrillator will demonstrate similar drawbacks.

SUPRAVENTRICULAR ARRHYTHMIAS

A variety of supraventricular arrhythmias may be seen following AMI, which although of little direct impact on the course of the disease often have prognostic implications. One of the more direct relationships is sinus bradycardia. The association of sinus bradycardia with inferior infarction seems the most likely explanation for the association of slow rate and improved mortality, compared to the overall outcome of myocardial infarction. Resulting from increased vagal tone, sinus bradycardia may protect the myocardium by decreasing oxygen demand. However, bradycardia does not always have such benign or potentially beneficial associations – it is known to predispose to escape (or bradycardia-dependent) ventricular arrhythmias and this may be of importance in the very early phase of infarction. Rarely, sinus bradycardia occurs as a result of SA block when it would seem to reflect direct damage to the sinus node or surrounding atrium.

Sinus tachycardia, by contrast, frequently indicates a grave prognosis. In fact a considerable number of all patients with infarction exhibit sinus tachycardia at some stage but it is in those in whom the heart rate remains persistently high that it indicates extensive myocardial loss. For this reason it is particularly common in anterior infarction, and desirable though attenuation with beta blockade may be, treatment is rarely tolerated, because of left ventricular failure.

Atrial fibrillation occurs in 10–15% of patients with acute myocardial infarction[28], is transient in the majority and may be due to a number of causes. Although the major cause is direct ischaemic injury to the atria or sinus node, other factors such as pericarditis or left ventricular failure may be relevant. Indisputably there is, however, a higher mortality in those with atrial fibrillation. It occurs both in those who are older and those with more severe infarction, and is also seen more frequently in patients with ventricular arrhythmias. Whether atrial fibrillation itself influences the prognosis adversely (via increased ventricular rate and loss of atrial transport) is not clearly established, but as the majority of episodes are transient (50% lasting less than 30 mins) it may be predominantly those with sustained atrial fibrillation who are at potentially increased risk.

AV CONDUCTION DISTURBANCE

First degree and second degree Type I atrio-ventricular (AV) block are the commonest of the conduction disturbances in acute myocardial infarction, sharing similar aetiologies and implications. Both are associated with inferior infarction, are due to disturbances at the level of the AV node (predominantly ischaemic injury, although a parasympathetic element may be relevant) and do not affect survival (particularly as the vast majority are transient). First degree AV block is seen in approximately 10% of all patients with myocardial infarction, a slightly lower percentage exhibiting second degree Type I AV block.

Second degree Type II AV block occurs much less frequently (10% of all cases of second degree AV block) but is of much greater importance. It is almost exclusively associated with anterior infarction, is usually due to interruption in conduction below the level of the main His bundle and frequently progresses to complete AV block. This form of block may be observed on exercise testing[29].

The importance and implications of complete AV block depend largely on the clinical setting in which it occurs. Following inferior myocardial infarction it frequently occurs after progression through first and second degree AV block and is associated with an adequate junctional rate as well as narrow QRS complex. The mortality is in the region of 20–25%, little different from the overall mortality. In those patients in whom haemodynamic collapse accompanies the appearance of complete AV block, temporary pacing produces an excellent response. In those already suffering haemodynamic embarrassment prior to AV block pacing appears to have minimal influence on the outcome.

The mortality in patients with anterior infarction who develop complete AV block is 70–80%. The septal necrosis usually necessary to impair AV conduction in these patients often produces intraventricular block prior to the appearance of complete heart block, which frequently occurs without antecedent first or second degree AV block. The escape rate is generally low, QRS complexes widened and haemodynamic deterioration profound.

Intraventricular block similarly reflects the distribution of thrombosis related to the blood supply of the 3 fascicles. As the right bundle and left posterior fascicle have dual blood supply from the left anterior descending and right coronary artery, it is clear why the prognosis is so grave when these conduction patterns are produced. However, not all conduction disturbances observed at the time of infarction are immediate complications – approximately half are present with the first ECG recording and appear to represent pre-existing conduction system disease. This is of clinical importance, as progression to complete heart block is less frequent with pre-existing block than with conduction disturbances that are newly acquired.

Left anterior hemiblock is the least adverse of the fascicular blocks, although the mortality is greater than in those with uncomplicated infarction. Compared to the 5% of patients whose infarction is complicated by anterior hemiblock, left posterior hemiblock affects only 1% and right bundle branch block approximately 2%. Both confer markedly increased mortality, the major difference being that AV block is uncommon with the former and not infrequent with the latter.

Bifascicular block in its various forms imposes the greatest increase in mortality predominantly because of the associated severity of coronary artery disease and ventricular function. Additionally, the risk of developing complete heart block is high. Left bundle branch block (the combination of anterior and posterior fascicular block) is associated with as high a mortality as the other forms of bifascicular blocks. As might be anticipated, the incidence of serious ventricular arrhythmia is high in these patients but appears to be related to the severity of infarction rather than any influence of the conduction disturbance.

References

1. Report of the Joint International Society and Federation of Cardiology/World Health Organization Task Force on Standardization of Clinical Nomenclature (1979). Nomenclature and criteria for diagnosis of ischaemic heart disease. *Circulation*, 59, 607–9
2. Reichenbach, L. D., Moss, N. S. and Meyer, E. (1977). Pathology of the heart in sudden cardiac death. *Am. J. Cardiol.*, 39, 765–72
3. Davies, J. M. (1981). Pathological view of sudden cardiac death. *Br. Heart J.*, 45, 88–96
4. Warnes, C. A. and Roberts, W. C. (1984). Sudden coronary death: relation of amount and distribution of coronary narrowing at necropsy to previous symptoms of myocardial ischaemia, left ventricular scarring and heart weight. *Am. J. Cardiol.*, 54, 65–70
5. Cobb, L. A., Baum, R. S., Alvarez, H. A., Shaffer, W. A. (1975). Resuscitation from out of hospital ventricular fibrillation: four years follow-up. *Circulation*, 51, 52 (Suppl. III) 223–8
6. Myerberg, R. J., Conde, C. A., Sung, R. J. *et al.* (1980). Prehospital cardiac arrest: early and long-term clinical and electrophysiological characteristics. In Kulbertus, H. E. and Wellens, H. J. J. (eds.) *Sudden Death*, pp. 219–31 (The Hague: Martinus Nijhoff)
7. Lawrie, D. M., Higgins, M. R., Godman, M. J., Oliver, M. F., Julian, D. G. and Donald, K. W. (1968). Ventricular fibrillation complicating acute myocardial infarction. *Lancet*, 2, 523–8
8. Vismara, L. A., DeMaria, A. N., Hughes, J. L., Mason, D. T., and Amsterdam, E. A. (1975). Evaluation of arrhythmias in the late hospital phase of acute myocardial infarction compared to coronary care unit ectopy. *Br. Med. J.*, 37, 598–603
9. Julian, D. G. and Campbell, R. W. F. (1983). Sudden death. In *Scientific Foundations of Cardiology*, Sleight, P., Van Jones, J. (eds) pp. 220–3 (London: William Heinneman)
10. Campbell, R. W. F., Murray, A. and Julian, D. G. (1981). Ventricular arrhythmias in the first 12 hours of acute myocardial infarction: National history study. *Br. Heart. J.*, 46, 351–6
11. Lie, K. I., Wellens, H. J., VanCapelle, F. J. and Durrer, D. (1974). Lidocaine in the prevention of primary ventricular fibrillation. *N. Engl. J. Med.*, 291, 1324–9
12. Noneman, J. W. and Roger, J. F. (1978). Lidocaine prophylaxis in acute myocardial infarction. *Medicine*, 57, 501–15
13. May, C. S., Furberg, C. D., Eberlein, K. A. *et al.* (1983). Secondary prevention after myocardial infarction. A review of short-term acute phase trials. *Prog. Cardiovasc. Dis.*, 25, 335–60
14. Koster, R. W. and Dunning, A. J. (1985). Intramuscular lidocaine for prevention of

lethal arrhythmias in the prehospitalization phase of acute myocardial infarction. *N. Engl. J. Med.*, **313**, 1105–10

15. Schaffer, W. A. and Cobb, L. A. (1975). Recurrent ventricular fibrillation and modes of death in survivors of out of hospital ventricular fibrillation. *N. Engl. J. Med*, **293**, 260–5

16. Ruberman, W., Weinblatt, E., Goldberg, J. D., Frank, C. W., Chaudhary, B. S. and Shapiro, S. (1981). Ventricular premature complexes and sudden death after myocardial infarction. *Circulation*, **64**, 297–302

17. Bruce, R. A., De Rouen, T., Peterson D. R. *et al.* (1977). Noninvasive predictors of sudden cardiac death in men with coronary heart disease. Predictive value of maximal stress testing. *Am. J. Cardiol.*, **39**, 833–40

18. Schultze, R. A., Strauss, H. W., and Pitt, B. (1977). Sudden death in the year following myocardial infarction. *Am. J. Med.*, **62**, 192–7

19. Weaver, W. D., Lorch, G. S., Alvarez, H. A. and Cobb, L. A. (1976). Angiographic findings and prognostic indicators in patients resuscitated from sudden death. *Circulation*, **54**, 895–900

20. Myerberg, R. J., Conde, C., Sheps, D. S., Appel, R. A., Kiem, I., Sung, R. J. and Castellanos, A. (1979). Antiarrhythmic drug therapy in survivors of prehospital cardiac arrest: Comparison of effects on chronic ventricular arrhythmias and recurrent cardiac arrest. *Circulation*, **59**, 855–63

21. Greene, H. L., Reid, P. R. and Schaeffer, A. H. (1978). The repetitive ventricular response in man. An index of ventricular electrical instability (abstr.). *Am. J. Cardiol.*, **41**, 400–405

22. Mason, J. W. (1980). Repetitive beating after single ventricular extrastimuli: incidence and prognostic significance in patients with recurrent ventricular tachycardia. *Am. J. Cardiol.*, **45**, 1126–31

23. Farshidi, A., Michelson, E. L., Greenspan, A. M., Spielman, S. R., Horowitz, L. N. and Josephson, M. E. (1980). Repetitive responses to ventricular extrastimuli: incidence, mechanism, and significance. *Am. Heart. J.*, **100**, 59–68

24. Denniss, A. R., Baaijens, H., Cody, D. V., Richards, D. A., Russell, P. A., Young, A. A., Ross, D. L. and Uther, J. B. (1985). Value of programmed stimulation and exercise testing in predicting one-year mortality after acute myocardial infarction. *Am. J. Cardiol.*, **56**, 213–20

25. Roy, D., Marchand, E., Theroux, P., Waters, D. D., Pelletier, G. B. and Bourassa, M. G. (1985). Programmed ventricular stimulation in survivors of an acute myocardial infarction. *Circulation*, **3**, 487–94

26. Stevenson, W. G., Brugada, P., Waldecker, B., Zehender, M. and Wellens, H. J. J. (1985). Clinical, angiographic and electrophysiologic findings in patients with sustained ventricular tachycardia after myocardial infarction. *Circulation*, **6**, 1146–52

27. Hamer, A. W. F., Rubin, S. A., Peter, T. and Mandel, W. J. (1984). Factors that predict syncope during ventricular tachycardia in patients. *Am. Heart. J.*, **107**, 997–1002

28. Hunt, D., Sutton, C., Slowman, G. and Srinivasen, M. (1982). The prognosis of atrial fibrillation with acute myocardial infarction. In *Atrial Fibrillation*, Kulbertus, H. E., Olsson, S. B., Schlepper, M. (eds) pp. 211–8 (Mölndal: AB Hassle)

29. Woelfel, A. K., Simpson, R. J., Gettes, L. S. and Foster, J. R. (1983). Exercise-induced distal AV block. *J. Am. Coll. Cardiol.*, **2**, 578–81

Index

INDEX